More praise for *Better than Well*

Scientific American Editor's Choice and a *Christian Science Monitor* Noteworthy Book of the Year (2003)

"[Carl] Elliott has produced a powerful meditation—moving, sardonic, humorous, and startling by turns—on the role the 'enhancement technologies' of American medicine have come to play in shaping our sense of who we are or wish to be. Ritalin, Botox, voice generators, sex-change surgery, nose jobs, uppers, downers, Viagra, growth hormones, breast implants, anabolic steroids, even penis studs, nipple rings, and voluntary amputations: all have been conscripted into the relentless pursuit of happiness, fulfillment, and self-realization—'The American Dream.' In the grand tradition of Thorstein Veblen, David Riesman, Walker Percy, and Erving Goffman, this is an observant, offbeat description of how we live now that is also a biting critique of it."

—Clifford Geertz, The Institute for Advanced Study

"Elliott . . . is able to tug on the thread of a single enhancement technique and unravel what seems to be the whole of American culture."
—*Mother Jones*

"Elliott, packing the book with intriguing examples of manifestations as well as cultural references, examines our self-consciousness and the roots of it. The writing is intelligent and thought provoking."
—*Publishers Weekly*

"Elliott grips the reader's attention all the way."
—*Scientific American*

"The path from Walden Pond to plastic surgery may be hard to discern, and seem completely off the map, until you read *Better than Well*."
—*New York Times*

"[*Better than Well*] is a rare piece of writing: part philosophical tract and part social commentary that is as engaging as a good novel. . . .

Elliott's absorbing account will make readers think again about the ways that science shapes our identities."

—*American Scientist Online*

"Engaging and provocative . . . a refreshingly quirky journey, its twists and turns dotted with cultural and literary references."

—*Christian Science Monitor*

"An ambitious and accessible look at how people use medical 'enhancement technologies' from Botox to beta-blockers in the seemingly endless struggle to look younger, feel better, and declare themselves happy and fulfilled." —*Atlantic Unbound*

"The fear of missing out on all that life could offer has given the quest for self-enhancement a powerful moral dimension. The novelty of *Better than Well* is that it makes the same case for such unlikely procedures as accent reduction, transsexual surgery and . . . a longing for amputation. One man's mutilation, it seems, is another's self-discovery." —*The Economist*

"*Better than Well* illuminates the questions central to our techno-medical era more lucidly, and elegantly, than anything I've come across in a long while. Elliott poses the perfect questions and then unravels their implications so, by the end, you see your plain old bottle of Prozac, your cosmetic array, your white-washed, shabby chic house in ways disturbing, surprising, and too true."

—Lauren Slater, author of *Prozac Diary*

"*Better than Well* is an impressive achievement on a par with other landmark works in social criticism, and it should lay the ground for further discussion of these enhancement technologies within medicine, medical ethics, the medical humanities, and among the general public." —*Metapyschology Online*

"[A] thorough and thoughtful book." —*New York Daily News*

"An absorbing read that probes our foibles and uncertainties with gentleness, wisdom, and humor." —*Kirkus Reviews*

"*Better than Well* is absorbing and entertaining, full of keen observations punctuated by humor, personal anecdotes, and references to literature and pop culture. Reading it feels a lot like a long, rambling conversation over coffee with an insightful and well-read friend."

—*Minnesota Monthly*

"*Better than Well* offers a wide-ranging, ironic, and gently mocking (while still very serious) consideration of the emerging partnership between American medicine and the biotech century."

—*Literature and Medicine*

"[An] engrossing book. . . . Highly recommended."

—*Library Journal*

"One might even argue that enhancement has been, historically, the unifying theme of medicine and the locus of its relationship to religion and moral philosophy. Such insights will enrich but also complicate ethical discussion; Elliott is to be congratulated for furthering that enrichment." —*Journal of the American Medical Association*

"This book is ultimately about the meaning of home: how and why we feel at home in our bodies, our selves, and thus in the world. It is, in short, a stunningly good book." —*Religious Studies Review*

"*Better than Well* shows why Carl Elliott has emerged as one of the most thoughtful and perceptive observers of American social life in bioethics." —*American Journal of Bioethics*

"[Elliott's] moral questions are important ones because they turn on the basic philosophical question of what it means to live a good life . . . with considerable aplomb, he makes historical, philosophical, and personal observations to buttress his points." —*The Lancet*

BETTER THAN WELL

AMERICAN MEDICINE MEETS

THE AMERICAN DREAM

Carl Elliott

with a Foreword by Peter D. Kramer

W. W. NORTON & COMPANY

NEW YORK · LONDON

For information about permission to reproduce selections from this book, write to Permissions, W. W. Norton & Company, Inc., 500 Fifth Avenue, New York, NY 10110

Manufacturing by Courier Westford
Book design by Chis Welch
Production manager: Julia Druskin

LIBRARY OF CONGRESS CATALOGING-IN-PUBLICATION DATA

Elliott, Carl, 1961–
    Better than well : American medicine meets the American dream / Carl Elliott ; foreword by Peter D. Kramer.
        p. cm.
Includes bibliographical references and index.
    ISBN 0-393-05201-X (hardcover : alk. paper)
    1. Social medicine—United States. 2. Medical innovations—Social aspects—United States. 3. National characteristics, American. [DNLM: 1. Self Concept—Popular Works. 2. Happiness—Popular Works. 3. Social Control, Informal—Popular Works. 4. Social Medicine—Popular Works. BF 697 E46b 2003] I. Title.
RA418.3.U6 E455 2003
306.4'61'0973—dc21

                                                                                                          2002015947

ISBN 0-393-32565-2 pbk.

W. W. Norton & Company, Inc., 500 Fifth Avenue, New York, N.Y. 10110
www.wwnorton.com

W. W. Norton & Company Ltd., Castle House, 75/76 Wells Street, London W1T 3QT

1 2 3 4 5 6 7 8 9 0

For my parents

CONTENTS

FOREWORD

Peter D. Kramer

Twenty years ago I held down a general hospital psychiatry job that included liaison with the medical and surgical wards. One of the duties was what today would be called "ethics consultations." Why these fell to psychiatrists is an interesting question—it was not because internists and surgeons felt insecure in their judgment. It was more that when patient care got sticky in a certain way, attending physicians threw up their hands and called in the shrinks.

Genuine moral dilemmas turned out to be rare. My standing challenge to students and residents was: Find me a case where what is at issue is a matter of ethics. What looks like an impasse is generally inattention to detail.

A typical consultation might involve an older gentleman of shaky mental status who adamantly refused to undergo a lifesaving procedure. If one took time to chat, it would emerge that the recalcitrant patient came from an ethnic group where important decisions were made by the family at large. He was not so much withholding consent as asking that relatives be called in. And then the data on the contemplated procedure would turn out to be ambiguous. Perhaps the attending physician's anxiety about the treatment had been translated into a hasty attempt at coercion. What psychiatry had to offer were patience and curiosity, and sometimes a sense of humor. They formed a solution in which ethical dilemmas dissolved.

Carl Elliott trained as a physician before becoming a philosopher. This combination, medicine and metaphysics, recalls the range of disciplines that once shaped psychiatry. I often think that Carl brings the profession's posture (I mean, when we are not stiff-necked) to the practice of medical ethics. He has a relaxed manner. He is simultaneously curious and reflective. He tolerates absurdity, loves odd and discordant facts. On occasion, a belly laugh will escape. But in Carl's hands, dilemmas do not disappear; instead, they ramify.

It is said that medical ethics has revived ethics altogether, for philosophy. In the second half of the last century, philosophers had become linguists, only without linguists' training in the particulars of language. And then medicine was transformed by consumerism, subspecialization, and a host of technical advances. Decisions once made in private between physician and patient became matters for public discussion, among strangers with differing values and viewpoints. Hospitals called in philosophers as arbiters—of matters of life and death. Speak about doing things with words!

And yet, medical ethics often remained a matter of words: competency, informed consent, quality of life. The practice of ethics sometimes seemed little more than attempts to define those terms operationally, in the hopes that real-world decisions could be rationalized.

Carl has moved in a different direction. He has seized the moment, the enlivening offered ethicists by medical dilemmas, to turn philosophy to its classical roots in moral psychology. For Carl, when we ask whether person X should undergo procedure aleph for condition zeta, we are covertly raising questions posed by the Skeptics, Cynics, Epicureans, and Aristotelians. What is identity? What is the good life? How far does autonomy extend? Who are we in our intimate relationships? What is it to be human here and now?

Carl does not hide behind jargon. He doesn't hide at all. He places himself in the picture: What does it feel like to be with this determined eccentric who claims he will not feel like himself unless he is permitted to cut off his leg? But that is an odd and extreme example. More characteristically, Carl asks what it is to be a television-watching American, a bit bored in his job and in his love life, and yet pleased, too, with the very goods and opportunities that are often said to be stultifying. That, after all, is the context in which the odd case occurs, our consumer culture, a culture of extremes of satisfaction and dissatisfaction, a culture of self-congratulation, self-discovery, and self-improvement.

I first met Carl Elliott in the fall of 1997, at the Hungry Mind (now the Ruminator) Bookstore, in St. Paul, Minnesota, where I was reading from *Should You Leave?*, my commentary on the state of intimacy in the culture of self-help. Carl has a decided presence. He is slow, contemplative, and prone to quiet statements whose humor and originality explode on you belatedly. He is also incurably social. He knows everyone in bioethics and has them working for him on one or another project. Carl's intention was to involve me in a group discussing enhancement technologies—techniques not for curing illness but for making healthy people better endowed in one or another capacity. In particular, the group asked how these technologies illuminate issues of identity.

The topic is one I had considered in *Listening to Prozac.* My observation was that the new antidepressants were less remarkable for their ability to ameliorate mental illness than for their tendency to inspire claims of personality change. What do we make of testimony that a person is "myself at last" on a new medication? Absent the discovery and marketing of that chemical, might he have lived his whole life and never been himself? And what of those on medication who claim not to be merely recovered—back to the baseline state, before they were ill—but "better than well"? Is that outcome credible? Desirable? Permissible? Perhaps it is the American ideal.

Carl thought that my misgivings about enhancement were insufficiently pronounced. I undervalued depressive traits. What if a medication could diminish a person's sense of alienation? Wouldn't we worry a great deal about that outcome?

In the long run, our debate turned out to be expensive. (In brief: We presented our views at a conference. A not-for-profit medical ethics institute published the papers in its journal . . . and a drug company dropped its funding for the institute. The debate and the detailed story will appear in *Prozac as a Way of Life*, edited by Tod Chambers and Carl Elliott.) But there in the bookstore café, we met on friendly ground. I had built the overtly philosophical sections of *Listening to Prozac* around questions posed by the Southern novelist Walker Percy, who had given me encouragement early in my career. It turned out that Elliott was editing a book on Percy, as a doctor and a moralist. (It appeared in 1999 as *The Last Physician*.)

We discussed one of Percy's less-known works, a pastiche of self-help called *Lost in the Cosmos*. Percy tries recapture issues of identity for philosophy, by asking questions firmly rooted in the culture. On a late-night television show, taped in Burbank, California, why do audience members from Chicago applaud when the host mentions their city? Percy wants to consider location and dislocation, the circumstances that color the sense of self.

That is Carl's project, too. He was convening philosophers, sociologists, anthropologists, psychiatrists, and geneticists—thinkers of any stripe who worried over the ways people try to improve themselves. The particular topics ranged from liposuction to the implantation of computer chips. In his own work, Carl was thinking about groups of self-improvers, from southerners who adopt midwestern accents to blacks and whites who alter their skin color.

This book is the result of those inquiries, and others. Carl has titled it *Better than Well*. I am honored that he should have done so. As philosophy, to my mind, *Better than Well* most resembles the remarkable work of Stanley Cavell on cinema screwball comedies. I mean in this sense: Carl takes products of the culture known to all of us, like television advertisements for shyness remedies, and makes them work to frame questions about human nature. And in this sense as well, that like Cavell (and like Cavell's intellectual forbears, Thoreau and Emerson), Elliott tells us about America. He writes of bowlers and billiard players, karaoke singers and pistol-shooting champions. Elliott's characters, in *Better than Well*, might be those of an indie road movie.

Like Walker Percy, I should have said as well when I was listing philosophers Carl resembles—especially since Carl writes with grace. He is a storyteller.

The would-be amputee seems less bizarre in the light of Carl's compassion and set within the range of Carl's vision. We are, even those of us who value life and limb, self-improvers, hoping to be or appear to be a bit braver or less awkward, hoping to live longer, to be truly happy, to be ourselves at last, and a bit more. The American Dream may seem strange in some of its manifestations, and coercive—Carl refers to the "tyranny of happiness"—but it is our dream. At best, as we approach it, we oscillate between irony and avidity.

This tolerance for mixed emotion—again, the psychiatrist's posture—is another of Carl's strengths. He is unafraid of the messiness of human nature, though perhaps a bit worried over the moment in which we find ourselves, when human nature may be changing, at our own hands.

INTRODUCTION

In the late 1960s, the pharmaceutical company Sandoz began marketing a new tranquilizer called Serentil. The ad for Serentil read: "The newcomer in town who *can't* make friends. The organization man who *can't* adjust to altered status within his company. The woman who *can't* get along with her new daughter-in-law. The executive who *can't* accept retirement." These problems often make people anxious and tense, the ad noted. But Serentil can help. Not just because Serentil eases tension, but also because it can fix "the disordered personality, who often responds with excessive anxiety." In large, capital letters at the top of the ad was the slogan, "For the anxiety that comes from not fitting in."[1]

This, in a nutshell, is the problem that follows enhancement technologies wherever they go: the American obsession with fitting in, countered by American anxiety about fitting in too well. The Serentil ad was not a success. In fact, the U.S. Food and Drug Administration forced Sandoz to withdraw it and publish a correction. The mistake Sandoz made was not that of offering Serentil as a medical fix for social problems; their mistake was making the offer so explicit.

Sandoz did not try to redefine the social problem into a medical problem, did not use medical language, did not hide behind technical-sounding diagnostic labels. They just said it out loud, for everyone to hear: here is a drug that will make people who can't fit in less anxious about not fitting in. And so all the American buttons were pushed: it's a crutch, it's a chemical lobotomy, it will suck away Yankee initiative and erode the work ethic. The FDA forced Sandoz to issue a correction stating that, contrary to its earlier ad, Serentil was useful only in "certain disease states," and that Sandoz did not intend Serentil to be used for "everyday anxiety situations encountered in the normal course of living."

The debate over the Serentil ad followed what has become a familiar pattern. Doctors begin using a new drug or surgical procedure that looks as much like a cosmetic intervention—or "enhancement technology"—as a proper medical treatment. This new technology promises to take the edge off of some sharply uncomfortable aspect of American social life (social stigma, childhood teasing, occupational stress, sexual inadequacy, racial discrimination, or suburban alienation). The technology takes off spectacularly, after which comes round after endless round of self-flagellation about social conformity, dependence, and treating social problems with pills. For a while there are the usual symptoms of public hand-wringing—anxious editorials, dispassionate debates in medical journals, an occasional congressional hearing or governmental task force—and then the issue takes a nosedive into obscurity. The technology is either consigned to the history books, like Miltown (a minor tranquilizer of the 1950s that no one remembers anymore), or accepted as part of ordinary life in America, like acne creams and diet drugs. Occasionally controversy will resurface a few years later, the way a public outcry over Ritalin emerged two decades after the initial Ritalin scare in the 1970s, but more often it is simply forgotten, except for the occasional physician who is old enough to recall what we used to worry about back in the old days. Cosmetic surgery, Valium, Ritalin, Prozac, Paxil, steroids, gene therapy, growth hormone, Viagra, Botox—all have their days in the headlines, and each time, the same debates are rehearsed. *Brave New World* is invoked; self-reliance and bootstrap pulling are encouraged; slavish conformity to the opinions of others is roundly deplored. "We have created in America a culture of drugs. We have produced an environment in which people come naturally to expect that they can take a pill for every problem—that they can find satisfaction and health and happiness in a handful of tablets or a few grains of powder."[2] The speaker? Richard Nixon.

"Enhancement technologies" is a relatively new term, but there is nothing new about medical enhancement. Strictly speaking, "enhancement" constituted a significant part of what my father, a small-town southern family doctor, has been doing in his office from the time he set up shop in the late 1950s: immunizing children, freezing warts, removing moles and cysts. When I was a teenager, back in the days before there were any good remedies for acne, my father used to mix homemade solutions of clindamycin and rubbing alcohol in his office for my friends and me. Nobody ever thought to call enhancement technologies like these morally troubling or beyond the scope of proper medicine. They were safe, effective interventions that made people feel better about themselves.

Bioethicists and clinicians began to worry about enhancement technologies in the late 1980s with the development of gene therapy.[3] Gene therapy refers to the prospect of treating genetic illnesses by manipulating genetic material. The first human gene therapy protocols were aimed at a metabolic disease called ADA (adenosine deaminase) deficiency, which results in a compromised immune system. Many gene therapy enthusiasts saw the ADA deficiency protocol as a first step toward treating genetic diseases that are far more common, like cystic fibrosis. Yet many of those same enthusiasts were troubled by the prospect of eugenics, the effort to improve human beings by altering their genetic condition. So a bright line was drawn between genetic "treatment," which was seen as ethically acceptable, and genetic "enhancement," which was not. Other writers have clung to this distinction as a way of determining not just which technologies we ought to have worries about, but also which technologies health services should fund: medically necessary "treatments" should be funded, while "enhancements" should not. And so the distinction between enhancement and treatment seems to be one that we are stuck with. Bioethicists now use the term "enhancement technologies" to designate a variety of drugs and procedures that are employed by doctors not just to control illness, but also to improve human capacities or characteristics.[4]

Not too long ago I gave a talk on enhancement technologies to an audience of doctors and medical students at a local hospital. During the question and answer session, a student raised the issue of cultural conformity. The danger that most people seem to see with things like cosmetic surgery and genetic enhancement, he said, is that the American people will use the technologies to conform to a narrow, restricted cultural ideal. Everyone will want to be young, white, thin, smart, athletic, and good-looking in a very conventional, Hollywood sort of way. But he thought this fear was unrealistic, even absurd. For example, he wore an earring, and his hair was pulled back in a ponytail. This made him stand out among his medical school classmates, he explained, but he liked it that way. In his view, there would always be people like him in America: people who wanted to stretch the limits of convention, who thrived on being different, who resisted cultural norms. America is a country of individualists. Conformity is the last thing we need to worry about.

It wasn't hard to see why he felt this way. In the sea of middle-aged white coats and suits that surrounded him, his earring looked like an act of rebellion. Yet if we had been talking not in a hospital auditorium but on the street a few blocks away, his outfit would have been passé. Standing outside the Condom Kingdom or Saint Sabrina's Parlor in Purgatory, where every second passerby is wearing dreadlocks, neck tattoos, and a tongue stud, he would have been far more likely to turn heads on the street wearing a blue blazer and a tie. He knew this, of course, but he was still able to see his appearance as a kind of existential act, a strike against conformity. He wasn't like those conservative, bow-tied midwestern guys in loafers. He was a rebel and an outsider. He didn't care what other people thought. He wore an earring.

What you see when you look at America may make all the difference to the way you approach the debate over enhancement technologies. Is America a country of rebels or a country of social conformists? A land of Huck Finns or a land of George Babbitts? Perhaps, as Tocqueville thought, it is both. Tocqueville believed that social conformity and social rebellion are merely different sides of the same coin. Both are consequences of the American preoccupation with the opinions of other Americans. This, he thought, is because Americans are so disdainful of authority and tradition. Americans don't look to their ancestors for guidance, and they don't see any obvious signs of superiority in their contemporaries, so they are "constantly brought back to their own judgment as the most apparent and accessible form of truth."[5] But Tocqueville also saw how this aspiration to self-sufficiency easily slides into social conformity. If you can't look up to any external authority to tell you what to think and how to act, then you are constantly looking over your shoulder at your peers. Authority is replaced by public opinion. "When the public governs," writes Tocqueville, "all men feel the value of public goodwill, and all try to win it by gaining the esteem and affection of those among whom they must live."[6]

Tocqueville put his finger on a tension that lies at the heart of the way Americans think about enhancement technologies. People who see America as a land of rebels are worried about individual rights being taken away. They are ever vigilant of the government, the law, the schools, and the churches depriving us of the right to do with our bodies what we wish. They may not be particularly interested in breast augmentation themselves, may have no use for Propecia or Botox or Viagra, but they want nobody telling them what they can't have. People who see America as a land of social conformists, on the other hand, worry about what people will do with these individual rights once they are guaranteed. They worry about a homogeneous cultural landscape, stripped of character and diversity, where everyone dreams the same dreams and aspires to identical futures. Both visions have some truth to them, of course. You can look at America and see a country of rebels and visionaries and lost souls: Wyatt Earp on his horse, Travis Bickle in his taxi, Charlie Parker improvising solos in a lonely hotel room. But you can also look at America and see a very different place: a land of generic shopping malls and chain restaurants, of fashion slaves and social strivers, of religious fanatics committing mass suicide like lemmings going over a cliff. You can look at America and see 240 million people watching cable TV in their basements.

Many of us feel some vague moral qualms about enhancement

technologies, but we are not quite able to say why. We feel uneasy about our children taking Ritalin, about aggressive marketing campaigns for antidepressants, about our own unspoken wishes to be thinner and brighter and more outgoing, yet we are not quite able to articulate the source of our uneasiness. Are we worried about treating social problems with medical interventions? Do we fear that enhancement technologies are a crutch? Or are these worries simply irrational gut reactions to technologies that, after all, may make our lives much better? On the face of it, it seems a little odd to worry about interventions that promise to make us happier, more attentive, and better looking.

My aim in this book is not to make an argument so much as a diagnosis. I want to try to put my finger on some of the reasons behind the uneasiness that many of us feel about these technologies, even as we embrace them. I also want to hazard a guess or two as to why Americans in particular produce and use enhancement technologies in quantities that are often, quite frankly, unprecedented anywhere else in the world. We need to place these technologies in a cultural and historical context that will help us to understand better the pressures that lead us to use them, but that goes beyond the clichés about fashion models and happiness in a pill that have characterized many discussions of these technologies in the past.

Although my ostensible topic is enhancement technologies, I want to use that topic as a lens through which we can examine a much larger issue: the nature of identity, at least as we have come to understand identity in the contemporary West. The issues at stake in medical debates over enhancement technologies are important, I believe, mainly because of what they can tell us about pathologies in the way that we live. The uneasiness that many of us feel about enhancement technologies can tell us something important about selfhood, authenticity, and the good life.

A thumbnail version of my diagnosis would go something like this. To understand our uneasiness with enhancement technologies, we need to understand something about the architecture of the self. We need to understand ourselves as inheritors of a cultural tradition in which the significance of life has become deeply bound up with self-fulfillment. We need to understand the complex relationship between self-fulfillment and authenticity, and the paradoxical way in which a person can see an enhancement technology as a way to achieve a more authentic self, even as the technology dramatically alters his or her identity. We need to understand something about the institutional structures in which enhancement technologies are provided, especially the way that our impatience with moral authority has given way to an embrace of technical expertise. We also need to figure out why self-presentation began to assume such importance in American life in the early twentieth century, and how it has been sustained by our particular culture. In short, we need to understand the complex relationship between enhancement technologies, the way we live now, and the kinds of people we have become.

BETTER
THAN
WELL

1

THE PERFECT VOICE

God talks like we do.
—Lewis Grizzard, *Atlanta Journal-Constitution*

I n 1985, the English physicist Stephen Hawking lost his voice. Hawking suffers from amyotrophic lateral sclerosis, or ALS, a degenerative neurological illness. Over the years Hawking's illness had left his voice increasingly slurred and difficult to understand, but it was not until an episode of pneumonia forced him to have a tracheostomy that Hawking lost his voice completely. After the tracheostomy, Hawking could not speak at all. He could communicate only by raising his eyebrows when someone pointed to the correct letter on a spelling card.

Several years later, a computer specialist from California sent him a computer program called Equalizer. Equalizer allowed Hawking to select words from a series of menus on a computer screen by pressing a switch, or by moving his head or eyes. A voice synthesizer then transformed the words into speech. The computer was a vast improvement on the spelling card system, and for the most part, Hawking was also pleased with the voice synthesizer. "The only trouble," he wrote in a 1993 essay, "is that it gives me an American accent." Yet Hawking then went on to say that after years of using the voice synthesizer, the American voice came to feel like his own. He started to identify with that voice, and feel as if it were really his. "I would not want to change even if I were offered a British-sounding voice," Hawking wrote. "I would feel I had become a different person."[1]

The anthropologist Gregory Bateson used to ask his graduate students if a blind man's cane is part of the man.[2] Most students would say no, that the limits of a person stop at his skin. But if Hawking is right, then the answer may be more complicated. For despite the fact that Hawking's "voice" was computer-synthesized, despite the fact that it came from a set of audio speakers rather than from his mouth, despite the fact that the synthesized voice sounded mechanical, robotic, and worse still, American, Hawking eventually came to feel that it was *his* voice. Hawking's identity, at least in his view, does not stop at the boundaries of his skin.

How exactly is a voice related to an identity? Many of us feel as if our voices are, in some vague and undefined way, *our* voices, an immutable part of who we are, but in fact our voices are changing all the time. The voice of a person at five years of age will sound different from the voice of the same person at age forty-five, and her voice will sound different again at age seventy-five. An Alabaman living in North Dakota probably will not speak with the same accent that he speaks with back in Tuscaloosa. A black American may sound different when speaking to other black Americans at home or at church than she does when speaking to white Americans at the office. Our voices even sound noticeably different to us from the inside, first-person standpoint than they sound to other people. For many of us, it still comes as a mild shock to hear our own voices on tape.

Hawking's remarks about his voice synthesizer reflect two tensions in modern identity that run through many debates over enhancement technologies. The first is a tension between the natural and the artificial, or more broadly, between what is *given* and what is *created*. The reason it initially sounds jarring to hear Hawking say he identifies so closely with a computer-generated voice is precisely because it has been generated by a computer, rather than by nature itself. Yet the fact that Hawking does identify with the computer-generated voice reflects something of the flexibility of modern identity. It is not uncommon these days for people to say they feel more like themselves while taking Prozac or typing in an on-line chat room, or that it was only after undergoing cosmetic surgery or taking anabolic steroids that their bodies began to look the way they were meant to look. Statements like these sound odd (and merit a deeper look) precisely because they confound what we expect to hear. We may expect to hear that an artificial technology makes a person feel *better* about herself, but we don't usually expect to hear that it makes her feel more *like* herself.

Related to this tension between the given and the created is a second tension, between the self as it feels from the inside and the self as it is presented to others. Most modern Westerners have some sense that there is a gap between self and self-presentation—between the self that sits alone in a room, thinking, and the self that hops up on stage to crack jokes and take questions from the audience. We also tend to think that the true self is the one that sits alone, a solitary self that endures over time, while the on-stage self is a mere persona, a type of useful role-playing that can be used or discarded as circumstances demand. But when Hawking the Englishman says he identifies with his American accent, and would feel like a different person with a British-sounding voice, he closes this gap between self and self-presentation. An accent is not a part of the self that sits silently in a room. It is a part of the self that is presented to others. By identifying so closely with his accent, Hawking is identifying less with his solitary self than with his self-presentation. This makes the gap between the two somewhat questionable.

The voice is a good place to start thinking about identity, because many of us don't even think about our voices until we are made self-conscious about them. Those occasions of self-consciousness usually come when our identities are in flux or subject to challenge. If I am an adolescent boy, I will become self-conscious when my voice begins to deepen and crack. If I move to England, I will become self-conscious when the natives roll their eyes at my American accent. If I get sex-reassignment surgery and become a woman, I will become self-conscious when I still sound like a man. My voice is always distinctly *my* voice, but often I will not think of it as such until someone calls attention to my identity.

IF YOU WERE listening to me speak these words, you would hear them spoken with a noticeable southern drawl. Some people might call it a twang, though I myself prefer the more flattering term "lilt," which was the term Lilli Ambro used when she heard me speak. Ambro runs an "accent-reduction clinic" in Greensboro, North Carolina called The Perfect Voice. Clients of The Perfect Voice come to Ambro for help in learning how to diminish, change, or erase their Southern accents. A speech pathologist by training, with a background in professional singing, Ambro is a southerner herself—a North Carolinian, educated at one of the very cradles of southern womanhood, Salem College. In fact, she speaks with more than a trace of a southern accent herself.

I had gotten in touch with Lilli Ambro after coming across a shelf of cassette tapes in a Berkeley bookshop aimed at helping recent Asian immigrants to the United States overcome their foreign accents. I had just spent several days with a research group talking about whether enhancement technologies were a form of liberation or self-betrayal, whether Prozac and sex-reassignment surgery help people change themselves or help them discover who they really are. Seeing these cassettes displayed in the bookshop, after walking out of the research meeting, the thought struck me that the purpose of an accent change is not really so different from many of the enhancement technologies we had been discussing. That thought eventually led me to The Perfect Voice, one of a number of accent-reduction clinics springing up throughout the South.[3]

Southerners have a complicated relationship with their accents, a complex mixture of pride and shame and fierce defensiveness. It's like a little brother who is a drunk or maybe a little crazy and therefore somewhat embarrassing—you are always shaking your head when his name is mentioned—but you can't really disown him because, well, damn it, he *is* family. Most southerners, when they talk to Yankees, will defend a southern accent as the most beautiful and melodic of all American accents, but deep down we are not really convinced this is true. Many of us modify our speech, often unconsciously, when we are around outsiders, and talk more southern in the company of one another. Some of us even learn to speak Yankee at work or when we are visiting up North. Many of us wish not so much to get rid of our southern accents as to get a *better* one, an accent that evokes a genteel, mythical old South rather than, say, *The Beverly Hillbillies.* Nobody explicitly teaches us this, but we somehow absorb the lesson that north of the Mason-Dixon line a southern accent generally codes for stupidity or simplemindedness. You can watch only so many movies and television shows featuring big-bellied southern sheriffs, sweaty fundamentalist preachers, and shotgun-carrying rednecks before the message sinks in. We learn early on that in certain settings, like universities, a southern accent needs to be moderated, if not effaced, or else you will not be taken seriously.

When I was growing up in Clover, our small corner of South Carolina, it would occasionally happen that someone in town would accomplish something worthy of attention from the local television news stations. The high school football team would make it to the upper state championships. A local preacher would accidentally burn down a church. Once, I remember, state law enforcement authorities staged an undercover sting operation and caught a local policeman stealing chocolate Easter eggs and frozen steaks from the grocery store. When these newsworthy events occurred, teams of television news reporters would make the trip down I-77 from Charlotte to investigate. Our moment of fame. In anticipation, we would all sit around the television and look at Clover through the lens of the television camera.

It was always a little embarrassing. The reporter would ask someone from Clover a question on camera, the Cloverite would answer, and my parents would immediately groan and shake their heads. "Why do they always pick these kinds of people to be on TV?" my father would say. "They sound like such hicks." It was true. They did sound like hicks. They would draw out their words in a country twang. They would say *in*surance, with the emphasis on the first syllable. Greenville became Grainville. Here became hair and hair became hay-ur. They sounded like one of those guys with overalls and a banjo on *Hee Haw.* Yet we never noticed this until we saw these people on television. Had we come across the very same people in the barbershop or the public library or in church, it would never have occurred to us that they had an accent. To be honest, their accents were probably no different from ours.

What interested me about this was the way the distinctiveness of our local accent was hidden from us until we pulled back and saw it—or rather listened to it—from the position of someone else. It was only by watching television, looking through the lens of the camera, that we were able to see what we ordinarily took for granted. What was most obvious to a television viewer, of course, was the way the local accents compared to the other ones on TV, which are all non-southern (that is to say, Yankee) accents. The television news reporters may well have been southerners themselves, but even southerners talk like Yankees when they are on TV. It is an unspoken convention: if you are on TV you talk like a Yankee. Everyone does. If you don't, you sound like a hick.

Lilli Ambro told me that most of her clients at The Perfect Voice are people who have to do a lot of public speaking, like actors or certain kinds of businesspeople. One was, unsurprisingly, a television news reporter. Another was an aspiring actress whose acting coaches had advised her that to have a successful career she would need to be able to switch her southern accent on and off. All were southerners except one. The exception was a man from Pennsylvania running for local public office who wanted to reduce his northern accent in order to improve his chances for election. (This knife cuts both ways. In the South, a northern accent codes for arrogance and bad manners.) Most (though not all) of her clients were white. It goes without saying, perhaps, that most of these clients felt they needed to change their accents in order to succeed at work, and felt strongly enough about it that they were willing to pay $45/hour to undergo a successful "dialect change."

What sort of accents were these people trying to change? In her book on cosmetic surgery, sociologist Kathy Davis notes how difficult it was for her, as an outside observer, to guess exactly what feature of themselves the potential clients wanted cosmetic surgery for—that many of the women who wanted nose jobs did not have obviously large or misshapen noses, or that many of those who wanted breast reductions did not have obviously large or asymmetrical breasts. The "defects" that bothered them so much seemed to be exaggerated in their own eyes.[4] So I wondered aloud to Ambro whether there was a parallel in her work—whether it was ever difficult for an outsider to see exactly why these people wanted their accents changed. "No," she replied immediately; it was not hard to see why these people wanted to change. They all had very "strong" southern accents, she said. When I pressed her on what she meant by this, it became clear that most of her clients sounded like country folks or hillbillies. They were worried not so much about sounding southern as about sounding like hicks. Which made sense: this was the South, after all, where most people talk with southern accents. The worry in the South is not to get rid of your accent, like an expatriate southerner trying to pass in the North, but rather to transform it to a better one (which generally means something closer to what Ambro calls a "standardized American" accent). Ambro told me that she does not generally get clients who want to rid themselves of a Tidewater Virginia accent, say, or an old Charleston accent, or any of the accents that sound especially well bred to southern ears. Yet she did admit that she occasionally tried to convince some of her clients that accents that sounded objectionable to their own ears were actually quite lovely.

I have to confess that when I called Lilli Ambro, I was skeptical about the notion of accent-reduction clinics, notwithstanding Ms. Ambro's good intentions and her charming manners. Expatriate southerners like me are likely to worry excessively that distinctive features of the South are going to disappear; that in a vast consumerist sea, an age of generic TV news anchors speaking standardized American, southern accents will go the way of the corner barber shop and the porch swing. (Or, possibly even worse, that a southern accent will become a curiosity piece to be marketed to Yankees, like small-batch bourbon and alligator farms.) But what worried me most was the sense that by trying to change your accent, you are rejecting something of who you are. Unlike a Chinese or Cuban immigrant who speaks English with an accent, we southerners are raised to speak the way we do. It is our mother tongue. It is the first thing that non-southerners notice about us when we open our mouths. To try to speak like a northerner, quite honestly, strikes me as phoniness—perhaps necessary phoniness on occasion, and a kind of phoniness to which we are all prone, but phoniness nonetheless. This is also what rubs me the wrong way about some enhancement technologies, especially those designed to efface markers of ethnicity. They look pretty close to fakery.

I once had a colleague at McGill University who spoke with a perfect upper-class English accent. It was only when I asked him what part of England he was from that I found out he was born and raised in Ontario. He had spent a couple of years at Oxford as a student many decades previously. Apparently he had adopted an English accent while he was there, and had hung onto it ever since. I can't remember ever having met a southerner who would affect an Oxford accent (where I come from, Oxford is a town in Mississippi), or who would even feel inclined to try, but many southerners do try to talk standardized American, or what they think is standardized American, saying "you" instead of "y'all" and articulating their words very carefully. In the United Kingdom, the BBC has made a nod toward acknowledging the legitimacy of regional accents by occasionally substituting Scots-, Irish-, and Welsh-accented newsreaders for the traditional Englishmen. But in the United States, the newsreaders all speak as if they come from nowhere—which to a southern ear, usually sounds like somewhere up North. (A Tennessean I once met in Chicago told me that all Americans should hang on to their native accents or else we would all sound like we come from Indi-goddamn-ana.)

The newspaper piece that led me to The Perfect Voice was written for the *Greensboro News and Record* by a reporter with the southern-accented name of Parker Lee Nash. She is a self-described "southern girl, raised by bootleggers and Baptists," and her attitude toward The Perfect Voice could probably be best described as ironic and gently mocking. (She writes that to talk like a Yankee, you have to "open your mouth big and wide and relax your tongue so it flops up and down like a dog lapping water.") What interested me most about her article was the lighthearted remark she concluded with. After spending a day in accent-reduction classes, learning things like how to say "ham" in such a way that it does not contain two syllables, she concluded, "All the accent reduction classes in America can't take the Southern out of me. Thank the Lord."[5]

Implicit in that offhand remark, it seemed to me, was both the worry about an accent change ("Am I trying to change who I am?")

and the reassurance that this worry is misplaced ("No, being southern is about more than having a southern accent"). And so I began to
wonder whether clients at an accent-reduction clinic had any mixed
feelings about their change—whether they felt that putting on an
accent was artificial, or a betrayal of their heritage.

When I put this question to Lilli Ambro, she proceeded (as southerners are inclined to do) to tell me a story. She once had a client who
was a preacher. Or more precisely, he was a sort of junior preacher,
an assistant to a more senior pastor in a local church. She wasn't sure
what denomination, but it wasn't Presbyterian or Episcopalian—
more likely it was Baptist, or some poor relation. This preacher was
from out in the country and he had an appropriately countrified
accent. His senior minister had told him that he needed to work on
the way he spoke, or else the congregation wouldn't take him seriously. Hence his visit to The Perfect Voice. Interestingly enough, he
did not last any longer than a lesson or two. The reason, he said, was
because he felt that the accent-reduction classes were changing his
personality. (Almost as an afterthought, Ambro added, "He never did
pay his bill.")

As odd as this preacher's reaction initially sounded to me, I think
I can understand it. To paraphrase Kurt Vonnegut, if you pretend for
long enough, you may become what you are pretending to be. Yet
when I mentioned the story to a colleague from the North, a philosopher at an Ivy League university, he was puzzled by the thought that
anyone could feel that his identity was bound up in anything as trivial and incidental as an accent. Southerners, of course, usually understand the connection between accent and identity right away. So does
anyone from the United Kingdom, where accent is a very public
marker of social class, perhaps even the most important one. The
British often confess to tremendous anxiety about accent, and what
it reveals about social standing. And indeed, expatriates of all sorts in
the United Kingdom are constantly made aware of their accents, and
what the accent reveals about their geographical origins. I suspect
that the thought that an accent is incidental to identity would occur
mainly to people who have never had attention called to their own.

In *Democracy in America*, Tocqueville contrasts the behavior of
Englishmen in foreign countries with that of Americans. If two Eng-

lishmen meet in a foreign country, he says, they will pay no attention to one another. "But two Americans are at once friends," he writes, "simply because they are Americans."[6] Tocqueville attributes this difference to the complexities of the English class system. Englishmen don't quite know how to behave with other Englishmen; until they begin to speak and listen carefully to one another, neither can immediately discern the other person's social class. Social class therefore becomes a matter for uncomfortable investigation. But Americans have no such class system to negotiate, and hence no need for investigation. The Americans are more comfortable with each other, because both know immediately where they stand.

Tocqueville sees very clearly the anxiety that uncertainty about social class can generate. What he did not anticipate was the way that Americans would replace anxiety about class with anxiety about status. Status does not demand uncomfortable investigation in quite the way that class does, because it is so obviously a matter for public display. Status is a matter of self-presentation. Europeans often assume that status in America depends on how much money you make, but money is only part of a complex equation. (As the transplanted Englishman Andrew Sullivan puts it, status has less to do with how much money you make than who returns your phone calls.)[7] Unlike class, status is crucially dependent on what other people think of you. More than that, in fact, in some ways it *is* what other people think.

Status in America can come from many things, of course: wealth, education, achievement, beauty, talent, celebrity, or the family name that you have inherited. At least part of the American anxiety about status comes from the pressure to put these markers of status right out in front, like a walking self-advertisement. You must dress for success, develop a dazzling personality, sell yourself, make a good first impression. For Sullivan, this helps explain why Americans are so obsessed with their bodies. Americans are constantly worrying: Too fat or too thin? Too tall or too short? Breasts too large or too small? Is having no hair on your head cool (the way it is for black men) or does it make you a candidate for Rogaine (as it does for white men)? In the British class system, the body is secondary—as Sullivan puts it, it is "an unchanging, clammy, misshapen blob that performs the task of conveying the accent from one geographical location to another." But "for status-conscious Americans," Sullivan concludes, "the body is a walking nervous disorder."[8]

American status contrasts sharply with British class, which is something that a person is born to, and which, as a consequence, is largely a settled affair. English people can't do anything about who their parents are, where they were sent to school, or how they came to speak the way they do. If an Englishman tries to change his accent, he may well be accused of class betrayal or, even worse, American-style social climbing. But in America, people are expected to try to change their status. We encourage people to make more money, get better jobs, and marry up the social ladder. The status system in America can be both empowering and terrifying: empowering, because you can actually improve your social position, but terrifying, in that you can fail, with no one to blame but yourself.

Yet American status is nothing if not local. What counts as a marker of status for university professors is nothing like what counts for corporate executives; and status on a Philadelphia basketball court is measured on a different yardstick than status at a New Orleans debutante ball. The fact that the yardstick of status can differ so dramatically from one place or community to another is part of what drives the tension some Americans feel about their accents. An accent may drive your status up at work, but down at home; up in Manhattan, but down in Natchez; up for your day job at the phone company but down for your night job at the bar. Even the lowly southern accent will count as a mark of status if you happen to be a bluegrass fiddler or a stock-car driver.

Or, for that matter, an airline pilot. In *The Right Stuff*, Tom Wolfe writes about that particular southern drawl that anyone who has traveled on American commercial airlines has heard over the public address system. It is always the same, writes Wolfe: an easy, down-home southern voice that seems to get even easier and more down-home when something alarming is happening to the plane. As the airplane shakes and rattles and jolts up and down a thousand feet a clip so that your stomach leaps up into your throat, a folksy voice will come on the intercom just as relaxed as a voice can be: "Now, folks, uh . . . This is the captain . . . ummmm . . . We've got a little ol' red light up here on the control panel that's tryin' to tell us that the *landin'* gears're not . . . uh . . . *lockin'* into position when we lower 'em . . . Faint chuckle, long pause, as if to say, *I'm not even sure all this is really worth going into—still, it may amuse you* . . . "[9] Later, after the plane has dumped its excess fuel into the ocean and the flight attendants are walking briskly and tight-lipped down the aisles asking you to remove all sharp objects from your pockets and put your head between your legs—to "assume the position," as the pilot puts it, with "another faint chuckle ('*We do this so often, and it's so much fun, we even have a funny little name for it*')," even as your heart pounds and your palms sweat and your mind races through all the things that could go wrong, you still cannot quite bring yourself to believe that the trouble could really be all that critical, otherwise how could the pilot, who surely would know better than anyone else if the plane is in real danger, keep on drawling and chuckling in that relaxed, aw-shucks southern voice?

That voice may sound vaguely southern, writes Wolfe, but in fact it is Appalachian in origin; specifically, it is West Virginian. That voice is the pilot's approximation of the accent of Chuck Yeager, the legendary test pilot who broke the sound barrier in 1948 at what is now Edwards Air Force Base. Yeager's legend among the brothers of the pilot fraternity has been so powerful—his thirteen kills as a fighter pilot at the age of twenty-two, his record-breaking test flight in 1948 (which he performed, effortlessly, with two broken ribs), his general shit-kicking, cool-as-ice demeanor—that every pilot who has gone through Edwards Air Force Base after Yeager has wound up talking like a West Virginian. Since the military is the training ground for so many pilots, the accent has spread even further, from test pilots to fighter pilots to commercial pilots. Today when passengers hear a voice coming out of the cockpit, chances are the voice will sound like some approximation of Yeager's West Virginia drawl.[10] In the world of airline pilots, suggests Wolfe, talking like a West Virginian is a marker of status.

Status is not everything, of course. Accents often mark status, but they are also a mechanism by which people demonstrate their solidarity with others who share their identity.[11] If you talk the right way, you show that you stand side-by-side with your fellow West Virginians, or Highland Scots, or African Americans. Educated speakers of a dialect often hang on to a trace of that dialect, even as they try to speak the standard version of the language. In this way, you can have your cake and eat it too: you get the status advantages of speaking standard English and the solidarity advantages of speaking with a slight southern drawl. You raise yourself in the eyes of those who see your accent as a marker of backwardness, but you also steel yourself against the complaint that you have betrayed your heritage.

In the vast museum of American consumerist oddities, accent-reduction clinics like The Perfect Voice probably merit little more than a small corner display. Yet there are at least two aspects to them that are worth thinking about more carefully, in light of the consumerist forces that drive the development of enhancement technologies. One is the way the language of illness is used to describe, however lightheartedly, the process of changing your accent. You do it at a clinic, and you are treated by a speech pathologist. In fact, you are not really changing your accent; you are "reducing" it, as if it had somehow ballooned out of control, like your weight or your blood sugar, and you need treatment in order to rein it back in.

The other thing to notice is just what is being sold at the accent-reduction clinic. Enhancement technologies are usually marketed and sold by taking advantage of a person's perception that she is deficient in some way. Accent reduction is no different. What is being sold at the accent-reduction clinic is old-fashioned, American-style self-improvement, and the yardstick on which the self-improvement is measured is social status and success at work. The accent-reduction clinic takes advantage of the perception (or perhaps the reality) that non-southerners see a southern accent as something to be hidden or overcome, and that even southerners themselves see certain kinds of southern accents as better than others. (The reason why it is better to talk like Scarlett and Rhett than those guys in the overalls in *Deliverance* is clear enough. But behind the more subtle gradations of accent is a peculiar sort of ancestor worship practiced by some white southerners that associates certain accents with a distinguished genealogy.) If The Perfect Voice is in any way representative, the people most inclined to change their accents are those whose success at work depends on the successful public presentation of themselves—actors, businesspeople, newsreaders, and the occasional minister.

It is the relationship between public performance and the inner life that produces the mixed feelings that I suspect many southerners would have about an accent-reduction clinic. Southerners are quite familiar with public performance, of course; there is a good reason for all those self-dramatizing southern women in the plays of Tennessee Williams. But self-dramatization is one thing, and pretending to be a Yankee is another. Talking like a northerner would strike many southerners as a necessary evil at best, and at worst, a form of selling your birthright. It is a form of "passing," of hiding what is distinctive about your cultural identity. (The proper southern response to being made to feel ashamed of your accent, of course, is to exaggerate it.)

KATE JIRIK IS an honors student at the University of Minnesota. She has a near-perfect grade point average and will very likely graduate from the university summa cum laude. Like Stephen Hawking, Jirik is severely disabled and uses a wheelchair, and she cannot speak in her natural voice. She communicates with a computer and voice synthesizer. Her disability makes her a slow, one-finger typist. I got to know Kate when she asked me to be a faculty advisor for the honors thesis she was writing on the eugenics movement.

When Kate was four months old, she aspirated on aspirin and suffered anoxic brain injury. Later she was overdosed on phenobarbital. At thirty months she was institutionalized and it was assumed that she was profoundly retarded. But as she got older, her adoptive mother and others taught her to communicate using Bliss symbols, an international communications system often used by the disabled. Later she learned English, and at the age of eighteen or nineteen years she got her first voice synthesizer. It was Kate who initially called my attention to the relationship between voice and identity. When we first met in person, Kate, like Hawking, told me how attached she had become to her computer-generated voice. She had even resisted upgrading her computer software because it would have meant changing her voice.

Yet Kate's predicament differs in an important way from Hawking's. Hawking has a degenerative disease that began when he was a university student. He was a fluent English speaker who lost his voice, then got a voice synthesizer. But Kate has never been able to speak English in her natural voice. She can make some natural sounds ("I babble," she says) but for complex communication her spoken voice has always been that of the voice synthesizer.

For most people, thinking and speaking are tied together in complicated and rather mysterious ways. We hold imaginary conversations in our heads. We "think out loud." We learn to read first by speaking the written words aloud, then suppressing the speech and "hearing" the words. Often we clarify our thoughts by articulating them to other people. This complex relationship between thought and speech is part of the reason why conversation is so important for intellectual work: not just hearing what people say to you, but the fact that you must respond, and hear yourself respond, and clarify your thoughts in response to what you hear yourself say. As I thought about Kate's predicament, and the way that she has been able to succeed academically despite her disability, I began to wonder about her inner life, and whether it has developed differently in response to her inability to articulate words in her natural voice. What is it like to think and speak without ever having spoken complex thoughts in your natural voice?

Because she communicated first nonverbally, then with Bliss symbols, and only later in English, Kate says it is almost as if she must interpret her inner life and translate it for the English-speaking voice synthesizer. This can be slow and cumbersome, and she finds some things very difficult to translate—personal feelings, for example, or ideas with strong emotional content. "With no voice for so long," she says, "I had to use nonverbal means first." Sometimes she still communicates this way, through gestures and other kinds of behavior, especially when she becomes frustrated with computerized communication. The idea of unspoken imaginary conversation, however, or clarifying a thought by speaking it aloud—ideas that seem completely natural to me—Kate finds very odd. "I organize things in my head," she tells me, "and then put them in English and then write them."

Kate says she realizes that she thinks differently than most people, and that she used to consider this a problem. Now, however, it sometimes seems like an advantage. "I'm starting to realize that it allows me to make connections that don't occur to most people, and that

that can be a benefit," Kate says. She is especially careful about preconceived conceptions of the world that most people take for granted, because she often did not learn the same things herself. "For example, I spent most of my first ten years in an institution for profoundly retarded children. None of the kids there could talk so I figured talking was something you learned to do as an adult, since the adults could talk." She admits that this seems rather bizarre to her now, but it fit the information she had at the time. "I think I can bring a different perspective to certain things," she says, "but that may also be wishful thinking on my part."

When I first met Kate, she told me she felt as if the computerized voice was *her* voice, and that comment intrigued me. What would it mean to identify so thoroughly with a voice that emerged from a machine? How would it feel to have your identity so intimately tied to a technology? As I talked more with Kate, however, I began to think that perhaps I had overinterpreted her comment. As important as her computerized voice is to her, the voice that is most closely tied to her identity is still the voice that comes from her throat. "The voice that is mine is not computer-generated," she told me. "But I will take this one since that one is not available." Despite her initial reservations, in fact, she has changed computer programs since the time of our first meeting, which has given her a new voice. The new voice sounds more feminine, which she prefers. "Plus," she says, "I can swear on this computer and be understood."

In some ways, Kate's experience with her voice is not much different from that of the rest of us: it balances the demands of self and self-presentation. Unlike a transsexual learning how to speak like a woman, or a recent immigrant to America trying to speak like a native, Kate does not have to "pass," at least as the notion of passing is conventionally understood. There is no community that she is trying to become a member of, no real tension between impersonation and authenticity. The identity that she feels the need to convince people of is simply the identity any American takes for granted—that of an intelligent person who can communicate in English—but which she says is not always apparent to others because of her physical appearance. The most important thing about her voice, she says, is that it be clear and understandable. She resisted her first voice synthesizer for that very reason. "It sounded stupid," she says. "I hated everything about it." As the technology improved over the years, however, Kate became more comfortable with the computer voices. She says, "I could change to a better computer voice pretty easily but it would have to be more understandable, less of a lousy pronouncer, have better intonation, and sound more feminine." When I asked her if the voice she was using now felt natural, she replied: "It's understandable." Written communication is still the most comfortable of all for her, however. She says she often prefers to communicate with people first by e-mail, because in person many people initially assume that she cannot communicate at all.

As Kate and I talked one afternoon about her synthesized voice, and her frustration with spoken conversation in the classroom, it occurred to me that a voice synthesizer might actually be an advantage over a natural voice in anxiety-producing situations. Many people worry about speaking in public, for example, because they fear their voices will betray them—that their voice will quaver, squeak, or sound choked-up and croaky. Some people use beta-blockers to prevent this from happening, which reduces their anxiety by masking it. But Kate says she has exactly the same fear when she speaks in class or gives a presentation. It's a different experience for her, of course, since she first types what she wants to say and then lets the program run. But her worry is the same: "It's hard to be in front of a group," she says, "because my computer can mangle English." In a way, her experience with the voice synthesizer is like that of someone taking beta-blockers. Just as beta-blockers hide what is going on inside a person by blocking the outward manifestations of his anxiety, a voice synthesizer hides what is going on inside Kate.[12] As she puts it, "I sound calm even when I freak."

The possibility of your voice sounding calm when you freak comes from the disjunction between the voice and the body that ordinarily produces it. From a historical standpoint, this disjunction has been a long time in the making. The radio and the telephone broke the link between voice and physical presence by allowing the voice to be transported over long distances. The phonograph broke the link between voice and time, by allowing the voice to be recorded and played back at a later period. Audiotape added a further wrinkle by allowing technicians to cut and splice sounds, creating new combinations that could be unfamiliar even to the original speaker. This created the technical conditions for a gap between voice and identity that was evident even by the mid-twentieth century. "Anyone who has made a BBC recording and been in on the editing session may emerge feeling that he can no longer call himself his own," said Roy Walker in the late 1950s. "You might have the feeling that if you went quickly out of the studio you might catch yourself coming in."[13]

In my conversations with Kate, however, I have been struck by her sense of connection to the customs and standards that govern ordinary speech, even as she uses a synthesized voice. She definitely prefers a voice that sounds female, for example, to one that sounds male. She also finds it a major problem that her voice synthesizer cannot really reflect her sarcasm or humor. "My synthesizer treats everything like a serious conversation," she says. "If I want to be sarcastic or funny, I have to put that at the end of my comment because I can't synthesize tone of voice. It sounds rather dumb. I have to say something like "I totally agree with you; I'm being sarcastic." While my own sense is that Kate underestimates the degree to which her humor comes through with her voice synthesizer (I found her offbeat humor one of the most striking things about her when we first met), her point remains. The synthesizer cannot really mimic the tone of voice that most of us depend heavily on to alter what we mean when we speak. (Think of the difference that tone of voice can make even with the simple phrase "No kidding.") Kate says, "Mostly I don't use sarcasm or other things that depend on tone of voice because it loses its effectiveness when you have to spell it out."

And then, of course, there is the accent. As it turns out, accent is very important even for a synthesized voice. When I asked Kate if she would feel comfortable using a voice that spoke with an upper-class English accent, she said no. Why not? "Because I am from Minnesota," she says. I point out that the synthesized voice doesn't have a Minnesota accent either, and she agrees. Then she pauses. "But it is a computer."

FOR MALE-TO-FEMALE transsexuals, one mark of a successful transition is getting "ma'amed" on the phone. "A few years ago a telemarketer called me 'ma'am' for the first time in a while," remarked one transsexual recently in an on-line forum, "and I felt really proud."[14] Phone conversations are especially important for a successful transition because you cannot depend on your appearance or your manner to communicate anything about your gender. You must depend entirely on your voice, and your voice can easily fail you. If you sound like a man, you risk being treated as a man, no matter how convincing your physical appearance.

A person who was born a woman and has undergone sex-reassignment surgery to become a man can count on hormones to deepen his voice. Androgens will add mass to the vocal apparatus, lower the pitch of the voice, and make him sound more masculine. But the reverse is not true. Estrogens taken by male-to-female transsexuals do not raise the pitch of their voices. Thus many male-to-female transsexuals spend an extraordinary amount of time and effort (not to mention money) learning how to speak like a woman. They undergo voice coaching, buy audio- and videocassettes, trade hints and tips on the Internet, even get surgery to raise the pitch of their voices. It can be a surprisingly difficult change.

From its very beginnings, sex-reassignment surgery has been tied to the idea of "passing." Most of us (at least in the West) live in societies where a person must be classified as either a man or a woman. Sex-reassignment surgery can help a person make the transition from one category to the other, but our society does not allow much space between categories. This makes passing very important. Transsexuals may feel like neither ordinary men nor ordinary women, but given the set of social structures that we have, they are forced to pass as one or the other.[15] A man who undergoes surgery and hormone treatment to become a woman must pass as a woman for the transition to be considered successful.

For postoperative male-to-female transsexuals, a lot rests on the success or failure of this effort to pass as a woman. Many Americans feel threatened, offended, or repulsed by the transsexual identity. Failing to pass can be physically dangerous. "Without a passable voice, it can be terrifying to find yourself in an elevator and to have a man try to chat you up," says Lisa Stewart, a male-to-female transsexual in Canada. "The risk of violence is very much on the forefront of my mind." Yet passing is important even in the most tolerant parts of the country, in that an identity always depends on the recognition by others. Your identity as a woman is legitimated by being recognized as a woman; you feel more like a woman if you are "ma'amed" on the phone.

Passing, however, always exists in tension with the moral ideal of authenticity. Passing as the authentic item is never quite the same as *being* the authentic item. (If it were, it would not be passing.) With passing, there is always the danger of being discovered, of being found out and exposed for what you "really" are. This tension is suggested in a story told by Melanie Anne Phillips, a male-to-female transsexual who markets a voice-training course on the Internet.[16] When she was making the transition from male to female, Phillips found herself unhappy with her female voice. She had tried raising the pitch of her voice, but that did not really work; her voice had simply come out sounding like a bad falsetto. One day she was trying out different voices, trying to sound female, and suddenly her voice "slipped gears." "I couldn't believe it!" Phillips writes. "I actually sounded female!" She tried saying one thing and then another, and everything came out sounding female. She says it was "almost like being magically transformed into a woman!"

The problem, Phillips says, is that she was not yet living full-time as a woman. At work she was Melanie. But at home she was still Dave, a married man whose children did not yet know that he was becoming Melanie. The day her voice slipped gears, it got stuck in the female mode. Try as she might, Phillips could not speak like a man again. When Phillips went home that evening looking like Dave but speaking like Melanie, his wife "flipped out." She demanded that Dave talk like a man, not like a woman. It took Dave an hour to get his old voice back. Only gradually did Phillips learn how to move back and forth between the old voice and the new one.

Which was Phillips's real voice, the old one or the new one? Clearly, any answer to that question is going to be problematic. One might as well ask: Is Phillips really a man, or really a woman? When sex-reassignment surgery was in its infancy, it accommodated the moral ideal of authenticity with the story of the "woman trapped in a man's body." According to this story, sex-reassignment surgery was a matter of finding yourself, of changing the mutable self-presentation to match the enduring inner self. But getting a new voice is harder to accommodate to this "true self" model, because it so obviously involves an act of impersonation. There is no true voice to uncover, at least in any obvious way. Changing your voice is a matter of hard training, of consciously finding and developing a way of talking that you are happy with, and that you can gradually, over time, accommodate as your own.

Most voice-training techniques for transsexuals involve some degree of self-conscious impersonation. The idea is to find a decent impersonation of a female voice that they are comfortable with, and which (eventually) they will feel to be their own. In a recent on-line discussion of voice training, one transsexual says she found her voice by imitating Helen Hunt. "The trick is to find an actress whose voice is similar to yours, and then try doing lines from the shows/movies she's in," she says. "I have several hours of Helen Hunt and cue up the VCR on a regular basis to do her lines along with her."[17] Even transsexuals who do not imitate a specific person often need to try out different voices until they develop one that feels comfortable. "Most transsexuals want a voice that suits them," says Anita Kozan, a speech-language pathologist who works with a number of transsexuals in the Twin Cities. "They want a voice that matches how they look." Matching how they look, Kozan points out, is not just a matter of finding a female voice; it is also a matter of finding a voice that matches their size and height.

Finding a voice involves a number of technical challenges. The most obvious challenge is finding a way to speak comfortably in a voice with a higher pitch. Most transsexuals get some kind of voice coaching to accomplish this, but some turn to surgery. Surgery cannot alter the resonance of the voice, nor will it give anyone a voice that they have never used before. But some surgeons claim that surgery can raise the pitch of a male-sounding voice to the point where it falls somewhere within the female register.[18]

The pitch of the voice depends partly on the vibrations of the vocal cords as air passes across them.[19] One way to raise the pitch of a voice is to increase the tension of the chords. Imagine a guitar string. If you turn the key on a guitar and loosen the tension of the string, then the pitch will be lower when you pluck it. If you tighten the key and raise the tension, then the pitch will be higher. The faster the string vibrates, the higher the pitch.

This is the principle behind the most common procedure to change the voice, the crico-thyroid approximation. The crico-thyroid approximation surgically mimics what ordinary people do when they naturally raise the pitch of their voices. When a person speaks or sings in a high voice, he or she naturally contracts the crico-thyroid muscle. This muscle contraction brings together the cricoid cartilage and the thyroid cartilage in the neck, which in turn raises the tension of the vocal cords. The same thing is accomplished with the crico-thyroid approximation. A surgeon makes a small horizontal incision in the neck and sutures the cricoid cartilage to the thyroid cartilage. This suture stretches and tenses the vocal cords. If all goes well, the patient will then speak in a higher voice. It will probably not be an entirely new voice, but the crico-thyroid approximation may raise the baseline pitch at which the person usually speaks.[20]

Laser-assisted voice adjustment (LAVA) is a newer, still experimental procedure to feminize the voice, and it operates on a slightly different principle. Rather than raising the pitch of the voice by tensing the cords, the idea is to raise the pitch by reducing their mass. Imagine guitar strings again. The bass string on the guitar has a lower pitch than others of the same length because of its thickness. If you could devise a way to thin it out, you could raise the pitch. This is what the LAVA procedure does. In the LAVA procedure, the surgeon uses a CO_2 (carbon dioxide) laser to remove some of the vocal cord tissue. By removing the tissue the surgeon accomplishes two things. She reduces the mass of the cords, and she makes them stiffer, because of the scarring and healing involved. The reduced mass and increased stiffness make the cords vibrate faster, and this raises the pitch of the voice. Unlike the crico-thyroid approximation, however, LAVA is irreversible.[21]

Surgery can raise the pitch of a voice, but pitch is probably not the most important thing about a feminine voice. Many women speak in low-pitched voices but still sound like women. Kozan points out that most Western cultures prefer breathier, lower-pitched voices, for men as well as women. (Compare Western singing voices to Chinese or Indian singing voices, which sound tense, high-pitched, and somewhat nasal to a Western ear.) For Melanie Anne Phillips, the key to sounding like a woman is learning how to adjust its timbre. (This adjustment is what happened suddenly when her voice "slipped gears.") Timbre refers to the resonance of the voice, and it is determined by the properties of the throat, mouth, nose, and sinuses. Timbre is the acoustic property that makes a trumpet sound different from a trombone or a tuba, even when they are all playing the same note. Women have smaller "resonators" than men, so a male-to-female transsexual may have a voice whose pitch lies within the female range, yet still sounds like a man because of its resonance. But Phillips believes that transsexuals can alter the timbre of their voices with vocal training. The aim is to make the voice not just higher-pitched, but "smaller"—less like a trombone and more like a trumpet. She advises clients to open their mouths more when they speak, and to carry their tongues higher in their mouths.

Near the end of her voice-feminization video, *Girl Talk: Melanie Speaks on Developing a Female Voice*, Phillips makes a casual remark that reveals something of the moral tension behind the voice-feminization techniques that she teaches. After a long exposition on the many differences in the way that men and women speak and gesture—the way that women wave their hands and let their voices move up and down in pitch while they talk, the way their speech is passive and indirect—Phillips acknowledges that some feminists might object that she is stereotyping women. "But the point of this video is not to challenge stereotypes," she says. "The point is to *become* a stereotype." That comment may be debatable, but the dilemma it points to is genuine. How do you pass successfully, speaking and behaving in an unmistakably feminine way, unless you become a stereotype?

Candace Myers, a speech-language pathologist in Winnipeg, says that some transgendered people tend to "over-amp" at first, with very exaggerated feminine gestures. "This actually attracts more attention to them as 'unusual' and makes people question and look further, rather than immediately accepting them as female," she says. Sometimes Myers uses video feedback to let clients see how they are coming across. But part of her job is also to help them understand what sort of self-presentation they would like to have. Myers says she now asks transsexual clients what sort of woman they would like to be. Their replies vary tremendously: "I'm a lesbian," "sort of butch," "like Martha Stewart," "sort of casual and tomboyish," "very feminine," or even, "I'd like to be like you!"

No doubt part of the reason *Girl Talk* has become so popular is Phillips's own feminized voice. Her voice is so convincingly feminine that it initially appears effortless. But Phillips has a background in acting, and in the course of demonstrating the voice-feminization techniques she advocates, she shifts voices so often and so easily that the appearance of effortlessness is undermined. After Phillips imitates Mickey Mouse, the Wicked Witch of the West, a Valley Girl, and a southern belle, her feminized voice comes to sound more like one among many possible impersonations. At that point, it also sounds like the product of an enormously stressful, time-consuming amount of work.

Given the work involved in acquiring a feminized voice, it is not surprising that some transsexuals initially hesitate to describe their female voice as their "true," "real," or "natural" voice. Some confess to discomfort with the impersonation involved. In a recent on-line discussion, one transsexual said, "The thing I hate most about my new voice is that it is fake. And I do not wish to be fake in any way."[22] Lisa Stewart told me via e-mail, "Producing a female voice does feel like an impersonation because you know it sounds funny. At the same time, a girly voice does feel like it's coming from me—it's a voice I feel I possess." Yet she also pointed out that her old voice was uncomfortable as well, although for different reasons. "My male voice is distressing—not from a passing factor, but it feels like a physical defect."

As false or as alien as a female voice may feel at first, however, many transsexuals eventually find themselves identifying with their new voices. Like Stephen Hawking with his voice synthesizer, they gradually become comfortable with the voices they are learning to use and to feel as if these voices are their own. "I think with the constant practice it becomes less 'fake' and more your own voice," writes Snowy Angelique Maslov, a male-to-female transsexual in Australia. "You personalise it; flesh it out and then slowly incorporate it within your normal life until you just don't notice."[23] "As my voice improves," Stewart wrote to me, "I identify more and more with it."

Given enough time, I suspect, some transsexuals probably come to feel as if their new voice is part of their "true selves." The self accommodates the changes brought about by the technology. Some transsexuals will even say as much. "I don't think your new voice is artificial when it reflects who you are inside," writes one. "Even with a different voice we are the same person, only one who is now more whole than before." Once the self-presentation matches the inner self, the new voice becomes the true voice. Another person explains, "My voice is not fake, it is my voice. And I think people hear that and accept it."

WHAT MANY MALE-TO-FEMALE transsexuals say of voice-feminization surgery could as easily be said of many other enhancement technologies. A technology may initially feel awkward or uncomfortable, but with enough time and practice it comes to feel natural, even an extension of the self. A new driver can hardly manage to shift gears and steer a car at the same time, but in time she can maneuver the car as easily and naturally as she can maneuver her own body. The same goes for wearing contact lenses, using a computer, or for that matter, piercing your ears or dying your hair. Feeling a sense of identity with a technology (and what it does for you) is often less a matter of what is "natural" than what you are used to. In fact, nothing feels less natural than trying to make your technology-free body do something to which it is not yet accustomed, as anyone knows who has tried to square dance or brush their teeth with their left hand.

When prosthetic technologies restore or simulate human capacities destroyed by injury or illness, it is one measure of the prosthetic's success if the patient comes to feel as if the technology is natural. It rarely occurs to us anymore to ask if an artificial hip joint or a pacemaker is unnatural or alien, and the same may soon be true of technologies that affect other human capacities. Hearing that is simulated by virtue of cochlear implants is not the same kind of hearing that most of us take for granted, but it does not seem unlikely that a person with a cochlear implant, over time, will come to feel that her simulated hearing is as natural as her sense of taste or touch. The same could be said for robotic limbs, night-vision enhancement, or computers wired directly to neurons. If technological restorations can come to feel natural, then so can technological enhancements.[24]

Is a blind man's cane part of the man? The question is confusing (and for that reason, philosophically interesting) precisely because of the ambiguity of the word "man." If "the man" means the man's body, then the answer depends on whether the cane is conceptualized as a bodily extension or an especially important tool. But if "the man" means his "self," his identity, then the answer must be mapped on an entirely different grid. Because the self, even in its peculiarly Western, late modern complexity, is by no means identical to the body, the mind, or even the soul. Yet it overlaps with all three. The Western self is (among other things) a moral concept, a locus of pride and shame. "Anything whose depreciation makes me feel resentful is myself, whether it is my coat, my face, my brother, the book I have published, the scientific theory I accept, the philanthropic work to which I am devoted, my religious creed, or my country," wrote sociologist Charles Cooley. "The only question is, Am I identified with it in my thought, so that to touch it is to touch me?"[25]

The term "enhancement technologies" suggests that what is morally important about such technologies is the fact that they are being used for self-improvement. But this suggestion is both unhelpful and misleading. Many enhancement technologies are interesting (and sometimes unsettling) not primarily because they enhance people, but because they affect something central to their identities. When a person undergoes surgery so that she can speak like a woman, or changes her nose with cosmetic surgery, or takes an antidepressant that transforms her from a shrinking violet to the life of the party, what is at issue is not simply whether the change is for the better or for the worse, or even whether the change has been mediated by technology, but the mere fact that the person has changed. She may not have exactly become a "different person," even in a figurative sense, but her identity may well have changed in a way that would strike many of us as morally significant. When Dave came home from work speaking in Melanie's voice, we can all understand his wife's distress.

This does not mean that there is necessarily anything wrong or distasteful about changing your identity. Some changes of identity are for the better, and others fall well within the range of what we accept as a matter of individual style. Nor does it mean that all enhancements involve changing your identity. Getting your teeth straightened or rubbing Minoxidil on the back of your head are probably no more life-changing than going to the barbershop. But identity is better than enhancement as a framework for thinking about these technologies, because our ambivalence about so many enhancement technologies is often ambivalence about the kinds of people we want to be. The question is not just whether there is any moral cost to the quest to become *better*, but whether there is any moral cost to the quest to become *different*. If we have mixed feelings about accent-reduction clinics, cosmetic surgery, or Prozac, this is partly because we have mixed feelings about the visions of the good life these technologies serve.

2

THE TRUE SELF

To be natural is such a difficult pose to keep up.
—Oscar Wilde

Tucked into a stone edifice in London's Red Lion Square is a
building, which, in the fashion of so many British structures,
manages to look both venerable and unassuming. It houses
the South Place Ethical Society. The South Place Ethical Society was
founded in 1793 by a splinter group of the Baptist Church called the
Philadelphians, in rebellion against the doctrine of eternal hell. Later
the society formed an association with the Unitarian Church, but it
broke with the Unitarians in the mid-nineteenth century. Today the
South Place Ethical Society is linked to no formal religious group
whatsoever. It identifies its ethical stance as humanist, and it sponsors
public lectures and courses on broad humanist ideals. The written
history on the bulletin board in its foyer mentions its past links with
luminaries such as Huxley and Russell. At the front of the main lecture hall, which looks very much like a sanctuary, a motto appears in
large script: "To thine own self be true."

If you were looking for a symbol of the moral direction of Western civilization over the past 200 years, you could not do much better than this. The South Place Ethical Society has gradually shifted its
moral vision from the Baptist God to the individual self, like an

astronomer turning away from the telescope to look at his own reflection in the mirror. "To thine own self be true" articulates perfectly the notion of authenticity as a moral ideal: the idea that we each have a way of living that is uniquely our own, and that we are each called to live in our own way rather than that of someone else.[1] This is not an ancient, time-honored ideal. Philosopher Charles Taylor argues that it emerged only in the late eighteenth century. But it has come to suffuse contemporary life so thoroughly that often we hardly recognize its presence until it is pointed out to us.

I pick up a parenting book; it promises to help parents guide their children in "discovering and expressing their true selves." I take my children to see a Disney movie; the heroine, a young girl in ancient China, sings, somewhat incongruously, that you "must be true to your heart." I walk into a library; on the wall is a poster that says the reason we travel is to "discover who we are." Put in the context of a children's movie or a self-help book, the notion sounds trite, but I don't intend to make it sound that way. I could equally well have pointed to the novels of Joseph Conrad or the philosophies of Hutcheson and Rousseau.[2] The fact is that it would be hard to find anyone living in the West today who has not absorbed something of the power of authenticity as a moral ideal. The idea of conscience as a moral guide, the concept of self-fulfillment, the democratic political commitment to our right to pursue our own vision of the good life, the notion of psychotherapy uncovering an inner truth buried deep within the unconscious—all these are part of the way in which authenticity has become a crucial part of modern identity.

By authenticity as a moral ideal, I have in mind the ideal Taylor summarizes when he writes, "There is a certain way of being human that is *my* way. I am called upon to live my life in this way, and not in imitation of anyone else's life." Taylor suggests that this idea "gives a new importance to being true to myself. If I am not, I miss the point of my life; I miss what being human is for me."[3] Taylor traces the ideal of authenticity to the eighteenth-century notion that each of us has a moral sense, or a feeling for what is right and wrong, good and bad. The notion of a moral sense suggests that understanding right and wrong is not just a matter of calculation, but rather is anchored in our feelings. We each have an intuitive sense of morality, a conscience that guides us. The ideal of authenticity, says Taylor, comes out of a displacement of this idea. The original idea was that you needed to be in touch with your feelings so that you can know how to do the right thing. It was an instrument for moral knowledge and right action. But soon being in touch with your feelings came to be a moral ideal in itself. Authenticity, says Taylor, came to be something we must attain if we are to be true and full human beings.[4]

The ideal of authenticity drives much of the language that patients and clients use to describe their use of enhancement technologies. Technologies from Prozac to face-lifts are routinely described as tools of self-discovery and self-fulfillment. "It costs me a lot to be authentic," says Agrado, the transsexual in Almodovar's film *All about My Mother*, as she recites the cost of all her cosmetic surgery. As Almodovar's script suggests, words like identity and authenticity provide us with a way to describe self-change without betraying a complex moral ideal. Or as Agrado puts it, "A woman is more authentic the more she looks like what she has dreamed for herself."

"I WAS THREE or perhaps four years old when I realized that I had been born into the wrong body, and should really be a girl." This is the opening sentence of *Conundrum*, Jan Morris's memoir of her transition from man to woman. For the first thirty-five years of her life Jan Morris was James Morris, a celebrated Welsh writer and foreign correspondent. Convinced that she was, despite appearances, really a woman, Morris began to take female hormones when she was in her mid-thirties. In 1972, at the age of forty-five, Morris underwent sex-reassignment surgery. Since that time she has lived as a woman.

The striking thing about Morris's memoir is the degree to which it is suffused with the vocabulary of identity and authenticity. Morris has been born into the "wrong body," she writes, a body at odds with her true self, and her medical treatment is a quest for authenticity. She tells of finding herself, of becoming her true self, of "achieving identity" through sex-reassignment surgery. Read today, from a distance of twenty-five years, these kinds of descriptions might seem unremarkable. But this is largely because the vocabulary she uses has come to seem so natural to us. We have become so accustomed to hearing these kinds of descriptions that they now seem like simple common sense, a natural way of describing the world, even when they are applied to a procedure as dramatic as sex-reassignment surgery. "I had been born into the wrong body," writes Morris, and we immediately understand what she means.

The narrative Morris relates in *Conundrum* relies on the ideal of authenticity for its moral justification as well as for its dramatic tension. Morris describes her early life as ordinary, even happy, yet it was also a time when she did not really know who she was. An American colleague once described James Morris as "so unobtrusive that one hardly knows he is there at all."[5] This unobtrusiveness was part of what made Morris such an effective journalist and travel writer. But Morris believes it was also the result of being "deprived of an identity."[6] The quality that others described as unobtrusiveness was to Morris a "detachment so involuntary that I often felt that I really wasn't there, but was viewing it all from some silent chamber of my own."[7]

From this silent, detached state, Morris moved gradually, hesitantly toward his authentic self. His first clue came to him in a bookshop in Ludlow, a small English market town. There he discovered a book called *Man into Woman. An Authentic Record of a Change of Sex,* which tells the story of Einar Wegener, a Danish painter who underwent sex-change surgery at a clinic in Dresden. Wegener never painted another picture after the surgery, and lived for only a year afterward, under the name Lili Elbe. Yet despite its bleak ending, the book gave Morris hope. He began to seek help from psychiatrists and sexologists.

From 1964 to 1972 Morris took female hormones, began to use the name Jan, and lived in what she describes as an androgynous state, neither unambiguously male nor female and apparently ageless. She describes this as less a feminization than a "stripping away of the rough hide in which a male is clad," the removal of "a layer of accumulated resilience."[8] Note her choice of words. Morris is not simply transformed; rather, her external male appearance is stripped away to reveal the true self that is underneath.

This stripping away is crucial, because the way others treat her is determined by what they see. What others see, however, varies tremendously from one culture to the next. The French, writes Morris, were curious about her androgynous state. Greeks were entertained. Americans usually assumed she was a woman. Scots were shocked, while Germans looked worried. The Japanese didn't seem to notice. "Are you a man or a woman?" a Fijian taxi driver asked her. "I am a respectable, middle-aged, English widow," Morris replied. "Good," said the taxi driver, "just what I want," as he put his hand on her knee.[9]

When Morris finally had the sex-reassignment surgery in Casablanca, she felt relief. "I felt above all deliciously clean," she writes. "The protuberances I had grown increasingly to detest had been scoured from me. I was made, by my own lights, normal."[10] Morris spent two weeks in the clinic recovering from the surgery. She found herself in the company of fellow patients from Britain, France, Greece, and America, a group that seemed to span the possible range of genders. What they all shared, according to Morris, was that they were all "gloriously happy." "Just for those few days of our lives, if never before, if never again, we felt that we had achieved fulfillment, and were ourselves."[11]

It is this kind of narrative that I have in mind when I suggest that authenticity serves as a moral ideal. At the start of a narrative of authenticity, the person is not really herself. She is unformed, ill at ease, lost in the world. She embarks on a quest, which may be dangerous and full of trials. Yet when it is over, she has found herself. She has achieved fulfillment. This is the kind of quest Morris describes. A previously rare and extraordinary transformation—from man to woman by way of surgery and endocrinology—sounds understandable, even ordinary, when Morris describes it using the language of authenticity. A woman trapped in a man's body: we can all immediately grasp what this means. We immediately understand the way that surgery becomes a means of remolding the outer body in conformity with the inner being, the way that it becomes a way for a person to achieve her true identity, the way that she may even feel called to do it. We understand all this because we have all so thoroughly absorbed the idea that hangs on the wall of the South Place Ethical Society. By getting sex-reassignment surgery, Jan Morris was being true to herself.

To an outsider who had grown up in a world unfamiliar with sex-reassignment surgery, Morris's claim might well sound preposterous. Here we have a person who was raised as a boy, who has been treated as male his entire life, who has married a woman and fathered children—yet who says he is really a woman, and that it is only by having his genitalia removed, taking hormones, and dressing as a woman that he can achieve his true identity. Put this way, it sounds rather implausible.[12] Even Jan Morris admits that she resisted the language of identity, finding it rather trendy and nebulous. Yet she can find no other words to describe her predicament. "I was not to others what I was to myself," she writes. "All I wanted was liberation, or reconciliation—to live as myself, to clothe myself in a more proper body, and achieve Identity at last."[13]

The language of authenticity may sound familiar to us, but authenticity is not an ideal that would come naturally to all people at all times. Contrast it, for example, with earlier Western views of how you come to be a true and full human being—the notion, for example, that you need to be in touch with God or, as Plato thought, with the Idea of the Good. Remnants of these early views remain with us still. But today the moral accent has been shifted from the external to the internal; today you must listen to the voice within you. The crowd might drown out that inner voice; you might find it difficult to hear because of all the other voices that are shouting all around you. But listening to it is crucial, because only that inner voice can tell you the person you are to be and the way you are to live. When Morris writes that all of her fellow patients in Casablanca were deliriously happy, having finally achieved fulfillment, she is articulating something of this ideal. True happiness cannot be attained without fulfillment, and fulfillment requires being true to that inner voice.

The crucial philosophical figures here, writes Charles Taylor, were Jean-Jacques Rousseau and, later, Johann Gottfried von Herder. Herder wrote that each of us has a unique way of being human. Each person has his or her own "measure." This was part of an altogether new idea, a shift Taylor sees as part of a massive inward turn in modern culture: the notion that people are beings with unique inner depths. Before the late eighteenth century, he writes, nobody had given individual human beings this kind of moral significance. Yet by the mid-twentieth century, the inadequacy of these "inner depths" was seen as the primary psychological problem afflicting Westerners. Psychoanalyst Rollo May could write in 1953 that "the chief problem of people in the middle decade of the twentieth century is emptiness." People living in the mid-twentieth century felt empty, May thought, because they did not know whether their inner lives were authentically theirs. "I mean not only that many people do not know what they want; they often do not have any idea of what they feel."[14] By May's time, the inability to understand what you really feel inside had become a barrier to living a full human life.

It is important to recognize the specifically *moral* pull of this ideal. Many people today have the sense that an authentic life is somehow a higher life, a more fulfilled life; they feel that if they do not discover a path that is true to themselves, to their own talents and desires and aspirations, they are missing out on what life could be. The fact that their lives are not being lived authentically means those lives are less vivid, less real, less fully lived than they might have been. Critics of the idea of self-fulfillment sometimes overlook this. They treat self-fulfillment as if it were simply selfishness. And sometimes it really is selfishness, of course, or narcissism, a cultivation of the self to the exclusion of anything outside it. What Taylor underscores, however, is the degree to which many people today feel *called* to pursue self-fulfillment—to devote themselves single-mindedly to a career, for example, or to cultivate their looks through severe diets and punishing workouts at the gym, even if it means ignoring their children, their partners, their friends, their God, or in fact any of the other things that people in other periods or cultures have thought essential to a good life.[15]

In her book *The Body Project*, historian Joan Jacobs Brumberg drew on the diaries of adolescent American girls as a way of understanding how the relationship of girls to their bodies had shifted over the past century. Prior to World War I, she found, girls rarely used the language of identity and self-improvement when they wrote about their bodies. In comparison to today, they were far less likely to mention their bodies at all. When they used moral language, it was usually directed not toward their bodies, but toward their character and behavior. When these girls wrote about self-improvement, they resolved to pay *less* attention to the self, not more, lest they be accused of vanity. Brumberg quotes the diary entry of an adolescent girl in 1892: "Resolved, not to talk about myself or feelings. To think before speaking. To work seriously. To be self-restrained in conversation and action. Not to let my thoughts wander. To be dignified. Interest myself more in others."[16]

Compare this, says Brumberg, to a diary entry of an adolescent girl in 1982: "I will try to make myself better in any way I possibly can with the help of my budget and babysitting money. I will lose weight, get new lenses, already got new haircut, good makeup, new clothes and accessories."[17] Not only is this girl concerned with her body and physical appearance in a way that would have been utterly alien to her 1892 contemporary, she also expresses her concerns using the language of morality. To lose weight and get a new haircut is to become a better person. Her physical appearance is an expression of who she is.

Self-discovery is crucial to this project. Finding yourself has replaced finding God. What is more, if you do want to find God, you find Him by looking inward. Writing in his characteristically cryptic, puzzling, and darkly solemn manner, philosopher Ludwig Wittgenstein observed, "You cannot hear God speak to someone else. You can only hear him if you are being addressed." Then, in parentheses, Wittgenstein added: "This is a grammatical remark." In their own odd way, these oblique remarks go straight to the heart of the ethic of authenticity. The ethic of authenticity tells us that meaning is not to be found by looking outside ourselves, but by looking inward. The meaningful life is an authentic life, and authenticity can be discovered only through an inner journey. By adding the parenthetical explanation—"this is a grammatical remark"—Wittgenstein tells us that he is not making a point about God, but about the way we *speak* about God. The voice of God comes not from outside us, but from within us; this is why we can hear him, as Wittgenstein puts it, only if we are being addressed. We may look to God for meaning, but even God dwells within us.

I N H I S M E M O I R, *Muscle*, Sam Fussell describes how, at the age of twenty-six, he finds himself working at a New York City publishing house. The Oxford-educated son of two university professors of English, Fussell has decided to spend a year in the United States while waiting to enter graduate school. He has a problem in New York, however. The city terrifies him. He is terrified of the crime, of the crazy people on the streets, of a place where deranged strangers seem to seek him out. Soon Fussell finds himself physically ill: pale, coughing, fever, colds. His doctors say it is pleurisy, then pneumonia, but Fussell knows the real problem. It is fear.

It is this fear that leads Fussell to what he, in retrospect, calls the disease of bodybuilding. He catches the disease when he ducks into a bookshop to avoid a man approaching him with a crowbar. Wandering through the aisles of the bookshop, like Jan Morris in Ludlow, Fussell picks up a copy of the Schwarzenegger biography, *Arnold: The Education of a Bodybuilder*. It is then that the thought hits him: why not turn himself into a walking billboard of invulnerability like Schwarzenegger himself? This resolution leads him to the local YMCA. Soon he is working out with free weights and reading bodybuilding magazines obsessively. He quits his publishing job to devote more time to bodybuilding, and moves from his Upper East Side apartment into a windowless basement flat with two refrigerators in Queens that he calls "the bunker." His parents are horrified, but Fussell is obsessed, and two years later, after a bodybuilding regimen punishing even by the standards of his fellow builders, he decides that he has outgrown New York. He moves to Southern California, the bodybuilder's mecca, and on his second day there he starts to take anabolic steroids.

The transformation in Fussell's appearance is astonishing. Photographs in his memoir show a shy-looking twenty-two-year-old young man, bony and long-haired, legs crossed and sitting in a lawn chair. Several years later, they show a man so changed it is difficult to imagine it is the same person: an enormous, oiled, steroid-enhanced bodybuilder with a buzz-cut, muscles bulging freakishly, eyes glazed, veins popping out all over his body, strutting and preening on a stage in Southern California. The transformation in his life is no less astonishing. His friends, once bookish types, are now a cultish and devoted set of muscleheads and gym bunnies, obsessed not only with their own bodies but with those of one another. His daily routine is a perpetual cycle of eating, dieting, and working out, buying seventy eggs a week at the supermarket and pumping his body to overflowing with enhancement drugs. His demeanor, once fearful and anxious, is by his own account transformed into a pose of hulking, aggressive arrogance. "I went from answering the phone meekly to shouting SPEAK! into the receiver on the first ring." He intimidates others behind the wheel of a car and in person, at one point physically picking up one of his publishing house coworkers and tossing him through an open door. "Without being fully aware of it myself, I became the kind of man I once feared and despised. I became, in fact, a bully."[18]

Fussell makes it clear that his quest is about identity, about his sense of himself, and most of all, his discomfort and anxiety with the person he perceives himself to be. Yet he alternates between the vocabulary of authenticity and that of self-invention. Early on in the memoir he writes about his bodybuilding regimen as if it changed him into someone else. He was once a reserved intellectual, Fussell writes, but his regimen transformed him. "I was no longer me. Gone was the cautious, passive, tolerant student, the gentle soul who had urged departing friends to take care and actually meant it. The new me was a builder. A builder who no longer had any time for anything that wouldn't help him grow. Who, in place of the words "thank you," barked "no kindness forgotten, no transgression forgiven." As my behavior changed, the smiles of my fellow workers disappeared, their greetings tapering off to a nervous nod of the head. There was fear in the air."[19]

Yet as he finds himself more and more obsessed with bodybuilding, more immersed in the bodybuilding subculture, Fussell begins to describe the changes using the vocabulary of authenticity—not as a transformation into someone else, not as becoming a new person, but as becoming *himself*. His true self, it seems, has become the musclehead. He justifies his choice to start taking steroids by saying that he needs them in order to become the person he really is. It ordinarily takes at least five years to get muscle maturity, he explains, the polished look that comes from deep muscle definition and separation. The only way to speed the process up is to take steroids, or "the juice." He decides to start taking steroids almost immediately after arriving in southern California, explaining that while he felt like a builder on the inside, his appearance (at least by southern California standards) did not match up. "I, for one, couldn't wait three or four or five more years to become myself," Fussell writes. "I was so uncomfortable not being me that I had to have it, now."[20]

The apparent ease with which Fussell is able to describe his self-transformation both as becoming a different person and, then later, as becoming himself, indicates the way in which authenticity can be as much an ideal as a self-description. Clearly what drove Fussell the sickly, reserved weakling toward bodybuilding was a desire to change. He wanted to become stronger, braver, more resilient to the terrors of daily life in New York. He wanted to be like Arnold. Being true to himself at that point would have meant being true to a self that he despised. Yet once Fussell has begun to remake his life—quitting his job, moving to the bunker, working out, changing his demeanor—he begins to see himself very differently. The diet, the juice, pumping iron, all become ways of shaping himself into a better, stronger, more complete version of himself.

Yet he cannot do this by himself. It is not enough for Fussell to like what he sees in the mirror. Others must like it too. Fussell's story shows the importance for identity of recognition: for Fussell, it was crucial that other people see him as a builder. Fussell's anxiety about his appearance became acute when he moved to California, where he was surrounded by bodybuilders far more buffed and polished than he was. "If who you are is what you do, and as a bodybuilder, what you do is what you look like, then in California I was distinctly in trouble, because I didn't look like a bodybuilder."[21] Because he was posing, walking the bodybuilder walk and delivering the lines without looking the part he was trying to play, Fussell was jittery and uncomfortable. "I was concerned far less with competition than with self-identity. As long as the part I played was simply interior, I felt like a fraud."[22]

A *fraud*. The word has a moral resonance that runs through many of these self-descriptions. The drive toward authenticity is not just a matter of desire. The feeling is that you *ought* to be true to who you really are, that there would be something wrong, something vaguely dishonest or unsavory, about turning away from your true self; that this would be kind of a betrayal, or fakery. This, as much as anything, helps to explain the pull of the language of authenticity for enhance-

ment technologies. It is a way of justifying them to yourself, counter-
ing the imagined criticism that they represent a kind of phoniness,
narcissism, or status-seeking. No, they are none of these, you say; it
was only when I got the face-lift, started on steroids, got a sex-change
operation, that I really felt like myself.

In her book *Reshaping the Female Body*, Kathy Davis describes a
Dutch woman named Sandra who recently underwent breast-reduction surgery. Explaining her decision, Sandra says she did not feel
comfortable being the sort of woman who has large breasts. "Large
breasts are *supposed* to be sexy," Sandra says. "So *you* get to be a sex
bomb, whether you want to or not."[23] Men were constantly staring
at her, and other women were jealous. For years Sandra had tried to
hide her breasts under bulky sweaters and coats. After she finally had
the breast-reduction surgery, all this changed. She became proud of
the way she looked. She felt more at home in her body, even though
her breasts were the handiwork of a plastic surgeon. By way of
explanation, she says, "I guess I just always was the small-breasted
type."[24] Behind Sandra's explanation lies the desire for recognition: it
was crucial for her to be recognized by others as "the small-breasted
type," in the same way that it was important for Russell to be recognized by others as a builder.

Some people are tempted to dismiss this kind of talk as empty self-
justification. I think that would be a mistake. For one thing, if people are drawn to use the language of authenticity it must have at least
some moral resonance for them, and to their imagined interlocutors.
For another, it would be to ignore the extraordinary amount of effort,
pain, and risk that go into these self-transformations. It is no small
thing to undergo major surgery, much less embark on a five-year
bodybuilding program or to change your sex. The pull to undertake
these transformations is often extraordinarily strong, and the ideal of
authenticity can be a large part of this pull. The ideal of authenticity
says that if you are not living a life *as yourself* you have missed out
on what life has to offer. You are squandering your short time on this
earth. This is not simply the sense that an authentic life is a happier
life; it is the sense that an authentic life is a *higher* life. Higher,
because it is a life of fulfillment, a life in which you know who you
are and live out your sense of yourself.

The moral pull of authenticity is not just a matter of individual identity. It is also part of group identity—the sense that there is a proper way of being a woman or a man, gay or straight, or of being Jewish or Xhosa or Irish. By identifying yourself in some way, either as a conscious choice or having been born to it, you become subject to certain moral constraints. My wife and her sisters often joke about what it is to be a good German—a good German loves uniforms, is obsessed with rules and bureaucracies, keeps her house scrupulously tidy, and drives like a maniac on the Autobahn. But jokes are funny only if there is an element of truth behind them, and that element of truth is often stronger than the joke implies. A German may well make fun of the German obsession with tidiness but still be unable to keep from feeling embarrassed at not keeping a tidy house. An American may well realize the illusory nature of the ideal of independence, yet still feel ashamed of having to accept help from someone else. An expatriate North Carolinian may realize that a diet of fried catfish, hush puppies, and pork barbecue is, from a health perspective, a tightrope walk over the abyss, yet he may still feel drawn to eat these things in gut-stuffing quantities when he goes home for fear of feeling like a traitor. Often these moral constraints are not played out within ordinary consciousness (not explicitly anyway) but they still play a tremendously important role in people's lives and the choices they make. When Sam Fussell started taking steroids, it was partly because that was what identifying himself as a bodybuilder required.

The recognition that was so important to Fussell is part of a much larger cultural shift that has made recognition critical for modern identity. For many Westerners it is now very important (in a way that it was not so important 200 years ago) that others recognize and respect them for who they are. A crucial development, according to Taylor, was the collapse of social hierarchies in the late eighteenth century. Public recognition of a person's identity was not an issue in hierarchical social systems because identity was based on categories that everyone took for granted. A person's identity was fixed by his or her social place. Recognition was built into the system. This is still true to some extent today, of course; people still derive their identities from their social roles, like being a doctor or a mother. But today we also have the expectation that a person generate an individualized identity, or an identity particular to a person. This is part of the ideal of authenticity. Recognition is critical, because the effort to generate an identity can fail. Others can refuse to recognize your identity, refuse to grant it equal moral status, or insist on seeing you in a way other than the way in which you see yourself. Others may insist you are Canadian while you see yourself as Québecois; others may insist that you are male or female while you feel you are neither. The notion that identity is something that you work out for yourself automatically brings about a certain tension, because identity can never be wholly inwardly generated. It must be developed in dialogue with others.[25]

Social hierarchies, as Taylor points out, were supported by a foundation of honor. In the same way that an honored prize would lose all meaning if it were given to everyone, the notion of honor becomes meaningless when everyone in a society is said to have it. Not everyone can win the Booker Prize or membership in Phi Beta Kappa; not everyone can belong to the British aristocracy. Honor rests on a foundation of inequality. But democratic societies have replaced social hierarchies supported by the notion of honor with structures of social equality supported by the notion of dignity. Dignity, unlike honor, is assumed to be universal and egalitarian. This is what we mean, for example, when we speak about the dignity of all human beings.[26]

The replacement of honor with dignity reinforces in a crucial way the importance of respect for individual identity. Dignity is something to which everyone in a democratic society has a right. But it is also something that a society can withhold. Withholding it can be a blow to a person's identity, because a society *shapes* the identity of its people by mirroring back to them an image of themselves. If that image is distorted—if it is not an image that accords a person a measure of dignity, and thus cannot serve as the basis for self-respect—then it can be crippling. This is what W. E. B. Du Bois was getting at in a famous passage from *The Souls of Black Folk*, when he described this sort of mirroring as "double consciousness." Black people in America always have the sense of "looking at one's self through the eyes of others," wrote Du Bois, "of measuring one's soul by the tape of a world that looks on in amused contempt and pity."[27] Black Americans always feel their two-ness, Du Bois wrote, because the way they see themselves is distorted by the way they are seen by others.

On a far looser and less systematic scale, the forces that Du Bois described are part of what motivates the desire for enhancement technologies. Technology has become a way for some people to build or reinforce their sense of dignity while standing in front of the social mirror. The mirror is critically important for identity; it is rare for anyone in a democratic society to be completely unaware of it. Most of us can keenly identify with the shame that a person feels when society reflects back to them an image that is degrading or humiliating. But the flip side to shame is vanity. It is also possible to become obsessed with the mirror, to spend hours in front of it, preening and posing, flexing your deltoids, admiring your hair. It is possible to spend so much time in front of the mirror that you lose any sense of who you are apart from the reflection that you see.

CARY GRANT WAS not ordinarily an easy man to interview, writes Jay Stevens in his popular history, *Storming Heaven*, but as reporters gathered around him for questions on the set of the movie *Operation Petticoat* in 1959, Grant was uncharacteristically forthcoming. "I have been born again," he told the astonished group. "I have been through a psychiatric experience which has completely changed me." The psychiatric experience to which Grant was referring was the result of LSD, which he used over sixty times. "I was horrendous," said Grant. "I had to face things about myself which I never admitted, which I didn't know were there. Now I know that I hurt every woman I ever loved. I was an utter fake, a self-opinionated bore, a know-all who knew very little." As he sat tanning himself on the deck of a pink submarine, an aluminum sheet attached to his neck, Grant described the way that LSD had put him in touch with himself. "I found I was hiding behind all kinds of defenses, hypocrisies and vanities," Grant said. "I had to get rid of them layer by layer. The moment when your conscious meets your unconscious is a hell of a wrench. With me there came a day when I saw the light."[28]

Experiences of the sort that Grant described account for much of the intellectual fascination with LSD and other psychedelic drugs in the 1940s and 1950s. Scientists saw psychedelic drugs as a window into the unconscious, a way to explore the inner life and perhaps even to control it. "Words like 'grace' and 'transfiguration' came to my mind," writes Aldous Huxley in *The Doors of Perception*. The same man who had cast soma as a chemical villain in *Brave New World* would become an evangelist for mescaline, gushing about its ability to give him "direct insight into the very Nature of Things."[29] People who took psychedelic drugs often had epiphanies about the self: the timelessness of the self, the interconnectedness of all selves, the genuine, authentic self, once its defenses and self-deception and hypocrisies have been peeled away. The actual content of these epiphanies often sounded like something less than profound, of course, at least when they were revealed to others who had not taken the drug. Nonetheless, some people, like Cary Grant, found them life-changing. LSD had shown him the grail.

What LSD did for Grant highlights yet another strand of authenticity as a moral ideal. This strand emphasizes the importance of introspection, of looking inward to discover who you really are. For it is only by discovering who you really are that you can see what you ought to be doing with your life. This is not necessarily a simple matter. You can be deceived about your own identity. You may believe what you see in the mirror and find yourself building an identity around a social role. Sartre famously described this kind of inauthenticity in *Being and Nothingness*: a man who is so wrapped up in the idea of himself as a waiter, so attentive to each nuance of his performance as a waiter, so invested in being a waiter in every way, that his identity has essentially *become* that of the waiter. There is no longer any difference between his identity and his performance of a social role. If authenticity is described in this way, then the search for authenticity becomes a search for an identity *apart* from a social role. You must look not outward to others but inward to the self, conceptualized as an interior space set apart from the expectations of society. This is what Grant said LSD helped him do. It peeled away all of the vanities and hypocrisies and playacting that his social role had encouraged him to develop and perform.

Like body modification, the promise of LSD as a tool for authenticity depends on a particular conception of the self. Both postulate a self that is divided into an inner chamber, home of the true you, and

an outer shell, which can be molded in response to social expectations. Jan Morris and Sam Fussell saw body modification as a means
of achieving authenticity because the modifications shaped their bodies in correspondence with a true self—the self that resided in this
inner chamber. Grant saw LSD doing something slightly different,
but similar nevertheless. By giving him a peek into the inner chamber, it allowed him to discover who he really was, and thus to alter
his self-presentation in response to what he saw. Not his bodily self-
presentation, of course; that much remained intact. What LSD
promised to change was his personality, his behavior, the face he presented to the world. Once he had used LSD, his self-presentation
could be shaped not by social expectations, not by what he saw in
the mirror, but by what he had learned about his inner self.

This first flush of infatuation with psychedelic drugs came at a
time when Americans were particularly concerned with the pressures
of social expectations. Mid-twentieth-century America is often
remembered as a time of rigid social conformity, but it was also a
time when Americans worried obsessively about becoming conformists. This was the era of William Whyte's *The Organization Man*,
Sloan Wilson's *The Man in the Grey Flannel Suit*, Rollo May's *Man's
Search for Himself*, and countless other books that worried, in their
various ways, that Americans were living their lives in slavish com-
pliance to the opinions of others—neighbors, bosses, the corporation,
the peer group, the anonymous public. This, it was felt, was mani-
festly a bad thing. And it was a particularly bad thing if what really
counted was being in touch with yourself, finding your own way, living your life as an individual. In the early 1950s, this comment
appeared in an American magazine editorial. "Conformity, it would
appear, is being elevated into something akin to a religion. Perhaps
Americans will arrive at an ant society, not through fiat of a dictator,
but through unbridled desire to get along with one another."[30] The
comment is remarkable not for its substance but for its source. When
the editors of *Fortune* magazine began to worry publicly about American social conformity, it is safe to say that the idea had hit the mainstream.

One of the most sophisticated expressions of this worry was David
Riesman's 1950 study *The Lonely Crowd*, the title of which has

become a virtual synonym for the alienation of life in mass society.[31] Riesman famously identified the "outer-directed" personality as the dominant personality type of mid-century America. Contemporary glosses on *The Lonely Crowd* often identify the outer-directed personality as a social conformist, but in fact, Riesman's analysis was subtler than this. Riesman did not argue that the outer-directed person was more conformist than the inner-directed one. What he and his coauthors tried to explain were the various ways in which a society *enforces* conformity, of which the outer-directed personality was only one example. Rather than looking inward to his own values as a guide to action, the outer-directed personality takes his cues from others. According to Riesman, the outer-directed personality responds to the demands of life with a sort of radar, an exquisite sensitivity to the signals sent off by other people. Riesman saw outer-directed traits emerging first in cities and bureaucracies. There the outer-directed person must always monitor what others think, registering their approval or disapproval, and manipulating his self-presentation to match.

What gave rise to the other-directed society, such as the one Riesman believed we were entering in the early 1950s, was other people. Not that Riesman thought, like Sartre in *No Exit*, that other people are Hell. Other people are, however, problems. In a world marked by contact with people of other cultures and ethnicities, and where society is centralized and bureaucratized, the problem to be solved is not how to deal with the material world but how to deal with other people. For moral and social direction, outer-directed people look not to their elders, as they would have in earlier times, but to their contemporaries. These contemporaries may be peers, but they may also be people unknown to them, such as those they encounter through the mass media.

Riesman contrasts this with the older, "inner-directed" personality, a more stable core of traits inculcated in children at an early age by their parents and other figures of authority. While the outer-directed personality was flexible and adaptable, the inner-directed personality was stable and unwavering. If the metaphor for the outer-directed personality was radar, the metaphor for the inner-directed personality was a psychological gyroscope—an instrument for remaining true to oneself despite the pressures of the external world. Parents and other authority figures set the gyroscope of the inner-directed person in childhood, and it responded to the external demands of a novel life course in order to keep the person on track.

What Grant was describing with LSD was, in effect, a way of using your gyroscope rather than your radar. It was a way of staying inner-directed in an outer-directed world. A decade or so later LSD would become wildly popular for this very reason: psychedelic drugs, like sex and communal living, were seen as expressions not merely of hedonism, but also of a desire to get in touch with more authentic ways of living. In this sense, the appeal of LSD was just the reverse of body modification. Body modification is one way of coping with the social mirror: adjusting yourself in front of it until the mirror tells you that you look okay. The other way to cope, however, is simply to get rid of the mirror. That was the promise of LSD. At a time when it seemed to many people that the mirror was everywhere, that Americans were constantly worried about the mirror, that all the American anxieties and obsessions and nightmares were about this overbearing image in the mirror, here was a drug that simply turned your gaze away. Not from yourself; the gaze was still on the self. But this was the self as it really was, the authentic self, and not simply the self that you performed for others.

Times have changed since the 1950s, of course. When Riesman wrote *The Lonely Crowd*, the emergence of a flexible, manipulable self was viewed with some alarm. The idea that people may have no stable core of identity conjured up images of glad-handing aluminum-siding salesmen and status-grubbing sociopaths. An outer-directed person who altered his or her persona to suit his circumstances was a phony, a suck-up, a shallow conformist trying to get ahead by shifting his very identity to win the approval of others. As late as 1970, Lionel Trilling could lecture at Harvard on the emergence of sincerity and authenticity as moral ideals, on the way they have come to seem essential to human virtue.[32]

Today, however, mainstream intellectual current tells us to rejoice in transient, changing identities. A flexible identity is not about wearing a mask, not about being a shallow actor, not about being a hollow man. It is all part of the postmodern self, the play of identities, the shifting shape of public presentation. Many theorists, under the influence of Erving Goffman and Judith Butler, argue that social life is *all* performance; that masks are, in essence, our true selves—a notion that dissolves completely the notion of a true self. To think that there is a true, core self apart from the social roles we play, they suggest, is at best wishful thinking and at worst pure delusion. Psychiatrist Arnold Ludwig writes, "all the distinctions between true and false selves, or authentic and inauthentic selves, or fulfilled and unfulfilled selves make little sense, and have no basis in reality."[33]

With this shift has come a far more positive take on the healthiness and morality of self-transformation. Not only *can* we change our identities, it is suggested, we *do* it all the time. And we ought to be glad, because this kind of plasticity is healthier, more honest, more apt to bring us happiness. Self-help guru Gail Sheehy writes, "the most healthy and successful [people] now develop *multiple identities*, managed simultaneously, to be called upon as conditions change."[34] The contemporary self is a "protean self," as psychiatrist Robert Jay Lifton puts it, capable of transforming itself into something new as circumstances demand.[35] We are all performers, this notion suggests; all actors, all in masks, all in drag. Better to recognize this and embrace it than to pretend it isn't so.

This shift began in the 1970s when theorists began to ask how the self could be conceptualized as unitary and fixed when a given person could behave so differently under different circumstances. Psychologists such as Kenneth Gergen demonstrated empirically the extent to which people (Americans, anyway) modify their own views of themselves in response to their social surroundings. Put us in the presence of others who compliment us and puff us up, and our self-esteem will soar. Jan Morris pointed out something similar when she described what it was like to begin living as a woman. "The more I was treated as a woman," she writes, "the more woman I became."[36] Her own sense of the person she was shifted in response to the expectations of those around her. If other people expected a case to be too heavy for her to lift, it became too heavy for her. If other people expected her to be incompetent at reversing a car, she became incompetent. If people expected her to be less talkative, or less informed, or less self-centered, that was what she became. Soon, she writes, it all "began to feel only natural, so powerful are the effects of custom and environment."[37]

The realization that people behave very differently depending on their circumstances helped turn intellectual fashion against ideas such as authenticity. To many people, the phrase "authentic self" brought to mind a core of identity whose attributes are fixed and immutable, cast in childhood and hardened by adulthood, stable and unwavering no matter who or what circumstances a person might encounter. The psychologist Jerome Bruner calls this the "essentialist self." According to Bruner, prior to the 1970s psychological theory had treated the self as if it were a real object that could be discovered and inspected. Psychoanalysis was the "principal essentialist sinner."[38] For psycho-analysts, the id, the ego, and the superego did not map conceptual constructs, but were real entities. Psychoanalysis was the tool by which the true self could be inspected. With the right guide, you could discover who you really were.

These days, however, intellectuals prefer to talk not about authenticity but about performance, masks, and postmodern play. We no longer have identities; we "perform" them. We do not live lives; we follow social "scripts." The concept of a "true self" has become entrenched in popular culture, but it has abandoned the scholarly journals. As Lauren Slater's friend Ian tells her in *Prozac Diary*, "You're thinking too much about a real self. At the very least, it's passé. The real self as a belief went out in the 70s."[39]

The notion that we all *perform* (rather than have) an identity has also become important in contemporary identity politics. Performing an identity that defies conventional social categories has become a way of challenging those categories. So if you feel confined by the rigidity of behavior expected within a given social category—that there is one and only one way of living as an African American, a woman, or a gay man—then you may embrace the idea of rebellion, of breaking the rules or inventing new ones. And if you feel oppressed by categories that seem to have no place for you—if, say, you are mixed-race, transgendered, or intersexed—then fluid, mutable categories, or even no categories at all, have the ring of liberation. The way to combat oppressive social structures, many people believe today, is to do away with them entirely. Thus, shifting your identity, seen in Riesman's day as an act of social conformity, is now seen as a tool of rebellion. Altering your identity has become a way of challenging the status quo, rebelling against social categories, subverting the idea that there is one and only one way to live out your identity.

Does this mean that the authentic self is, as Arnold Ludwig suggests, an illusion? I don't think so. Part of the confusion here is philosophical. You can buy into the idea of an authentic self without buying into the idea of an essentialist self. An authentic self need not be defined by a single essential characteristic, in the same way that a family need not be defined by any single essential characteristic. Some members of the family have blue eyes, but others may have brown or green eyes. Some members of the family are genetically related to one another, but others are not. Some members of the family have the same high forehead, the same dimpled chin, the same hot temper, but others have none of these traits. Yet we have no problem admitting that the family exists, and these people are all members. In a similar way, the mere fact that people behave differently under different circumstances, or for that matter, over time, does not mean that they are constantly transforming into different people, or that they have different selves. It simply means that the self has many aspects. These aspects may show themselves in some circumstances but not others, like a family trait that emerges among some cousins but not others.[40]

There is nothing remarkable about this. The ordinary, modern Western view of selfhood—what people *mean* when they talk about the self—is flexible enough to take account of the fact that people can be duplicitous, that they can change over time, that they can behave erratically or inconsistently from one situation to the next. The fact that Anna can behave differently when she is with Vronsky than she does when she is with Karenin does not mean that there is no authentic Anna. It simply means that any account of the authentic Anna will need to be rich enough to take account of the complexities of her character. Our language has accommodated these complexities with words such as self-betrayal, fakery, and insincerity. The ordinary Western notion of selfhood is flexible enough for us to make sense of Kurtz's descent into darkness, or Gatz's transformation into Gatsby. Stories of transformation are part of our modern linguistic and cultural repertoire.

And remember: they make good stories only because we can ordinarily expect a person to have a relatively stable and coherent set of mental and physical attributes. Radical self-transformation is the exception, not the rule. When people do undergo such radical transformations—brain injury, madness, psychological trauma, a profound religious conversion—we often find ourselves at a loss to describe what has happened. Which is the true self now? Which is the real person? Yet the fact that it is so difficult to speak of such a person's "true self" here simply points to the degree to which we take for granted the notion that people do, in the ordinary run of things, have true selves.[41]

In fact, it would be hard to make sense of our contemporary Western moral vocabulary if we gave up entirely on the notion of a true self. The notion of self-betrayal collapses when there is no self to betray. Being true to your ideals makes no sense if those ideals are in a constant state of flux. Psychologist Kenneth Gergen, for example, argues that there is no such thing as a core identity—that we all put on masks and discard them as we wish. These masks are not even masks, because we are, in effect, what we pretend to be. "Once donned," writes Gergen, "mask becomes reality."[42] As a metaphor, this is lovely. But as a philosophical argument, it is dead wrong. The very concept of mask presupposes that there is something underneath. Otherwise a mask is not a mask. It is a face. The very idea of pretending presupposes that there is a difference between the real and the fake, between acting and the real thing, between performance and being natural, between sincerity and insincerity. A child has to *learn* to pretend, to act, and to be insincere. The concepts do not make sense without a background of constancy and authenticity against which they can be contrasted.

WHEN PSYCHIATRIST Peter Kramer published *Listening to Prozac* in 1993, he touched off an ongoing debate over medical enhancement that is strikingly different from earlier debates. In earlier debates, the issue was whether there was anything wrong with transforming external appearance in accordance with a felt inner identity. (Is cosmetic surgery a kind of fakery and, if so, is there anything wrong with that?) But with Prozac the issue changed. Prozac seemed to transform inner identity itself. A shy person might take Prozac and become outgoing and extroverted. A rigid, obsessive person might take Prozac and become flexible and easygoing. We are used to transformations from illness to health, from clinical depression to psychological well-being. But what should we make of a transformation from one normal state to another?

Even more striking than the transformations themselves was the language in which some of Kramer's patients described the changes. These patients would report not that Prozac made them feel like new people, but that it made them feel like *themselves*. "This is who I am," said one patient after taking Prozac. "I just feel strong. I feel resilient. I feel confident."[43] Kramer's most widely discussed patient was a divorced, middle-aged woman called Tess, whom Kramer was treating with Prozac for depression. After Tess recovered from her depression, Kramer tapered and then discontinued the medication. Eight months later, Tess came back and said, "I am not myself." Kramer was intrigued by this remark. Tess had returned to the very state in which she had been for most of the past forty years, her entire life apart from the brief period she was on Prozac, and yet she said she did not feel like herself. She felt like herself when she was on Prozac.

The Prozac debate was complicated still further by the fact that people respond to antidepressants in ways that are anything but uniform. Some people say that they feel like a fake on the drugs, others like the person they always wanted to be, still others like the person they really are. Kramer and others began to wonder: Are these transformations chemical makeovers or chemical self-discoveries? If a person undergoes a striking transformation on medication but feels more like himself, is this a metamorphosis to a new, better self, or the restoration of a true self that had been masked by pathology?[44]

To put the question this way, however, is to speak about the self as a fixed, concrete, unitary entity. It is as if changing your self is no different from changing your shirt, and finding yourself is like finding a penny on the sidewalk. But the self has many aspects to it. We all have parts of ourselves of which we are proud or ashamed, aspects of our characters that emerge only at some times and under some circumstances. If a drug makes us feel or behave in ways that are new and alien to us, it may seem natural to say that the drug makes us feel phony.[45] But if a drug brings out some aspect of ourselves that time and circumstance have heretofore kept hidden, it might feel right to say that the drug has restored our "true self"—by which we might mean that part of ourselves that we wish had been allowed to grow and flourish. When psychologist and memoirist Lauren Slater began taking Prozac, she found that old memories began coming back to her—the smell of horses, the taste of wild grapes, a memory of leaping gracefully into the air on ice skates, and her mother clapping again and again. This was not exactly a matter of Prozac creating a new self, writes Slater. "(W)hen I take Prozac I am not being made over so much as I am being remembered."[46]

The debate over Prozac sometimes made it sound as if stories of self-transformation were unique to a handful of people taking anti-depressants. In fact, however, we were hearing similar stories from ex-hippies about LSD and Ecstasy, from transsexuals who had undergone sex-reassignment surgery, from struggling businessmen who had started taking Ritalin, from all manner of people who were using medical interventions as a means of self-transformation. The changes experienced by some people on Prozac were dramatic, but the language they used to describe the changes was predictable. Today, ten years after *Listening to Prozac*, a GlaxoSmithKline television ad features a woman with "generalized anxiety disorder." She smiles at the camera and says that with Paxil, "I feel like myself."

If vocabulary of authenticity was novel in the time of Rousseau and Herder, today it has become almost trite. The moral ideal of self-fulfillment has become a commonplace, and the language of identity is inescapable. Talk of the self permeates ethnographies, interviews, autobiographies, and memoirs. It appears on Web sites, in chat rooms and electronic discussion groups. Patients use it in support groups. Advertisers use it when they pitch their products. This is the way we talk now. This is the way we think. This is the way we picture our lives. This is even the way we talk about medical technologies and the problems that they cure. The conceptual apparatus of identity has become a natural way of describing our psychopathologies, our ideals, and our aspirations.

Enhancement technologies have become part of "the governance of the soul," as Nikolas Rose puts it, the management of meaning through the management of the self.[47] As our culture has shifted the locus of meaning in life away from God and onto individual psychology, we have created a moral yardstick that measures the success of a human life in terms of psychological well-being. As Rose points out, it is within this moral framework that jobs become a locus of self-fulfillment, social interactions become "relationships" that are healthy or pathological, and the tragedies of life become opportunities for therapy and psychological growth. It is also within this framework that enhancement technologies get their moral purchase. Today, enhancement technologies are not just instruments for self-improvement, or even self-transformation—they are tools for working on the soul.

3

THE FACE BEHIND
THE MASK

Glory fades, but humiliation lasts forever.
—Britt Elliott

In the spring of 1999, the U.S. Food and Drug Administration approved the first drug treatment for "social phobia" or, as it is now sometimes called, "social anxiety disorder." The drug approved to treat it is Paxil, the trade name for paroxetine. Glaxo-SmithKline, which manufactures Paxil, has launched an aggressive marketing campaign aimed directly at consumers. A recent ad for Paxil in the *New York Times Magazine* showed a set of contrasting photographs. Each photograph pictured a young man delivering a business presentation. The first picture is soft and brightly lit, and the young man sits at a table of friendly, benignly smiling colleagues. This is the reality of social interaction, the photograph suggests; it has the header, "What it is." The contrasting photograph, which has the header, "What it feels like," shows the same setting transformed into an inquisition scene. The room is dark, the people around the table look menacing. The young man is bound with heavy ropes like a torture victim, and a bright light shines directly into his face. "Over 10 million people suffer from social anxiety," the text says, "and a chemical imbalance could be to blame." Paxil works to correct this chemical imbalance. The slogan for the ad reads: "Your life is waiting."

It's not a bad advertisement. It would be a better ad if the general tone were changed from hostility to humiliation. My brother Britt has a recurring dream where he is talking to someone, then looks down to discover he is wearing no pants. The situation varies—public lectures, parties, weddings, high school exams, family gatherings—but the theme is always the same: self-recrimination. "It made perfect sense when I was getting dressed; pants didn't seem necessary, but now it's so clear: My God, what was I thinking? Of course I was supposed to wear pants." And there's no point in explaining the mistake to other people because it makes no sense. Who would understand? He comes off like some kind of sexual deviant. Everyone is embarrassed for him; how will he ever face them again?

Now *that* is a commercial for social phobia. If GlaxoSmithKline could somehow harness the sense of humiliation suggested by that dream, they could sell a lot of Paxil.

The hallmark of social phobia, according to the latest edition of the American Psychiatric Association's *Diagnostic and Statistical Manual of Mental Disorders (DSM-IV-TR)*, is the fear of humiliation or embarrassment. But this general fear of embarrassment often attaches itself to very specific actions. People with social phobia often worry desperately that their hands will tremble while they are eating or writing, or that they will blush and sweat while giving a public speech, or that they will tense up in a public bathroom and be unable to urinate. The anxiety of anticipating these situations may lead them to avoid social situations obsessively, so that they will go to great lengths to avoid eating with other people, making small talk in hallways, or speaking in front of a group. The diagnostic criteria for social phobia distinguish it from ordinary shyness by stipulating that the distress of social phobia must be so severe that it interferes with a person's job, social activities, or everyday routine. An example commonly given in the psychiatric literature is a person who turns down a promotion at work because it would mean he or she would have to give public presentations.

Psychiatrist John Marshall, at the University of Wisconsin, tells the story of a patient he calls David, a fifty-five-year-old neurologist who could talk comfortably to his patients or to other physicians but dreaded going to dinner parties. "They scare me to death," David said. "My wife seems to think it's a crime to stay home on the weekends. Every Friday night she has something lined up for us to do—dinner with this couple, dinner with that couple, we owe them one, they owe us one. . . . I don't know. I just can't stand it." David dreaded Friday evenings so much that by Wednesday he was tense, by Thursday evening he could not sleep, and by Friday afternoon he was so agitated he could not see patients in his office. Often his shirt would be soaked with sweat by dinnertime on Friday, and he would toss back several drinks in anticipation of the evening. "I'm afraid I won't know how to act," he told Marshall. "I'm just afraid I'll make a tremendous fool of myself. I sweat, tremble, flush . . . With each bite I think the food is going to go down the wrong way, and just can't stand the idea of choking and coughing and turning red while everybody's just sitting there, paralyzed, staring at me and seeing my face all contorted."[1]

Marshall prescribed an antidepressant, a monoamine oxidase inhibitor (MAO inhibitor) called phenelzine, or Nardil. After a few weeks on the drug David said he felt "like a new person." He felt more confident, and began to enjoy initiating conversations with other people. After several more weeks on the drug David even enjoyed the Friday dinner parties. "My wife is calling me a social animal," he said. "I'm actually looking forward to those Friday evenings at the country club, and we've begun to have small dinners and large cocktail parties at our house." Even his office nurse noticed the changes in David's personality. "Patients now comment on how much more outgoing and friendly he is," she said. "He is a completely different person."

IN THE PSYCHIATRIC literature, social phobia is commonly said to be the third most common mental disorder in the United States, after depression and drug abuse. Studies show that over 13 percent of Americans will suffer from it at some point in their lives, and it is still frequently called an underrecognized disorder.[2] Yet fifteen years ago, social phobia was seen as a rare problem, and was hardly mentioned in the psychiatric literature. When I ran a computer search using the key word "social phobia" on Medline, the most comprehensive medical database, I found only 16 articles published from 1966 to 1984. But the same search run from 1984 to 1998 turned up 653 articles. I ran another search in PsychInfo, a database that covers more of the psychological literature, and the disparity was even more striking: from 1967 to 1983 only 17 articles on social phobia were published, but from 1984 to 1998 the number shot up to 1137.

What happened in the mid-1980s to bring about such an explosion of interest in social phobia? Two things. First, in 1987 the revised third edition of the *Diagnostic and Statistical Manual of Mental Disorders (DSM-III-R)* was published, and for the first time it included a diagnosis of social phobia. This gave legitimacy to the term "social phobia" and shape to the entity itself. When the *DSM* was revised again in 1994, it gave "social anxiety disorder" as an alternative designation—a much softer, patient-friendly term.

Second, and perhaps more crucially, evidence began to emerge in the mid-1980s suggesting that patients with social phobia would improve on antidepressants. Initially, studies showed that social phobia responded to MAO inhibitors, such as the one that Marshall prescribed. MAO inhibitors had been available since the early 1950s, when researchers noticed that patients in tuberculosis clinics who were treated with iproniazid (Marsilid) experienced a psychic boost.[3] But MAO inhibitors were never very popular as antidepressants, because they require strict dietary restrictions. (In 1962 a patient taking an MAO inhibitor went into a hypertensive crisis and died after eating cheese rich in tyramine, and the drugs were temporarily withdrawn from the market.)[4] Studies showed that the MAO inhibitor phenelzine (Nardil) was useful for social phobia as early as 1986.[5] Shortly thereafter came the first stirrings of the SSRI revolution: the development of the class of antidepressant drugs known as selective serotonin reuptake inhibitors (SSRIs), of which Prozac was the earliest and most well-known example. During the 1990s, studies suggested that some of these antidepressants worked for social phobia; that, in fact, they worked better than Nardil. The SSRIs are also (arguably) easier to use, and were widely perceived to be less likely to cause serious side effects. The most convincing studies were for Paxil. One well-known study in *JAMA (Journal of the American Medical Association)* showed that on Paxil, more than 50 percent of subjects with social phobia had improved.[6] In 1999, the year the Food and Drug Administration approved Paxil for social phobia, GlaxoSmithKline spent $91.8 million advertising it directly to consumers.[7]

Before psychiatrists started using antidepressants for social phobia, they did not have a lot of other good options. They could prescribe beta-blockers for stage fright, but beta-blockers do not really work for other kinds of social anxiety. They could prescribe benzodiazepines like Valium and Librium (the so-called "minor tranquilizers"), but these drugs often leave people feeling drugged and sedated. They can also be habit-forming. So antidepressants, especially the SSRIs, filled a gap—a gap, in fact, that nobody really even saw before it was filled. The SSRIs have side effects too, of course—sexual dysfunction, the most widely noticed example, and in rare cases, a heightened risk of violence or suicide.[8] But many people taking SSRIs say the drugs make them feel more clearheaded, more confident, and importantly, more extroverted and outgoing.

For cynical observers, this is the end of the story, and not an especially new story anymore, that is, once it becomes evident that some aspect of character or behavior can be altered with a drug, we medicalize it and turn it into pathology. In this case we are medicalizing a personality trait called shyness, which has been with us for quite a while but has not previously been called a mental disorder. Psychiatrists have been quick to anticipate this objection, and many have emphatically rejected the notion that social phobia is just a technical word for shyness. Most stress the importance of diagnosing and treating social phobia promptly. An editorial in the *Medical Journal of Australia* calls social phobia a "legitimate pathology," while a review in the *British Medical Journal* points out that unless it is promptly treated, "a burden is placed on society."[9] Murray Stein states in a *Lancet* editorial that social phobia "is not a character trait to be cherished as part of the range of normal human diversity. It is a disabling disorder to be diagnosed and treated."[10]

Yet social phobia still sounds a lot like shyness. Anxiety about giving public speeches or making small talk with strangers, the worry that you will blush or your voice will tremble or that your palms will get sweaty—to shy people, this all sounds pretty familiar. Even the less familiar forms of social phobia, such as anxiety about setting off electronic alarms as you leave a shop, or the worry that your hands will shake so much that you will be unable to sign your name or hold your wine glass without spilling it, sound more like extreme forms of shyness and self-consciousness than like discrete medical disorders. While the *DSM-IV* distinguishes social phobia from ordinary shyness by stipulating that it must be so severe as to interfere with a person's job or social life, these stipulations have a rather arbitrary ring to them. They may provide clinicians with an agreeable cut-off point, but if shyness can be fixed with an antidepressant, the fact that the official guidelines do not call it "social phobia" will make little difference to the way most people think about it.

Perhaps shyness is being medicalized, perhaps not. That question, however, is ultimately less interesting than the question of how the possibility of medicalizing it has arisen. What is it about the way we live now, especially in America, that makes the notion of shyness as a pathology sound so plausible? And what is it about our current social and historical situation that makes a person's heart go into a pounding tachycardia at the mere thought of saying his name out loud to a group of strangers sitting around a table? Psychiatrists have tended to emphasize the biological roots of social phobia, pointing out just how universal it is. "Fear of being stared at is common to most animals," writes J. A. Den Boer in the *British Medical Journal*, "including humans."[11] But rabbits do not stay awake at night obsessing about how to avoid taking a pee in front of other rabbits. The biology of social phobia is (for me, at any rate) a lot less intriguing than its cultural substrate, the social and historical forces that produce all these sweaty palms, shaky voices, and tense bladders. Why are Americans such nervously enthusiastic consumers of Paxil?

S OMETIME AROUND THE turn of the twentieth century, Americans developed personalities. Before that time, we did not have personalities; we had characters. The word "personality" did not appear in the English language until the late eighteenth century. It did not come into common use until the early part of the twentieth. These days the words "personality" and "character" are pretty close to synonymous, at least in everyday American usage, but a century ago, having character was quite different from having personality. Character was bound up with your inner life. It was about the depths beneath the surface, about what is on the inside as well as what other people see. Character had moral dimensions; it concerned virtue and vice. Something of this sense remains today, of course. To praise or condemn a person's character, as we are constantly reminded in presidential politics, is to say something about a person's moral standing.[12]

Personality, though, is different. Personality, as the concept began to be used a century ago, was bound up with the idea of self-presentation. Historian Warren Susman looked at self-help books that were being published in America around the turn of the twentieth century, and he found that at a certain point they began to instruct readers on how to develop "personality": how to make yourself interesting and attractive to other people, how to make them like you and respect you and want to be around you. When these new self-help authors described the kind of personalities to which someone ought to aspire, they used adjectives like "magnetic," "stunning," and "masterful." These were very different kinds of adjectives than the ones used to describe character. One writer made the point that character is either good or bad, while personality is famous or infamous. You want your personality to be "dazzling."[13]

What was becoming important during this period was a distinction between the inner and the outer, or between self and self-presentation. As the idea of personality took hold, Americans started to take on the idea that we all put on a mask for the world. Everyone is a performer. Every self-help book Susman studied, for example, mentioned the importance of the voice and proper methods of public speaking and conversation. They stressed clothing, personal appearance, and manners. They taught proper breathing, proper eating, good complexion, beauty, grooming. Most important were poise and charm. The idea here is that in order to be socially successful, not only do we have to behave in certain ways, we have to *be* certain ways as well—which may or may not be the way we really are inside. If it isn't, we have to fake it.

Or perhaps faking it isn't quite the right phrase, because the idea of personality seemed to be more than just pretending to be interesting and charming and funny; you could really become that way. You could transform yourself. It seemed to be a staple of the self-help literature around this time (not to mention the present, as well) that personality really was something that you could develop through hard work. You might have been given a certain kind of personality, but with the right kind of help you could change. You can control your personality. Like a bodybuilder at the gym, you can beef up your personality, buff it and polish it and display it before the mirror. If you don't like what you see—or more importantly, if you suspect that others won't like it—you can always head back to the squat thrust machine.

There has always been a minor cult of self-improvement in American life, since Benjamin Franklin's self-help homilies. What changed at the beginning of the twentieth century was the nature of that self-improvement. Self-improvement began to be measured against the outward success of others. The work ethic of the nineteenth century, for all its obsessive concern with industriousness, did not really stress competition. Success was measured against abstract ideals of discipline and self-denial rather than against the things that other people accomplished.[14] But in the twentieth century this began to change. Advancement in business became a competition between peers for a limited number of spaces, and success came to depend on winning the approval of your superiors. Advancement depended more and more on interpersonal skills, and the advice industry took notice. In 1907, *Success* magazine and the *Saturday Evening Post* introduced departments giving instruction in conversation, fashion, and culture. By the early twentieth century, Americans were being told that the keys to personal success were salesmanship, self-promotion, and "personal magnetism."[15]

The problem addressed by self-help writers at the beginning of the twentieth century, Susman points out, was the problem of individuality in mass society. When you are surrounded on all sides by strangers, how do you stand out from the crowd? This is why such importance was attached to self-presentation. It was thought that we could learn to present ourselves to others as a way of making them take notice of us, of persuading them to see us as special. "Personality," as one self-help writer of the day put it, "is the quality of being Somebody."[16] But "being Somebody" could not be a mere act. To be Somebody, we must master and control the qualities we already possess in order to gain the good opinion of others—to make them say, as one writer put it, "he's a mighty likeable fellow."[17]

It was an impossible act to pull off, of course. For at the same time that the self-help manuals exhorted a reader to play to the audience, to eliminate the personal traits that might annoy other people and to develop the traits that will please them, they were also telling the reader: "Be yourself." To "be Somebody" you needed to be an individual, to stand out from the crowd and go your own way; but you also needed to be painstakingly attentive to how other people were reacting to you, and to eliminate the things that they disapproved of. As Susman points out, you were instructed to ignore the advice of others, but this instruction came from a best-selling advice manual.[18]

As sociologist Richard Sennett has written, public space in the nineteenth century was becoming a place where individuals were objects of obsessive public scrutiny—their clothing, their manners, the way they carried themselves and behaved, but especially their personalities. Personalities were not just facades but outward indicators of a person's idiosyncratic, individual traits. Your personality *revealed* something about you—about "you" as you really were, not just the "you" that you showed to others. This, in turn, brought about a new kind of social anxiety, one that arose from self-consciousness. Like a poker player worried about his tells, people became obsessed that they were giving themselves away inadvertently through their actions, their dress, and their facial expressions. People became fearful of acting spontaneously or unselfconsciously—imprisoned, as Christopher Lasch puts it, in self-awareness.[19]

This is the moral universe we have inherited, into which Paxil made its official entry in 1999. Not that the universe hasn't changed considerably, of course. We can laugh now at Dale Carnegie's hokey *How to Win Friends and Influence People*, or at Willy Loman's worries about being liked but not well-liked. But the fact is that Americans still see shyness as a social handicap. We devour self-help books like *How to Start a Conversation and Make Friends*, or *How I Overcame Shyness: 101 Celebrities Share Their Secrets*. Shyness is seen as a handicap that can be overcome—and not just with medication, but also with self-discipline and the right kind of training. "How to talk to strangers about anything," these books promise; "How to be the life of the party." "I conquered my shyness," say Michael Jordan and Richard Gere and Elvis, like 440-pound fatties who have slimmed down on a miracle diet. "And so can you!"

ONE NIGHT NOT too long ago I sat with two friends in a London bar talking about the ambiguity of appearances. We talked about role-playing, sincerity, and the subtle cues and codes that lie behind social masks. It was a good spot for the conversation. For one thing, it was a gay bar, populated partly by straights, and all manner of social cues were being sent out and returned. For another, above our table was a giant screen showing video clips of catfights from the television show *Dynasty*. This gave a conversation about role-playing a kind of surreal glow. As we spoke earnestly to one other about sincerity, above us a screeching Joan Collins executed precise karate chops to Linda Evans's clavicle and banged her head violently against a refrigerator door. Here, I thought, is role-playing squared. The acting is so exaggerated and turned in on itself that it takes on a kind of half-intentional comedy. It is camp, of course, and at the source of the camp aesthetic is this ironic hyperawareness— insincerity with a wink to the audience. "To perceive Camp in objects and persons is to understand Being-as-Playing-a-Role," writes Susan Sontag. "It is the farthest extension, in sensibility, of the metaphor of life as theater."[20]

If camp is the furthest extension of this sensibility—acting so exaggerated that it no longer aims at the illusion that it is not acting—then at the other end of the spectrum is absolute sincerity. This is the sincerity of a child, in whom there is no artifice, no acting, no gap between external presentation and internal feeling. Sincerity, to use Lionel Trilling's formulation, is "congruence between avowal and actual feeling." And as Trilling points out, it is probably no accident that the concept of sincerity, which dates to Elizabethan times, arose during a period that also saw a flowering of the theater.[21] The idea that there might be something fishy about pretending to have emotions that you don't really feel took on greater importance at a time when actors were doing this very thing professionally on the stage. Today, many scholars have latched onto the idea that all of social life is a performance. Erving Goffman used it most famously in *The Pre-*

sentation of Self in Everyday Life. Life is but a stage; we are all poor players, and the part we play is that of ourselves.

Yet life's theater often turns out to be a lot more complex than actual theaters. Sincerity (as anyone with small children knows) is a very tricky moral concept. On stage, an actor is expected to fake it, and the better she fakes it the more successful her performance is. We expect no congruence there between avowal and actual feeling; we do not expect an actor to be sincere. But in ordinary life things are different. We sometimes expect a performance, but we often frown on insincere performances. We teach small children that they must pretend to like presents they actually do not care for, that they must act as if they are happy to see uncles and cousins for whom they actually do not have much use, that they must appear to be paying close attention to the sermon even if they are daydreaming. These are all performances, all occasions where we know external avowal does not match up with inner feeling. Yet we expect a certain kind of performance—a *sincere* performance. When they tell their grandmother that they really like the sweater they dislike, they must say it as if they mean it. Not only must they fake their feelings; they must also fake sincerity.

Sincerity is also dependent on a particular conception of the person. In a famous essay on selfhood, the anthropologist Clifford Geertz contrasts our own Western concept of the person—as a "bounded, unique, more or less integrated motivational and cognitive universe"—with the concept of personhood in Java.[22] The Javanese sense of what a person is, says Geertz, turns on two sets of contrasts. The first of these contrasts is between the "inside" and the "outside." This inside/outside contrast refers to, on the one hand, the "felt realm of human experience," and on the other, to the "observed realm of human behavior." These are not surrogate terms for soul and body, Geertz takes pains to point out. The inside/outside contrast—*batin* and *lair*—refers to the contrast between the inner, subjective, emotional life that people experience, and the external behavior that they show to the world—their movements, postures, speech, and so on. Both realms, inside and outside, are seen as, in their essence, invariant from one person to the next. That is, they *efface* individuality rather than (as here in the West) express it. Nor are the two realms seen as functions of one another (as they are in the

West), but instead as independent realms that need to be put in proper order independently.

It is in the relationship between the inner and the outer that the second set of contrasts comes into play—the contrast between the "refined" and the "vulgar," as Geertz puts it. The goal of the civilized Javanese person is to be refined—pure, or polished, or smooth—in both of these separated realms of the self. In the inner realm this is achieved through religious discipline, such as meditation. In the outer realm it is achieved through etiquette. This code of etiquette is not only extraordinarily elaborate; it also has something like the force of law. Often this rigidly enforced etiquette comes across to others as a "predictable, undisturbing, elegant and rather vacant set of choreographed motions and settled forms of speech." The result, writes Geertz, is a kind of bifurcate self: "half ungestured feeling, half unfelt gesture." To appreciate the force of this conception of the self, you must see, as Geertz once did, a young man whose wife had suddenly and inexplicably died, yet who greeted people at the door of his house with a fixed smile on his face and formal apologies for his wife's absence. He explains to Geertz, "This is what you have to do to be smooth inside and out."[23]

At least part of the reason this conception of proper behavior seems so alien to us in the West is our notion of the moral importance of sincerity. We, unlike the Javanese, actually *worry* that the mask might be hiding our true selves underneath. Unless we are sociopaths, we suspect that there is something wrong with faking it, with pretending to feel one thing while actually feeling another. Of course we believe that this kind of fakery is sometimes necessary, that sometimes we must issue vacant compliments and feign pleasure at unwanted gifts and pretend to enjoy meals we find distasteful in order to avoid hurting another person's feelings. But this sort of insincerity comes at a cost; we find it uncomfortable even as we practice it. In fact, many of us think we *ought* to be a little uncomfortable when we are insincere. If insincerity becomes too easy, then we worry that we are becoming too superficial, too glib, like a Vegas lounge singer or a used-car salesman.

The Javanese, presumably, will see this man's smile neither as faking it (since the outer self-presentation does not necessarily reflect what is going on inside) nor as something that ought to make him uncomfortable (since this kind of outer performance is what is expected.) If a Westerner finds the Javanese smile puzzling, it may be partly because of a different sense of what is proper behavior, but it is also because of a different sense of how the self is put together. Before you can have anxiety about insincerity, before you can be nervous about an incongruity between your external self-presentation and your inner feelings, you must have a sense that (1) there is a *relationship* between your self-presentation and your inner feelings, (2) that your self-presentation should ordinarily *reflect* your inner feelings, (3) that in a particular situation there is a *difference* between your self-presentation and your inner feelings, and (4) that there would be something embarrassing or shameful about an incongruity between your self-presentation and your inner feelings being publicly *exposed*.

It would be misleading to imply, though, that Westerners all speak in one voice when it comes to sincerity, because even across different Western cultures we can see noticeable differences. The difference is typically one of cultural style: how much of your inner life is appropriate to reveal, under what circumstances, and how it should be accomplished. The three of us talking in the gay bar in London, for example, were English, German, and American, and each had spent a fair amount of time in the countries of the others. And though we disagreed on some things, one thing that my German friend and I could agree on was that to us, the British social presentation is especially difficult to read. Sometimes it comes off as insincerity, sometimes as careful politeness, and sometimes simply as inscrutability. Certainly I can say from experience that an American living in Britain may well find himself baffled by the face the British present to him. It often appears as a deeply complex, impenetrable mask of manners and social presentation that is practically impossible to see through. My impression was that no matter how long I were to study it, there is no way I would ever come to understand it fully. What the British say is not always what they mean, or not exactly; there are all sorts of cues and gestures and hints that take an enormous amount of decoding, and which another British person might be able to decode but which would always remain incomprehensible to outsiders. In fact, I have been told more than once that many of these cues are incomprehensible even to British people of another social class. *Gatsby* could never have taken place in Britain, because James Gatz would have never been able to fake it so convincingly.

If the British are masters at constructing this sort of social mask, they are also masters at articulating the anxiety of the mask falling off. It is only a slight exaggeration to say that the great themes of post-war British fiction are embarrassment and humiliation. Kingsley Amis's *Lucky Jim* is a model of the genre. It is the story of Jim Dixon, a young university lecturer whose main ambition is to avoid losing his job, despite the fact that he thoroughly despises it. His efforts to avoid the sack involve shamelessly sucking up to the department chair, half-heartedly romancing a more senior woman lecturer, and pretending that his scholarly article on medieval shipbuilding techniques is something other than an inflated product of "frenzied fact-grubbing and fanatical boredom."[24]

Amis's narrator highlights the gap between Dixon's self and his self-presentation by showing us the internal commentary that is running through Dixon's head, which is spectacularly at odds with his external behavior and speech. As he tries to reconcile with his girlfriend, Dixon fantasizes about knocking her over and pushing a bead up her nose. He is constantly screwing his face into some contortion or another, depending on the effect he wants to achieve. He makes smilingly vacant conversation with the pompous Professor Welch, yet at the same time, we are told, Dixon "pretended to himself that he'd pick up his Professor round the waist, squeeze the furry grey-blue waistcoat against him to expel the breath, run heavily with him up the steps, along the corridor to the Staff Cloakroom, and plunge the too-small feet in their capless shoes into a lavatory basin, pulling the plug once, twice and again, stuffing the mouth with toilet paper."[25]

At the end of the academic term Dixon has to deliver a public lecture on "Merrie England," the anticipation of which has been a source of tremendous anxiety to him for months. In his nervousness he drinks so heavily that when he finally wobbles to the lectern, he is so drunk that he can scarcely control what emerges from his mouth. He seems unable to speak in his own voice, and to his horror, hears himself imitating the accent and speaking style of Professor Welch, who is sitting in the audience staring at him in horror. Dixon realizes his mistake and tries to change his voice. He succeeds only to find that the voice that emerges from his mouth next is the voice of the principal of the university. The audience murmurs and laughs nervously. Dixon raises a drink of water to his lips with a trembling hand. He considers pretending to faint, but decides that the audience will think it is the result of the alcohol. Eventually he finishes the speech not by speaking in his own voice, which seems to have deserted him, but in an "alien, sarcastic tone which implies that every word he speaks is deluded, tedious rubbish." Within quite a short time "he was contriving to sound like an unusually fanatical Nazi storm trooper in charge of a book-burning reading out to the crowd excerpts from a pamphlet written by a pacifist, Jewish, literate Communist."[26] It is as if Dixon's external self-presentation has somehow disengaged itself from his inner self and is flying away on autopilot, oblivious to his desperate internal commands to return.

The German aesthetic, on the other hand, is often just the reverse. If to a blunt American the British often seem overly subtle and evasive, occasionally to the point of appearing insincere, the Germans can seem just the opposite: earnest, candid, sometimes refreshingly direct, sometimes embarrassingly so. If (to an American) the British self looks opaque, the German self looks transparent. What you see is exactly what is there. It is as if there is no mask at all. There is formality, of course, famously so, but it is formality without artifice: what is said is exactly what is meant. At its best it comes off as deep sincerity, so that you always feel that you know where you stand. At its worst it comes off as startlingly impolite directness. Reading accounts of the Austrian philosopher Ludwig Wittgenstein at Cambridge University, for example, where he spent most of his academic career, it is hard to avoid the thought that at least some of the reason for his unhappiness at Cambridge was the stark contrast between his blunt Germanic earnestness and the subtlety of his English colleagues. Wittgenstein constantly complained about the phoniness of Cambridge academic life, refusing to eat at High Table because of the dreariness of the conversation, while the English found Wittgenstein intolerably rude.[27]

My own aesthetic comes not merely from America but also from the American South, where insincerity has been elevated to a high art. Like the British, southerners wear a public mask of manners that hides the inner life. Unlike the British, however, our mask of manners is one of down-home relaxation and casualness. Southerners like formal occasions—debutante balls, elaborate weddings, dressing up for church—but we do not as a rule like to be seen in any way as rigid or excessively formal. The richest and most well born southern man will often make a show of driving a pick-up and showing off his coon dogs. Southern manners are often of the "y'all come see us, make yourself at home" variety, which are no less rigid than British manners, but which masquerade as informal or even nonexistent. British manners don't pretend to be anything but formal. In this sense, we southerners are doubly insincere, because our manners are insincere. The manners mask what is going on inside, but they also mask themselves by pretending that they are not there. Southern manners are all about pretending, but also about pretending that you are not pretending.

Americans in Germany (and perhaps especially southerners in Germany) typically complain that German social life is excessively formal, which they assume translates into social anxiety. And it is true that social relationships between strangers in Germany (as opposed to intimates) can appear quite cold. But it is a mistake to think that formality necessarily translates into anxiety. German social life often seems very formal and ritualized by American standards: ceremonious birthday parties, *Kaffee und Kuchen* on Sunday afternoons, the formal Herr Doktor, etc. But the rules are simple and known to everyone; there is no complexity involved in translating and interpreting them. For me, at any rate, German social occasions are far less anxiety-producing as a rule than their American equivalents (and certainly less so than in Britain) even as they are more formal. In Germany, it is as if the agreed-upon social rules are out in the open and recognized by everyone, and within those rules there is no deception and no artifice. You may get uneasy about the prospect of breaking a rule, or when someone else breaks the rules—forgetting a birthday, using *Du* instead of *Sie*—but this is a simple matter: an agreed-upon social rule has been broken. The anxiety inherent in many American and British social events, in contrast, comes not from their formality

(I can imagine few events less formal but more anxiety-producing than the feigned casualness of an American singles bar) but from the dissonance between outer self-presentation and the inner self. The anxiety comes not simply from the rigidity of social life but from uncertainty about the degree to which self-presentation is supposed to express or hide the inner life.

The view from the other side of the window is just the reverse. To Germans (I am often reminded), Americans often appear superficial and glib. Germans often complain to me that they can never tell if Americans really mean what they say, that even though Americans are superficially friendlier than Germans, Germans can never tell if the friendliness is genuine or if the Americans are just pretending. In Germany, warmth and friendliness imply social intimacy, not just neighborliness. So friendliness of the backslapping American variety doesn't seem to go very deep. One German friend told me that when she lived in Chicago it took her the longest time to get used to the phoniness of American cocktail party conversation. Someone would come up and start chatting as if he wanted to talk to her, ask her questions and wait expectantly for a response; but when she began to answer, he would soon sneak a look at his watch or glance around the room to see who else was there. She says that eventually she began to realize that people did not really want to *talk* about anything; they were just making polite conversation.

A T LEAST PART of the reason American social phobia takes the form it does is connected to the particular architecture of the American self. We attach a very high value to the individual, encouraging people to develop and express the things that make them who they are psychologically, biographically, and physically; we are highly conscious that these individual characteristics are being observed and judged by others, whose good opinions we crave; we attach great importance to individual self-presentation, and consider barriers to self-presentation, like shyness, to be social handicaps. All this is partly a matter of American cultural style. But it is also a consequence of the way we believe the self to be put together. Different cultures, different selves, different social anxieties.

Japanese psychiatrists, for example, have long been familiar with a disorder called *taijin kyofusho*. People with *taijin kyofusho* have an intense fear of offending or embarrassing other people. They may be afraid that they will stare inappropriately, or blush, or smell bad, or simply that they are ugly—and that as a result, others will be embarrassed. At its worst this anxiety can reach delusional proportions: the absolute conviction that you smell so badly that others are coughing or covering their noses, or that your gaze is so offensive that other people are forced to turn away in embarrassment. *Taijin kyofusho* is a Japanese preoccupation with the proper public presentation of the self, but turned outward and then folded in on itself. Like Americans, the Japanese fear being embarrassed, but they fear being embarrassed about offending other people.

Unlike North America, where social phobia is a relatively recent psychiatric phenomenon, psychiatrists in Japan have been diagnosing and treating *taijin kyofusho* for over a century. The term *taijin kyofusho* literally translates as the "disorder" (*sho*) of "fear" (*kyofo*) of "interpersonal relations" (*taijin*).[28] It is very common in Japan, and even has its own specialized form of treatment: Morita therapy, a type of psychotherapy developed by Shoma Morita in the 1920s.[29] *Taijin kyofusho* also enjoys minor celebrity among transcultural psychiatrists as an example of a "culture bound" syndrome, a psychiatric disorder whose parameters are drawn by a specific culture and which rarely occurs elsewhere. In its general outlines, of course, *taijin kyofusho* strongly resembles social phobia: people with *taijin kyofusho* are intensely anxious about social interaction with other people. But *taijin kyofusho* is called "culture-bound" because of the specific form it takes. While social phobia in the West involves a core fear of humiliation or being made to seem ridiculous in a public setting, *taijin kyofusho* involves the fear that one's behavior or appearance will make *others* uncomfortable. A nineteenth-century Western observer, quite understandably, called *taijin kyofusho* an "altruistic" anxiety.

Japanese psychiatrist Ryoei Takano points out that one of the most common obsessive acts in any country is blasphemy—the urge to profane the sacred, the ceremonial, or the taboo. The anxiety of the obsessive urge comes from the social prohibition against carrying it out. In *taijin kyofusho*, this anxiety often centers on inappropriate eye contact. Direct eye contact may be regarded as forthright and self-confident in North America and Britain, but in Japan it is seen as offensive. Japanese children are taught to fix their gaze at throat or shoulder level. People who look others in the eye are seen as excessively bold and aggressive. In Japan this kind of behavior may be something close to blasphemy—the equivalent, Takano suggests, of exhibitionism. The anxiety of social interaction in Japan, says Takano, is anxiety about being thought "indecent."[30]

This Japanese concern with the feelings of others has often been understood, quite plausibly, as a cultural marker of Japanese interdependence and emphasis on social harmony, as opposed to Western individualism.[31] We worry about being embarrassed, while the Japanese worry about embarrassing others. We prize cultural dissent and individual rebellion, while the Japanese are taught to efface their individuality and to put the group before the self. Personal rebellion in Japan, writes anthropologist Ruth Benedict in *The Chrysanthemum and the Sword*, is seen as a sign of weakness. Strength means resisting your own desires and interests and putting those of society first.

To Western eyes, even ordinary Japanese concern looks like an exquisitely tuned sensitivity to the opinions of other people. Benedict explains this sensitivity by distinguishing between cultures of guilt and cultures of shame. Guilt is bound up with a private sense of responsibility for one's actions. "Shame," she writes, "is a reaction to other people's criticism. A man is shamed either by being openly ridiculed or by fantasizing to himself that he has been made ridiculous. In either case it is a potent sanction. But it requires an audience or at least a man's fantasy of an audience. Guilt does not." If this characterization of Japan is any way accurate (it has been often criticized as an exaggeration), then it would help to explain this finely tuned sensitivity to what the audience is thinking. The power of shame in Japanese culture means that, as Benedict puts it, "any man watches the verdict of the public upon his deeds."[32]

The anxiety of *taijin kyofusho* is often compared to the anxiety of a stage performance. But as transcultural psychiatrist Laurence Kirmayer points out, this comparison risks understating the care with which a Japanese person must attend to the reactions of the people with whom he is interacting. A stage performer must attend to the reactions of her audience only in the broadest and most collective way. But social performance—that is, ordinary Japanese social interaction—requires a delicate set of perceptual instruments, finely calibrated to detect nuances of hierarchy, social distance, and etiquette. In Japanese society a person is expected to be able to read other people's faces, their gestures, the subtleties of their speech and behavior. Parents tell children, "You should understand what other people are thinking before they say anything by merely looking at their faces."[33] Yet these very people whose faces you are expected to read have been taught to keep their inner feelings hidden, to avoid expressing their will directly, and to couch their personal opinions in misdirection and innuendo. So not only must you be, in effect, a mind reader; you must read the minds of experts trained to keep the contents of their minds hidden, all the while worrying that your own mind might be read.

It is not yet clear how people with *taijin kyofusho* respond to antidepressants. While SSRI prescriptions in Japan are reported to be rising quickly, in part because of the aggressive marketing efforts of the pharmaceutical industry, until very recently Japanese psychiatrists did not prescribe antidepressants very widely. SSRIs were not even available in Japan until 1999.[34] This is not because of any shortage of psychiatrists to prescribe the drugs; Japan provides one of the highest levels of psychiatric service in Asia.[35] Nor is it because of a cultural resistance to pills. Japanese psychiatry is very biologically oriented, and Japanese patients have long been enthusiastic consumers of antianxiety drugs, such as benzodiazepines. According to the Japanese psychiatrist Toshi-Hiro Kobayakawa, the Japanese enthusiasm for benzodiazepines over SSRIs may be partly because the Japanese object less to sedatives than to stimulants. Comparing the stimulant action of the SSRIs to that of amphetamines, Kobayakawa says, "(W)e are much more sensitive to the changes, the exaggerations of behaviour, produced by the amphetamines." Stimulants may be less of a problem in the West, says Kobayakawa, because "the behaviour of people in the West is already more exaggerated."[36]

As Kobayakawa suggests, SSRIs often make people feel energized, self-confident, and less inhibited. But some people on SSRIs find their inhibitions loosened so much that they behave in ways that they later find humiliating or embarrassing. There is the case, for example, of a thirty-five-year-old businesswoman who began taking Luvox for panic disorder and then had to be prevented by friends from serving cocktails at a company party in her bra, "like Madonna."[37] It was only after decreasing the dosage of the drug that she found her behavior in any way unseemly or unwise. Another case report tells of a shy ten-year-old girl who was given Paxil for obsessive-compulsive disorder. Off medication she was described as quiet and sensitive, but once she began taking Paxil she stopped doing her schoolwork, lost her social inhibitions, and began to ask "inappropriate questions" and have problems with "interpersonal boundaries."[38] An unusual report from Germany tells of a fifty-three-year-old man with a long-standing enthusiasm for young boys but no previous sexual experience. After fifteen days on Paxil, he was having "frequent contact with young rent-boys leading to serious financial troubles." On Paxil, he said, he felt "alive for the first time."[39]

Other people taking SSRIs sometimes say that they no longer experience grief, anxiety, or sadness quite so deeply. Occasionally they will realize that circumstances *call* for sadness—that they are expected to share in another person's grief, or that they should be worried about their financial problems—but they are unable to call up the appropriate emotional reactions. A psychotherapist says she found it "hard to worry about anything" while taking an SSRI "because nothing mattered."[40] A graduate student says that rather than working on her dissertation she would rather "stay home and bake cookies."[41] Writer Ian Penman describes sitting entire days in his "Prozac Chair" staring out the window, "just being this nice new neutered, frozen, prone, Prozac me."[42] A fifty-year-old illustrator on an SSRI put it this way: "This must be what it feels like to have a lobotomy."[43]

Lauren Slater describes something similar in her memoir, *Prozac Diary*. Shortly after starting on Prozac, Slater found she could no longer read books in quite the same way. She would read Kierkegaard or Victor Frankl on meaning and the dignity of suffering, sentences that once she had clung to for dear life, and found that the writing no longer moved her in nearly the same way. "I had a cerebral appreciation for the sentence," she writes, "or perhaps, an appreciation based in memory, the way one remembers with fondness a past partner whom one no longer loves." The world as she had known it had changed, even disappeared. Prozac had removed her pathologies, but it seemed to have removed part of her as well. "Who was I?" Slater asks. "Where was I? Everything seemed less relevant—my sacred menus, my gustatory habits, the narratives that had so much meaning to me. Diminished. And in their place? Ice cream."[44]

How common are these reactions? Remarkably, the psychiatric literature has little to say on the issue. It is probably safe to say that an extreme loosening of inhibitions (like, say, the desire to serve drinks in one's bra at a company party) is pretty rare. But the phenomena of emotional blunting, apathy, and a general loosening of inhibitions ("disinhibition," as clinicians term it) are common enough to be familiar to most doctors who prescribe SSRIs, and to many patients who take them. In fact, there is a real ambiguity as to whether disinhibition and emotional blunting should be considered side effects of the drugs or, at least in some cases, their very point. If an American is taking an antidepressant because she is too shy, becoming less inhibited is exactly what she wants. In a culture that values an aggressively outgoing personality, disinhibition may well be a social advantage.

The tag line for Paxil on the GlaxoSmithKline Web site says, "Relieve the anxiety, and reveal the person." The assumption there is that gregarious extroversion is the natural state of the human being, which, were it not for social anxiety, would be evident to everyone else. We are all Americans under the skin, the line suggests, or least under the mask: we are all uninhibited, open-handed, cheerful, and outgoing. Were it not for your social phobia, you could talk fluently to new acquaintances, strike up conversations with alluring strangers, dazzle your friends on the dance floor. But your true self, the extrovert within you, is frozen with self-consciousness.

Perhaps Japanese people with *taijin kyofusho* will feel this way too. But we should not be surprised if they see things differently. For an American, who is expected to wear a mask of cheery extroversion, an SSRI might be just the thing. But for a Japanese person, who is expected to wear a mask of shy deference and modesty, an SSRI could be a social disaster. If you are worried that you will offend other people, then a drug that loosens your inhibitions is probably not going to help. In fact, it may make things worse. A lack of social inhibitions may be an advantage in a culture that values animated conviviality and the "sparkling personality," but it may well be a handicap in a culture that requires an exquisite sensitivity to matters of etiquette and social hierarchy.

David Plath, comparing the American sense of self to that of the Japanese, says that the American archetype "seems more attuned to cultivating a self that knows it is unique in the cosmos, the Japanese to an archetype that can feel human in the company of others."[45] If this is true, it would not be surprising if GlaxoSmithKline used a different ad to sell Paxil in Japan. The commercial appeal of revealing the true self depends not only on the idea that you have a true self that can be revealed by a drug, but also that you will be happier and better off for revealing it. This may be a uniquely American idea.

4

THE LONELINESS OF THE LATE-NIGHT TELEVISION WATCHER

> Celebrities have an intimate life and a life in
> the grid of two hundred million. For them,
> there is no distance between the grids in
> American life. Of all Americans, only they are
> complete.
>
> —George Trow

I do not enjoy giving public lectures. In fact, ten years ago it would probably have been fair to say that I dreaded public lectures. I am happy writing books, teaching small seminars, and talking philosophy with colleagues and students, but given the choice between a formal public lecture and a particularly complicated root canal, it would take me a while to decide. My confession might seem odd in light of the fact that I am, by profession, a university lecturer. And I will admit that over the years, my dread of lectures has given way to mere discomfort. I don't lose all that much sleep anymore. Still, I can't help but envy my colleagues whose public performances do not resemble those of a jack-lighted deer.

The peculiar mystery of American self-consciousness is how eighty-four million citizens of a country famous the world over for its brash, open self-confidence could identify themselves as shy. Foreign visitors have commented for two hundred years on the outgoing friendliness of Americans. Yet one out of two Americans claim to be shy, and of those who don't claim to be shy, three out of four say they have been shy at some point in the past.[1] This paradox has had some strange consequences. Despite the startling demand for shyness drugs, shyness self-help groups, shyness books, and shyness psychotherapies, a growing number of Americans are broadcasting their lives over the Internet twenty-four hours a day and lining up to appear on confessional talk shows where they can reveal their most embarrassing secrets to a national television audience. Some people call this a loss of intimacy, the death of the private, but in fact something stranger is going on. It is as if the only way an inner life gets any meaning is by this kind of self-revelation.

Sociologist Charles Cooley hinted at an explanation a century ago with his notion of the "looking-glass self." As the metaphor suggests, Cooley thought that our sense of ourselves is formed by our social reflection. Cooley thought the looking-glass self had three elements: the imagination of the way we appear to others, the imagination of their judgments about us, and some sort of reaction to that judgment—pride if we're lucky, mortification if we're not. Especially interesting to Cooley was the way that the private self was supported by this social reflection. "In the days of witchcraft," Cooley wrote, "it used to be believed that if one person secretly made a waxen image of another and stuck pins in the image, its counterpart would suffer tortures, and that if the image was melted the person would die."[2] So it is with the private self and its social reflection. Dress up the image and the person prospers; melt the image and the person melts as well.

What Cooley could not have understood in 1902 was the shape that the looking-glass self would take over the next one hundred years. Photography, motion pictures, television, computer technology, and the replacement of character by personality and fame by celebrity have altered the image Americans see in the looking glass. Not only do we worry about what we see in the mirror, we also worry about how we look when we are looking in the mirror. If excessive self-consciousness were not bad enough, now we are excessively self-conscious about being self-conscious. Today the looking-glass self has a camcorder, a big-screen TV, and a home page on the World Wide Web.

A RECENT PUBLIC opinion poll asked Americans to name their greatest fear. According to this poll, the thing Americans fear most of all is public speaking. Public speaking was number one; death was number seven. This finding has been consistent over years, not just for Americans but for Canadians and the British as well. More than snakes, heights, spiders, suffocating in enclosed spaces, or plunging to a fiery death in a plane crash, we fear the gaze of other people.

As anyone knows who has been called on to make an impromptu wedding toast or a speech at the Rotary Club and had it all go horribly wrong, the thing that makes public speaking so unnerving is the sense of exaggerated self-consciousness it produces. You become hyperaware of each little gesture you make, every pause in your speech, each slight catch in your voice. Your throat feels dry, so you pause, your hand trembling, to take a drink: the pause stretches into an eternity. You make a joke; nobody laughs. You cannot forget yourself and act naturally, and the harder you try, the more self-conscious and unnatural you become. Public speakers are expected to maintain a pose of relaxation, so if you are obviously uncomfortable in front of an audience—if, in fact, you are so nervous that you are speaking very rapidly in a high-pitched reedy voice that keeps cracking at inopportune moments—then you make the audience uncomfortable (much fidgeting, clearing of throats, aversion of eyes), which in turn makes you more uncomfortable still. Uncomfortable, in fact, to the point of near-panic. You get so caught up in this twisted, convoluted feedback exercise, conscious of every movement you are making and how it is coming across to your listeners and what their behavior says in turn about you, that you become paralyzed by self-consciousness.

What makes the fear of public performance unusual is this particular characteristic of the fear. Of all the things that we reluctant public speakers are afraid of—the fear that our minds will go blank, that we will say something foolish, that we will deliver a sixty-minute lecture with our pants unzipped—the most common fear is this: the fear that our fear will become apparent to the audience.[3] The most humiliating possible result would be to stand up at the podium and have your face turn pale, your voice quiver, your forehead drip with sweat onto the papers in front of you. That is what must be avoided at all costs. Naturally, the fact that this is so crucial to avoid makes it all the more likely that it will happen. This particular fear, then, results in a double handicap. Not only are you afraid of public speaking, the very root of your fear is that your fear will become public.

This particular characteristic of the fear is also what makes it receptive to treatment with beta-blockers. Beta-blockers (such as propranolol, trade-named Inderal) are ordinarily used to treat high blood pressure. They work by blocking particular sympathetic nervous system receptors. These are the receptors that get activated in times of fear or anxiety (the so-called "fight or flight" response). Beta-blockers do not alter consciousness in any way, like Valium, and they do not make people less inhibited, like Paxil. But they do block the outward signs of anxiety. The result is that, as you stand there looking nervously out at your audience, the beta-blockers mask your nervousness. You can maintain an artfully constructed pose of relaxation. The beta-blocker keeps your heart from racing, your hands from trembling, the sweat from pouring down your forehead. And this, as it turns out, can be very reassuring. The beta-blocker does not actually relax you in any direct way. But it relaxes you nonetheless, because it masks the very thing that you are most nervous about: having your nervousness become public. It keeps your mask of easy relaxation from falling off.

As sociologist Erving Goffman pointed out in his studies of "face-work" in the 1950s, Americans apparently see it as only natural to be relaxed and at ease during social interaction. Embarrassment is seen as a deviation from this natural state. So when a person becomes flustered during a social interaction, whether it is in front of a crowd or one-to-one with another person, we see it as a sign of weakness, low status, or defeat. As Goffman writes, "He who frequently becomes embarrassed in the presence of others is regarded as suffering from a foolish, unjustified sense of inferiority and in need of therapy."[4] This is what makes the public admission of embarrassment so difficult, and what gives beta-blockers their special appeal. Easy embarrassment is itself something to be embarrassed about, and hence, something to be treated with medication.

Beta-blockers were introduced in the early 1960s, but it was not until the mid-1970s that anyone thought to see if they would help stage fright. In one early study, a group of British researchers went to London music academies and recruited twenty-four string players intent on professional careers. These were talented musicians whose careers could be damaged or even ruined by an involuntary tremor or slip of the bow during an important performance. To insure that the musicians would be performing under sufficiently terrifying conditions, the researchers booked a concert hall where a solo debut is regarded as a "testing experience," invited the press, and recorded the performance with a battery of very obvious microphones. Each player performed four times over a period of two days, twice on beta-blockers and twice on placebo, in each case unaware of what he or she had taken. The study showed that not only did the musicians tremble less on beta-blockers, they also played better—usually by a small margin, according to the scores of professional judges, but in some cases quite dramatically.[5]

Studies have shown similar results for public speaking. Another group of British researchers recruited a group of unsuspecting volunteers, stood them in front of a video camera, and then, diabolically, asked them to give an extemporaneous speech on a topic such as "my feelings about giving electric shocks to human volunteers." Not only did the volunteers given beta-blockers show fewer outward signs of anxiety, they also *felt* less anxious. Diminish the outward signs of anxiety, and you diminish anxiety itself.

When I first began asking students in my classes how they felt about the ethics of the use of beta-blockers for performance anxiety, I was surprised by the intensity of their objections to the drugs. To me, beta-blockers looked harmless compared to many of the other technologies we had been discussing, such as extreme body modification, long-term antidepressants, or sex-reassignment surgery. Beta-blockers are safe and inexpensive, available to the poor as well as the rich. They take only an hour or so to work, wear off quickly, and do not result in dependence, personality changes, or surgery scars.[6] But many students saw beta-blockers as the academic equivalent of doping in sports—a pharmaceutical tool that could be used to competitive advantage in class presentations and dissertation defenses. That American students should see college education as a competition is not surprising, of course. (Americans tend to see almost everything as a competition.) But from a competitive standpoint, the notable characteristic of beta-blockers is their leveling effect: they help the nervous more than they help the relaxed. In the British public speaking study, it was the people who were most terrified by having to give an impromptu speech who experienced the most benefit from the beta-blockers. Those who were not anxious in the first place saw no benefit at all. In the London study of musicians, the player who experienced the greatest benefit was the one with the worst tremor. This player's score increased by 73 percent.

Of course, many anxious performers simply look for relief the old-fashioned way: with two or three fingers of Jack Daniels. But when alcohol has been subjected to the rigors of double-blind clinical trials, it has not usually come up to scratch. A few years ago a research group at the University of Michigan asked volunteers to give impromptu ten-minute speeches. Before the speech each volunteer was given what looked like a potent mixed drink, but only half the drinks actually contained any alcohol. The others were plain grapefruit juice and ice, with a little vodka rubbed around the top for effect. Contrary to conventional wisdom, the speakers who got the drinks with alcohol in them (equivalent to two or three mixed drinks) were no less anxious before or during their speeches than those who got the dummy drinks. They didn't feel any less anxious, and their heart rates didn't go down. What did make them less anxious was the *belief* that they were drinking alcohol. Volunteers who thought they were getting real drinks felt less anxious, whether their drinks had any alcohol in them or not.[7]

In contrast to alcohol, beta-blockers work for performance anxiety even when anxious performers don't know whether they have gotten the beta-blockers. Beta-blockers do not work for ordinary shyness or full-blown social phobia. They are effective only for performance anxiety. A trumpet player might use them to prevent an involuntary tremolo, and a nervous news anchor might use them before the evening broadcast, but in situations where the person's anxiety is not rooted in the fear that their anxiety will become apparent to an audience, beta-blockers do not work nearly so well. Not to have to worry about your heart pounding like a jackhammer or your hands turning clammy would be a relief in all sorts of social situations, of course, and to this extent a beta-blocker may be useful. But it is when all the eyes in the room are upon you that it provides you with real shelter.

Because beta-blockers produce better public performances, it is probably fair to call them an enhancement technology. Yet the "enhancement" produced by beta-blockers is different from that of most such technologies. Beta-blockers don't exactly improve a natural human capacity, like anabolic steroids for strength or speed, and they are not restorative, like face-lifts or baldness drugs. In some ways they are closer to Viagra, in that they bring an involuntary bodily response under the control of a pill. Yet beta-blockers accomplish this not by helping the body do again what it used to do naturally, but by preventing the body from doing what it naturally does. Beta-blockers help the person with performance anxiety give better public performances by preventing his body from betraying his inner mental state. They give him a mask of unself-consciousness whose chief attraction is that it does not look like a mask.

In SINCERITY AND AUTHENTICITY, Lionel Trilling contrasts the heroes of Greek tragedy with the men of Rabbinical literature. The Greek hero, says Trilling, is always conscious of the fact that he is behaving as a hero. Being a hero is a role that he consciously inhabits. The gods favor the hero, and the hero knows it; it is evident in the way he comports himself, the way he speaks and acts. "[T]he hero is an actor," writes Trilling, "he acts out his own high sense of himself."[8] But we see nothing like this in Rabbinical discussions of how a person ought to act. These men have none of the same sense of self-consciousness about their behavior. It is this sense of consciously inhabiting a role, of playing to an imaginary audience, that Trilling is getting at when he says, "What is especially to the point is that, as ethical beings, the Rabbis never *see themselves*—it is as if the commandment which forbade the making of images extended to their way of conceiving the personal moral existence as well."[9]

If our own self-consciousness seems closer to that of the Greek heroes than to the men of Rabbinical literature, it is because we, unlike the Rabbis, live in a world devoted to the making of images. Television was developed in 1948. Within seven years, it was present in 75 percent of American homes. To get an idea of just how fast the diffusion of television was, compare it to the telephone, which took sixty-seven years to reach 75 percent of American homes, or the car, which took fifty-two years. Even the radio took twice as long as television.[10] Today there is scarcely a single American who does not have access to a television, and there are very few households that do not own one. In fact, three out of four American homes have more than one television. Seventy-seven percent of American sixth-graders have a TV in their bedrooms.[11] The average individual American watches television for roughly four hours a day, and the average American household watches over seven hours of television a day. According to one study, television accounts for nearly 40 percent of the average American's free time.[12]

What all this time in front of the television has done to the American psyche is anyone's guess, but we know at least two things. One is that people who are shy and lonely spend more time watching television than those who are not. I think we all realize this, but like most things we already know, this has been empirically verified by academics with grant money. Grade-school children, college students, single people, senior citizens living in nursing homes: all are more likely to watch television if they are shy and lonely.[13] It is not clear, of course, whether they are shy and lonely because they watch so much TV, or whether they watch TV because they are shy and lonely. But the two phenomena go together. Heavy television watchers spend less time visiting friends, go to fewer dinner parties, and write to friends less regularly. They send fewer e-mails and greeting cards. They make fewer long-distance calls, entertain at home less, and work on community projects less often. In fact, according to sociologist Robert Putnam, there is no more consistent predictor of civic disengagement than dependence on television for entertainment.[14] This should not be all that surprising. We do not need sociologists to tell us that even four hours per day is a lot of time spent in the company of no human being other than the small, flickering simulacra on the TV screen.

The other thing we know about television is the way it has helped create an alternate reality that seems both more and less real than reality itself.[15] The television screen is the window through which we are allowed to see a parallel universe of supernatural beings called celebrities, who look and act like us, but who are as superior to us as the Greek gods were to ordinary mortals. As with the gods, we don't exactly envy them, but we want very much to be like them. We imitate the manner and styles of the celebrities we especially admire. Their world looks roughly similar to ours, but the television screen that divides it from our world is usually impermeable. If a celebrity were to knock on our front door, it would be almost as astonishing as Jesus turning up for the 11:00 A.M. service at the Presbyterian Church. On the rare occasion when the barrier breaks down and we actually spot a celebrity in the flesh, it feels as if the ordinary laws of physics have been violated. Either we are elated, as if we had witnessed a miracle, and we are compelled to share the news with our friends, or we feel self-conscious and embarrassed, as if we are unworthy to be in the presence of a deity.

To suggest that we have become increasingly aware of our self-presentation over the past century or so is hardly a radical thesis, of course. It is not even radical to suggest that visual technology has helped make Americans more self-conscious, even hyperaware, of the way we appear to others. In fact it would be very odd if, after mirrors, photographs, films, television, home video, and the World Wide Web, we were *not* more self-conscious about the way we come off to other people. What is worrisome about this self-consciousness is the strange loneliness and alienation that comes from watching people perform on television and in the movies, but which also drives the lonely person to watch more of them. If you are a shy and lonely TV watcher, as the novelist David Foster Wallace puts it, you spend your days getting unconscious reinforcement that genuine human worth dwells in the phenomenon of being watched.[16] You temporarily lose your self-consciousness by watching these luminous people whose particular genius lies in being able to convincingly fake unself-consciousness.

Movies and television did not create the phenomenon of celebrity, but they gave it a tremendous lift. Celebrity in its modern sense dates to the mid-nineteenth century, when the Industrial Revolution made possible the quick, inexpensive publication and distribution of printed literature.[17] This literature not only made celebrities out of writers, it also helped to create the idea of celebrity itself. Unlike fame, which suggests wide public recognition, celebrity requires an additional element of self-consciousness about that recognition, even the conscious manipulation of it.[18] Celebrities cultivate their recognition, sometimes to the point where their celebrity threatens to overtake the genuine accomplishment for which they initially gained recognition. Hence Daniel Boorstin's famous remark that celebrity is the quality of well-knownness for being well known.[19]

Yet celebrity also has an element of intimacy to it that is absent from fame. This is what gives celebrity its peculiar mystery, and what made literary celebrity in the nineteenth century feel like something new. As readers of novels and stories were transported into the minds of authors, they came to feel as if they actually knew something about those authors' personal lives. This connection between reader and author felt very different from the connection between an ordinary person and other famous public figures, such as politicians or military heroes. As Boorstin points out, conventional heroes actually become *less* interesting as they become more famous. Their personal characteristics and quirks get rubbed away, and they become dull and lifeless. But celebrities are celebrated precisely for their individual quirks of personality.[20]

If the mass production of print literature made celebrity possible, movies and television made possible its modern form, in which intimacy sits side by side with public performance. Literary celebrities such as Charles Dickens may have been skilled public performers, but their public readings were very similar to the theatrical performances to which audiences had long been accustomed. The distinctive characteristic of the movies and television, in contrast, is the intimacy they can bring to the performance itself. When D. W. Griffith began juxtaposing crowd scenes with close-up shots in his early films, he produced a connection between viewer and performer that differed from anything that had come before. It gave the audience the illusion of having penetrated the performer's inner life—not in the way that the novel had, by merging the inner consciousness of two individuals, but by bringing a sense of intimacy to a performer's outer self-presentation. As historian Warren Susman observed, the close-up shot was emblematic of the culture of personality being preached by the self-help manuals of the day.[21] Here was personality itself, on a fifty-foot screen. At the same time that the movies were reinforcing the importance of personality and self-presentation, they were also making experts in self-presentation seem intimately knowable to those who were watching them. Movies were the first step toward the creation of what George Trow would later call the "grid of intimacy and the grid of 200 million."[22]

There is a scene in Walker Percy's 1961 novel, *The Moviegoer*, where Binx Bolling and his cousin Kate go to see the movie *Panic in the Streets*, which happens to be set in the very neighborhood in New Orleans where they are watching the movie. After they have watched Richard Widmark race through the streets of New Orleans for two hours, Binx and Kate leave the theater and pause to look around the neighborhood. Kate says, "Yes, it is certified now." The neighborhood, simply by virtue of having appeared in the movie, has taken on a heightened reality. Its value has increased. The movie has certified it, and as a result, the people who inhabit the neighborhood are certified as well. Binx says that "if a person sees a movie which shows his very neighborhood, it becomes possible for him to live, for a time at least, as a person who is Somewhere and not Anywhere."[23]

Percy saw how the camera could transform everyday experience into something remarkable, even exhilarating. It can make an ordinary neighborhood look extraordinary even in its very ordinariness. What Binx felt as he exited the theater and walked in the path traced by Richard Widmark is the same feeling that drives spectators at basketball games to wave and point their fingers in the air whenever a television camera pans their way, or that drives audience members to applaud whenever their home town is mentioned on a talk show. The attention of the camera validates their existence. "I am seen, therefore I am," says the news reporter Daniel Schorr, but this gets at only part of what is going on.[24] Even the slightest contact with the world of the media can bring about an existential charge, like the woman who touched the hem of Jesus' robe.

Today, of course, many ordinary people are thrust into the media spotlight and experience the world of television up close—in talk shows, game shows, reality television, or news programs. The result is often a strange mixture of exhilaration and disappointment. Patricia Priest interviewed forty-three people who had appeared as guests on television talk shows, a group that included an organ donor, a rape survivor, a drug-using preacher, and a "sex priestess" who claimed to have had sex with over two thousand partners. These talk show guests were often disappointed with the experience of actually taping the shows. One man compared it to the letdown he felt when he lost his virginity. Yet once the shows aired, this initial disappointment gave way to elation. The talk show guests found that they had not merely rubbed shoulders with celebrities; they were treated like celebrities themselves. Old friends and acquaintances called them up. Strangers recognized them on the street. They were treated with a newfound respect that sometimes verged on awe. One young man, describing a couple that saw him on the street a week after his show appeared, said, "They stopped like they had seen God."[25]

The pursuit of celebrity is easy to mock, but there is a sense in which its roots are built right into our moral system. The moral ideal in which celebrity is rooted is "recognition." Recognition is less important in times and places where a person's identity is seen as fixed and given—as part of the natural order, the social hierarchy, the grand scheme of things—because it is not subject to question or change. But recognition is important for us precisely because it is *not* fixed and given. Recognition can be withheld. Nations can refuse to recognize populations as legitimate nations; populations can refuse to recognize individual members as full human beings, labeling them deviant, sick, or subnormal. The shame and anger felt by so many American minority groups is possible only because recognition has taken on such crucial moral importance. A distorted reflection in the looking glass does not merely fail to represent a person adequately; it builds a distorted identity.[26]

The lust for celebrity comes out of a deformation of this moral idea. If recognition is a moral good, then why shouldn't more recognition be even better? In a social system where success is measured on the yardstick of status, recognition takes on even greater significance, because a person's status can rise or fall according to the way that other people see her. Yet once recognition is treated as a moral good in itself, rather than a measure of anything deeper (such as dignity or accomplishment), this moral idea becomes deformed. Recognition is cut loose from its roots, and it becomes an end to be pursued for its own sake. People are encouraged to seek recognition for pursuits that are criminal, freakish, or simply trivial. Leo Braudy, in his social history *The Frenzy of Renown,* writes that shyness and the lust for celebrity are two sides of the same coin.[27] Shyness comes from the fear that recognition will be denied, while celebrity represents the ultimate fantasy of success.

T. S. Eliot called television "a medium of entertainment which permits millions of people to listen to the same joke at the same time, yet still remain lonesome."[28] His remark hints at both the attraction and the danger of television. Before television, Americans usually had to venture out into public space to be entertained—to the ballpark, the theater, the roadhouse, the concert hall. Today, not only do shy Americans not have to venture out into public space to be entertained, we do not even need to venture out into public space to get the buzz of human contact. With television we get that tingle of social contact, just enough to take us out of ourselves for the period of time that we are watching, without any of the anxiety of worrying about how we are coming across. We don't have to worry about our balding heads, our fat thighs, our nasal whining voices, or whether we are boring anybody by telling them the same story that we told them last month. When we watch television, we have the sensation of becoming invisible. We watch people perform, but they can't watch us. We can listen without saying anything. For the shy person, it looks like the perfect social arrangement.

Here, of course, is the great illusion of television and movies: performers are unaware of the fact that we are watching. As Wallace says, these people are geniuses at being watched and shrugging it off. They are watched by millions of people every week. As we sit there staring at the television, under the temporary illusion that we are voyeurs into their lives, they are sweating under klieg lights, their faces caked with makeup, cameras jutting into their faces, surrounded by people with clipboards and complex machinery who watch their every move to make sure it looks "natural." Voyeurs? We are the *audience.* They know we are there. We are their reason for existing. Yet we are also an *anonymous* audience. We can hiss at the television screen and the performers will never know it.

It is this combination of performance and nonchalance that makes good performers such dangerously seductive figures. What the shy person fears most is self-conscious performance. The shy person wants to be able to forget, for the few minutes he is in face-to-face contact with another human being, how he is coming across. Yet this very fear leads the shy person to spend four hours of television a day in the company of people who have gotten where they are by virtue of their special talent for being watched by lots of people, while at the same time looking impervious to the fact of being watched.[29]

One of my favorite scenes in Percy's *The Moviegoer* comes when Binx Bolling spots the actor William Holden walking unnoticed down Royal Street in New Orleans' French Quarter. Binx watches Holden for a while, and he sees him pass a young couple, maybe twenty or twenty-one years old, walking unhappily down the street, arm-in-arm. They are on their honeymoon, but neither of them is having a good time. The boy is afraid their honeymoon is too conventional, surrounded as they are by tourists down from Memphis and Chicago. The girl is unhappy too, but for a different reason: her new husband is unhappy and she doesn't know why.

Then they see William Holden. The girl pokes the boy; they both brighten for a moment—but only for a moment, because the boy can "only contrast Holden's resplendent reality with his own shadowy and precarious existence." This makes him more miserable than ever. The couple watch Holden; he needs a light for his cigarette. He stops and asks some ladies down from Hattiesburg shopping for iron furniture. They shake their heads no, they don't have a match, and then suddenly they recognize Holden and blush. But to their embarrassment, they still can't find a match. By this point the couple have caught up to Holden, and as they pass, the boy holds out a light without any sign of recognition. Holden nods his thanks, walks along between the two of them for a while. He and the boy look up at the sky and shake their heads. Holden pats them on the shoulders and walks on.

Binx exclaims, "The boy has done it! He has won title to his own existence, as plenary an existence as Holden's, by refusing to be stampeded like the ladies from Hattiesburg. He is a citizen like Holden; two men of the world they are. All at once the world is open to him . . . His girl is open to him too. He puts his arm around her neck, noddles her head. She feels the difference too. She had not known what was wrong nor how it was righted but she knows now that all is well."

What Percy understood was not just the way that the camera has led us to believe that celebrities are more complete, more of a piece, than ordinary human beings. He also understood the way that our own existence seems meager and impoverished in comparison to theirs. This is the flip side of the certification that Binx and Kate felt when they saw their neighborhood appear in *Panic in the Streets*. It is the *loss* we come to feel when comparing our own lives to those that have been certified by the camera. Holden's celebrity has elevated him to a point so high that it no longer even occurs to ordinary people to envy him; they feel nothing but self-consciousness in his presence. No wonder the ladies from Hattiesburg blush.

The antidote to celebrity, as Percy knows, is not sincerity. Sincerity is the mistake of the ladies from Hattiesburg, whose blushes reveal their awe of Holden, and it is also the mistake of autograph seekers, who acknowledge their own inferiority, both to the celebrity and to themselves. The antidote to performance is more performance. The boy must pretend that he does not know who Holden is. Holden may know the boy is pretending, and the boy may know he knows, but neither lets on. This shared pretense allows them to amble down the street together, not in self-revelatory sincerity, but in a kind of mutual irony. This is the kind of irony that says, "We both know what's going on, and we both know not to take it too seriously." Only then, as a fellow man of the world like Holden, can the boy win back his existence. He must see Holden, light his cigarette, and pretend not to recognize him.

I RECENTLY TRAVELED to Indianapolis to meet former television broadcaster Christine Drury.[30] For a number of years Drury was a news anchor and reporter with local Indianapolis television stations. She was very good at her job, except for one devastating problem. If she became self-conscious or made a minor misstep on camera, it would trigger an episode of blushing. Drury would feel the heat rising up from her chest, her mind would go blank, and she would begin to stammer. Even the heavy makeup she used on television did not help. The blushing was not as obvious under the makeup, but she could still feel her face going red, and she would become flustered. Just the thought of blushing made her anxious.

For as long as she can remember, Drury has blushed easily. Sitting in an uncomfortable chair, stepping on a rock, even being greeted by a friend could set off an episode of blushing. Her face, she says, would turn the color of red wine. Yet unlike many easy blushers, Drury has never considered herself shy. Nor was blushing ever fun or playful for her, the way it might be for some easy blushers. She never blushed when she laughed. Often she would abruptly break off conversations and rush from the room when she felt a blush coming on. She was constantly covering her mouth with her hand. At Mass on Sundays, when she had to walk to the front of the church to take communion, she would become so anxious that her teeth would chatter and her hands would tremble, making it hard to hold the chalice. Her blushing got so bad that she could not see the point of living anymore. "It controlled every decision I made," she told me, "and when severe blushing controls your life and your self-esteem, most of the decisions you make are bad ones."

I had read about Drury in an intriguing *New Yorker* profile by the surgeon Atul Gawande, and she has also appeared on various television and radio programs to raise public awareness of a nonprofit group she founded, The Red Mask Foundation. The purpose of the Red Mask Foundation is to provide information and support for severe, pathological, or chronic blushers. Some people use the term "red mask syndrome" for this condition, or the even more arcane term "idiopathic craniofacial erythema," but this is really just a complicated way of saying that some people's faces get red ("erythematous") and the cause is unknown (or "idiopathic"). Whether chronic blushers blush any more often than ordinary blushers is unclear, but they are obviously a lot more troubled by the blushing. Usually (but not always) their blushing is provoked by anxiety or self-consciousness. Nobody really knows how many chronic blushers there are.

Chronic blushing is a puzzle partly because ordinary blushing is so puzzling. What is the point of it? Does it have a biological purpose? We all blush from time to time, but some of us blush more than others. Many fair-skinned people blush easily, but dark-skinned people blush too. We often associate blushing with embarrassment or humiliation, but people also blush when they are complimented. Some people blush in private. Blushing is especially sensitive to eye contact. It is easier to make people blush by staring at them than by calling attention to them in other ways, such as pointing. Blushing can be a cause of embarrassment as well as a sign of it: A good way to make a blusher blush even more is to call attention to her blushing. All of which makes blushing seem very mysterious. Is any purpose served, biologically or socially, by a reflexive mechanism that makes other people aware of one's embarrassment?

Many psychologists believe that blushing is a response to public scrutiny. The trigger may not be that the scrutiny is negative, but that it is unwanted. If you do not want attention from others, then you are more likely to blush when you get it, even if the attention is positive. There also seems to be something special about *social* attention, as opposed to impersonal attention. People are more likely to become self-conscious when others are attending to their social characteristics—their appearance, personality, thoughts, and so on—than when others see them in an impersonal or utilitarian way. Thus exchanging pleasantries with a neighbor or colleague can be a more nerve-wracking experience than an impersonal exchange with a tollbooth operator or a bank teller, or even a scripted encounter with a barber or a dentist.[31]

Some evidence suggests that blushing is triggered more easily when there are more people around to see it. To test this hypothesis, a research group in Colorado instructed subjects to sing "The Star-Spangled Banner" while making vigorous arm movements. They videotaped the subjects singing, then had them watch the videotapes in three different situations: alone, with one other person, and with four other people. The researchers measured the redness of the subjects' cheeks with photoelectric color probes. They found that subjects were no more likely to blush in the presence of one other person than they were while watching the video alone, but when they were joined by four other people, their blushing increased dramatically.[32]

No surprise there, of course. The puzzle is whether their blushing would have increased even further with more people around. Blushing is associated with embarrassment, and while it is often assumed that embarrassment is a form of social anxiety, the two phenomena seem to involve subtly different sets of physiological mechanisms.[33] People with performance anxiety, for example, usually do not blush, even when they are being watched by lots of people. Instead, their faces turn pale. When they do blush, their blush is often of a different kind: not the sudden redness of the face and ears that appears within seconds, but a creeping blush that looks streaky and splotchy. It starts on the upper chest, then makes its way upward to the neck, cheeks, and jaw.[34] Unlike an ordinary blush, which comes on quickly and suffuses the entire face, the creeping blush appears slowly and looks like a rash. Since the physiology of blushing is so poorly understood, doctors do not know how to prevent it with medication, or the circumstances under which medication might work. Chronic blushers often take beta-blockers, but it is not clear how much they help, partly because it is not clear how beta-receptors are involved in blushing.[35] When beta-blockers block the sympathetic nervous system effects that kick in during anxiety, they typically prevent the constriction of peripheral blood vessels. This is why they keep an anxious person from getting clammy hands. But blushing is not caused by the constriction of facial blood vessels; it is caused by their dilation. The vessels get larger, blood rushes in, and the face flushes red.

Drury's blushing was quick and full, not splotchy and creeping, and beta-blockers did not prevent it. Nor did self-help books, antidepressants, or psychotherapy. Once she took a tablet of lithium prior to a broadcast. This was, she told me, one of her worst performances. In 1999, desperate for help, Drury traveled to Sweden to undergo a surgical procedure for excessive blushing called an endoscopic thoracic sympathectomy (ETS). The surgery can be tricky, but the idea behind it is strikingly simple: the surgeon simply snips through all the branches of the sympathetic nerves leading to the patient's face, except for those leading to the eye. The procedure is done endoscopically, using small scopes inserted through incisions made in the armpit. Once the nerves are cut, the patient no longer blushes. The ETS procedure was originally done for people with hyperhidrosis, or excessive sweating on the upper body, hands, and face. But surgeons discovered that not only did many of these heavy sweaters no longer sweat after the surgery, they didn't blush either. So surgeons began performing the procedure on chronic blushers as well. It seems to work. Some studies have reported that over 85 percent of patients are satisfied with the surgery.[36]

ETS is not free of risks. The most serious risk is Horner's syndrome, symptoms of which include a drooping eyelid, constricted pupil, and a sunken eyeball. It occurs when a surgeon accidentally cuts the nerves leading to the eye. One in one hundred patients undergoing ETS will get Horner's syndrome, and one in ten will find their heart rate decrease by about 10 percent, which may cause them to weaken physically. But the most common complaint after surgery is "compensatory sweating." After ETS, most patients find that their faces and upper bodies no longer sweat at all, and as a result their lower bodies sweat even more. About a third of ETS patients experience an odd side effect called "gustatory sweating"—sweating (or perceived sweating) in response to tastes or smells. When people with gustatory sweating eat, they can feel sweat bead up on their foreheads, the way it might if they were eating spicy food.[37]

These are risks that many chronic blushers are perfectly willing to take. The striking thing about the testimony of many chronic blushers is just how shameful and disabling they find their condition. Many see blushing as a sign of weakness or vulnerability. They will avoid any situation that is likely to bring it on. Because blushing is involuntary, many people feel that a blush will betray something that they are ashamed of but are trying to hide.[38] Blushing works like a lie detector that is unreliable and erratic, and apt to go off by accident at the most humiliating times. People who blush easily often fear they will blush even when they are *not* self-conscious or uncomfortable, and this possibility makes them anxious even in situations where they would otherwise feel right at home. On the Red Mask Foundation's Web site, a member recently posted a testimonial that read, "Tonight I will be going to church as I do every Wednesday night with the growing fear and anticipation of total humiliation for virtually no reason as I sit with my best friends."[39]

Drury says that ETS surgery liberated her. When she got home from Sweden she immediately began doing all the things that she had previously avoided. She could talk to people much more comfortably, and look them straight in the eye without blushing. She found herself noticing things about other people, even friends and family, that she had never noticed before, simply because she had never been able to look carefully at their faces without worrying that her own would turn red. Her performance on television improved, and her confidence soared. Friends noticed a difference in her immediately. "People would say, 'You look so skinny!'" Drury says. They could tell she was different, but they could not put their fingers on what had changed. She had told no one outside her family about the surgery.

The psychic mechanism at work with ETS is not all that different from that of the beta-blockers for performance anxiety. Because blushing can be both a marker of embarrassment and something to be embarrassed about, the surgical treatment of blushing removes the source of a person's anxiety. It eliminates the possibility of blushing at the wrong time (and on television, every time is the wrong time). Like a person with a new face-lift, people who have undergone ETS sometimes find themselves more confident and talkative than before. One ETS patient wrote on an electronic discussion list, "I need to be careful what I say, because I have just been blurting things out in public like I have never done before."[40]

Even though blushing is involuntary, it may have subtle social functions that ETS could erase. For example, some psychologists think blushing is a sign to others that you have broken a social rule or done something shameful. According to one pair of theorists, a blush serves as "an acknowledgment, a confession, and an apology." It tells others that you are sorry for what you have done, and implicitly asks for their forgiveness.[41] Some studies suggest that if you were to lose the ability to blush, you might occasionally forfeit the good opinions of other people, by blunting your ability to show embarrassment. In one study, researchers had subjects watch a videotape of shoppers in a supermarket who accidentally knocked over a stack of toilet paper. In response, the shoppers did one of two things: either they picked up the toilet paper and rebuilt the stack, or else they simply walked away. More importantly, some of them acted obviously embarrassed, while others acted unaffected. The subjects watching the videotape were then asked their opinions of the shoppers. The results were revealing. The subjects watching the videotape had higher opinions not only of those who repaired the display, but also of those who showed embarrassment. The fact that the blunderers were embarrassed about their blunders elevated them in the eyes of observers.[42]

Why would a chronic blusher choose to become a television broadcaster? When I asked Drury this question, she just laughed. "I have always been an extrovert," she says. She has never felt socially awkward, apart from her blushing, and has always made friends easily. As a high school student she admired the poise and glamour of television performers, especially the women who anchored the news. She majored in telecommunications at Purdue, and after graduating Phi Beta Kappa, got a job as production assistant at a local station. From there she worked her way up to a job as a newswriter, then became the overnight anchorwoman. It would have been an important step toward fulfilling her ambition, if not for her severe blushing.

When Drury talks about her blushing, she tends to speak of it as a problem external to her identity, an unexplainable affliction that interfered with her vision of herself. She emphasizes that severe, chronic blushing is a medical condition. Shy people might feel that blushing is natural for them, given their temperament, but Drury found blushing a visible contradiction of the person she felt she was. Other chronic blushers echo this sentiment. One chronic blusher, describing the change in his personality after he underwent ETS, writes, "My wife says I am one person now. Not the two like I was before one at home and one in public."[43]Some chronic blushers feel that their self-consciousness forces them to put on an act for strangers, a piece of social fakery invented solely for public display. They cannot be themselves, as they might be among intimates, but neither can they put on a convincing show of extroversion: their blushing gives their self-consciousness away. So they are stuck, neither themselves nor convincing fakes.

If chronic blushing is a medical condition, what exactly is the pathology, the blushing itself, or the psychic distress the blushing brings about? Chronic blushers seek out surgery because they are deeply troubled by their blushing, but none of us really knows for certain when we are blushing and how severe it is, unless we look in the mirror. Blushers can feel their faces getting hot, but subjective facial temperature does not match up all that reliably with facial color: a face can feel hot but not get red, and it can get red without getting hot. In fact, chronic blushers are often poor judges of whether they are actually blushing. In one recent study, researchers recruited three different groups of subjects. One group consisted of people who met the criteria for social phobia and were troubled primarily by blushing. The second group consisted of people with social phobia who did not have a blushing problem. The third group consisted of ordinary people without social phobia, who served as the control group. The researchers then tried to embarrass the subjects in a variety of ways—by making them give impromptu speeches, strike up conversations with a stranger, or sing in front of a video camera and then watch themselves on tape. While the chronic blushers *felt* as if they were blushing more, they did not in fact blush any more often than the other socially phobic people. Nor did the socially phobic people as a whole blush more than the ordinary control group. In fact, in two of the three situations the people with social phobia blushed *less* than the control group. Only when forced to watch themselves singing on videotape did the group of socially phobic blushers actually blush more often.[44]

Nor do chronic blushers seem to blush any redder than ordinary people, though they often believe they do. A group of Dutch researchers asked women identified as chronic blushers to sing in front of a video camera, and then watch the video in the presence of two men. As anyone who has had an unhappy experience in a karaoke bar might have guessed, the chronic blushers were easily humiliated by this experience. They felt far more embarrassed than women who were not easy blushers, and when asked to estimate how intensely they blushed, they consistently ranked their own blushing as far more intense than did the other women. But on *objective* measures of blushing, such as physiological tests of skin temperature and skin color, they scored no higher than the other women. They were not actually blushing any redder or more often. They simply believed they were.[45]

Drury is an ETS success story, yet even for her, the adjustment to life after ETS was not easy. At first the liberation from fear was exhilarating. She got a better news job as an evening anchorwoman for another station. But over time she began to feel ashamed that she had resorted to an artificial means of overcoming her self-consciousness. She eventually told a friend about the surgery, and he was horrified. Her self-confidence began to disintegrate, and she became depressed.

Her body had changed, but her mind could not quite catch up. "I could not get used to the new me," she told me. Before the surgery she was worried about blushing, but afterward she began to worry about *not* blushing. She was afraid that people would notice that she did not blush, and that her secret would be revealed. It was only after she went public about the surgery and founded the Red Mask Foundation that her confidence began to return.

I had traveled to Indianapolis partly because I was interested in the Red Mask Foundation, especially the social dynamics of their support group meetings. If most easy blushers (like me) blush because they are anxious about social encounters or public performances, what would these people make of a support group meeting? What would they make of a support group leader who not only relished public performances, but who was extraordinarily good at them? I did not get any answers that evening. As Drury walked into the room and shook my hand, she explained that some of the regular members of the group had canceled, and that the only people attending that evening would be she and her husband, Mike. She remarked that it was too bad I had not come to an earlier meeting. A crew from *48 Hours* had flown in to tape a session for television in February, and the room had been packed.

5

THE IDENTITY BAZAAR

Become who you are.
—Friedrich Nietzsche

Expressing your inner Spirit through your
outer image.
—advertising slogan for reVamp! Salon Spa

Experienced users of psychedelic drugs tell me that the kind of experience the drug gives you will depend on your surroundings. Given an atmosphere of warmth and security, you may get a sense of cosmic brotherhood, a feeling of deep intimacy with your fellow human beings. You may be at one with the universe. But in the wrong setting, a setting of apprehension or fear or hostility, you can be transported into an icy hell of paranoia and terror, a cold sterile coffin of anxiety, a psychic experience more terrifying than Edvard Munch could ever have imagined. My friends, I have been to such a place. I have been Christmas shopping at the Mall of America.

I have seen caravans of buses and vast prairies of cars. I have passed armies of exhausted shoppers laden with plastic toys, their eyes bleary from combat fatigue, their knees buckling under their loads. I have walked in the shadow of an inflatable Snoopy the size of a Greyhound bus. I have been assaulted by advertising jingles, wall-sized video screens, and perfume with the intensity of tear gas. I have seen an indoor roller coaster, an artificial rain forest, and a voluptuous mannequin wearing lingerie made entirely of white fur. I have been to Lego Land and the Limbo Lounge and a shop that sells nothing but magnets. I have heard John Schneider, the star of the television show *The Dukes of Hazzard*, sing the theme song to *Oklahoma* to a throng of admiring shoppers. I have seen Santa Claus surrounded on all sides by robot bears.

The Mall of America is the largest shopping mall in the United States. It houses literally thousands of shops, and it is built on an astonishing scale. In addition to the usual array of theme restaurants and multiplex cinemas, it has its own bus station, an Underwater World walk-through aquarium, and a full-scale indoor amusement park called Camp Snoopy. It is located in a suburb just outside the Twin Cities, where I live, and is only a short drive from the international airport, making it convenient for the tourists who fly in from Europe for the express purpose of shopping there. You might think that it is possible to enjoy the Mall of America in the same kitsch-laden way it is possible to enjoy seeing a Wayne Newton extravaganza in Las Vegas, yet even this is difficult, because despite its vast scale it remains, in the end, just a very big shopping mall. I rarely go to the Mall of America, quite frankly, because I can see myself in the faces of the shoppers there. We have that look of desperate happiness that you see on a dog in the physiology lab once the anesthetic starts to kick in.

It is significant that the Mall of America is located in Minnesota. Minnesotans are a prosperous people, but unlike many Americans, they do not really trust their prosperity. Prosperity sounds too much like having a good time. In fact, I suspect this is why the Mall of America has been so successful here: it turns pleasure shopping into an ordeal. Minnesota, it so happens, has been home to three of America's most perceptive critics of the pursuit of happiness in a consumerist age. Two were novelists: Sinclair Lewis, who made Babbitry a synonym for the petty small-mindedness of the American middle class, and F. Scott Fitzgerald, whose novels of doomed heroes and dazzling social climbers read like parables of the American obsession with status and wealth. But the name of the third, Thorstein Veblen, is less well-recognized outside academic circles. Veblen was trained in philosophy, wrote on economic theory, and it is from his deeply eccentric book published in 1899, *The Theory of the Leisure Class*, that we have inherited the famous phrase, "conspicuous consumption."

What Veblen saw, nearly a century before the Mall of America was constructed, was how people will buy things for the sake of public display. Conspicuous consumption is Veblen's name for buying not in order to acquire what you need, nor even to acquire what you want for utilitarian purposes, but in order to acquire public esteem. This is not merely a matter of trying to impress other people. Consumption is also the basis of *self*-esteem, or as Veblen says, self-respect—since self-respect depends on the respect of others. In Veblen's world, the point of buying things is not to satisfy your needs but to outrank your friends and neighbors.

It is not yet possible to buy many enhancement technologies at a mall, not even at the Mall of America. But this may be coming. Over the past decade Americans have witnessed the transformation of an extraordinary number of pharmaceuticals into items of mass consumption. Antidepressants are advertised in magazine and Web ads with slogans like "The Zoloft Saturday," "Paxil . . . Your life is waiting!" or "I got my playfulness back with Effexor". A thriving black market for lifestyle drugs has emerged on the Internet. Eli Lilly markets Prozac Weekly with cut-out coupons.[1] In 1999, the U.S. pharmaceutical industry spent $13.9 billion in promotions. In 2000, it spent $2.4 billion solely on direct-to-consumer advertising, mainly television ads. This represents a remarkable tenfold increase since 1996. Schering-Plough spent more money advertising Claritin than the Coca-Cola Company spent advertising Coke.[2]

At a time when Prozac is shilled in women's magazines and the success of Viagra is measured by the upward rise of Pfizer on the stock exchange, Veblen's words about conspicuous consumption sound prophetic. If Veblen is right, then understanding the forces guiding the production of Ritalin, synthetic growth hormone, and Paxil means trying to understand the forces that have guided the production of other items of mass consumption. Enhancement technologies, like cosmetics and hair coloring, have become a way for consumers to shape an identity.

READING VEBLEN NEARLY a century after he wrote *The Theory of the Leisure Class*, it is not easy to know which parts of the book to take seriously. It comes off as equal parts intellectual theory, social satire, and crackpot polemic. When Veblen writes in dispassionate academic prose that the fashion for walking sticks comes from the sense that the sticks can be used as weapons, or that consumers prefer dogs to cats because dogs are more useless, and thus emphasize the ability of the owner to waste economic resources, it is hard to figure just how he intended these passages to be read. Social satire? Theory? Parody of theory?

Even the unifying theme of the book, from which its title comes, veers dangerously close to highbrow parody. Veblen argued that the lower classes tended to emulate the styles and tastes of the leisure class, who do not have to work for a living. Consumers thus covet markers that show that they do not need to work or that they are incapable of work. This is the reason for the social preference for women to have small hands and feet; they "show that the person so affected is incapable of useful effort and must therefore be supported by her owner. She is useless and expensive, and she is consequently valuable as evidence of pecuniary strength."[3] The same goes for a thin waist, which, like a bound foot in China, showed a woman's lack of fitness for labor. Veblen is especially scathing when it comes to dress, and once again he sings the same caustic tune: the point of elegant apparel is to demonstrate publicly that the wearer does not engage in any productive labor. For example, about the woman's skirt, he writes: "The substantial reason for our tenacious attachment to the skirt is this: it is expensive and it hampers the wearer at every turn and incapacitates her for all useful exertion."[4]

Where Veblen is prescient, however, is his sense that in a consumption economy, consumer goods would become markers of who we are. Or perhaps more precisely, markers of whom we want to be. The goods we consume demonstrate to others, and to ourselves, our place on the social ladder. For Veblen this ladder signified class, but the point is apt no matter what it signifies: you can climb higher up the ladder by consuming more, and more wisely, than your peers; conversely, you can slip down the ladder by consuming foolishly, or failing to consume much at all. Consumption is the engine that powers the climb.

The phrase "conspicuous consumption" may be slightly misleading, however, if it suggests that consumers are buying in order to stand out from the crowd. Most people, says Veblen, do not consciously try to excel in their visible consumption. Rather, they try to live up to a conventional standard of decency in the amount and quality of what they consume. This is not to say that consumers are satisfied simply to live up to the average level of consumption. Instead, they are always striving for an ideal of consumption that is always just beyond their reach, like a monkey grabbing for one more coconut. The motive for this striving, says Veblen, is not greed but emulation: consumers are always trying to outdo those with whom they are in the habit of comparing themselves.

Veblen also saw that in a consumption economy, a person would be expected to become a great connoisseur of consumer goods—in the way that, for example, most college-age American men today are capable of making fine distinctions between the merits of near-indistinguishable mass-market brands of beer; or to take a case a little closer to home, the way middle-aged male American academics are expected to be knowledgeable about things like computers, wine, or single-malt whiskey (what Veblen calls "manly beverages and trinkets").[5] According to Veblen, in fact, academics are particularly slavish to the norms of conspicuous consumption, because their scholarly credentials often place them in a higher social grade than their earnings merit. Thus, academics are constantly comparing themselves to others who make more money than they do. They are constantly aiming higher in their consumption than they can reasonably afford, and so, Veblen says, "there is no class of the community that spends a larger proportion of its substance in conspicuous waste."[6]

If the picture Veblen suggests seems a bit simplistic—a pack of social strivers frantically buying useless goods in a futile effort to catch up with the lead dog—he did show an uncommon feel for the cultural position that consumer goods were beginning to hold in American life. Even in his eccentric polemics about skirts and walking sticks he is hinting at an important idea: ownership is not all that it seems to be on the surface; even the simplest of consumer items represents something far more complicated. For Veblen, buying and selling is not the simple exchange of money for goods in order to satisfy needs or wants. Consumption is part of a larger moral system, with a symbolic place in that system that transcends any simple exchange.

What Veblen and others saw at the beginning of this century was the way that the place of consumption in that moral system was being transformed.

In his memoir *Exile's Return*, Malcolm Cowley describes this as a transformation from a production ethic to a consumption ethic, the effects of which were apparent to him and other young men returning home from World War I in Europe.[7] The production ethic was the ethic of a young capitalist society, says Cowley, and stressed the values of thrift, foresight, personal initiative, and industry. He calls it a "business-Christian ethic," represented then by magazines like the *Saturday Evening Post*. You may have to suffer, this ethic taught; you may have to deny yourself luxuries so that you can put your money back into your business; but you will be rewarded for this self-denial in heaven. Your duty on earth is to produce more goods, and accumulate more wealth, with no thought to where the goods you are producing will eventually wind up. This production ethic worked well as long as markets continued to open up—in the West, overseas, or in the bank accounts of frugal working people who had saved their money. But in the period after the war, production of goods began to outstrip demand. New domestic markets had to be found, and so it was necessary to encourage Americans to buy rather than save. An ethic of consumption did just that.

As accustomed as we are today to the idea of consumption as a middle-American phenomenon, situated primarily in the shopping malls and car dealerships of suburbia, it comes as a slight shock to read that Cowley locates the consumption ethic in the bohemian values of Greenwich Village. A subculture of artists and intellectuals, Greenwich Village represented the alternative to middle America; it was, says Cowley, "not only a place, a mood, a way of life: like all bohemias, it was also a doctrine."[8] Village doctrine stressed the values of self-expression and living for the moment. Why spend your life piling up wealth that you cannot enjoy until you are very old? Better to enjoy life while you can. The Village also taught the equality of the sexes. Women should have the same pay and working conditions as men, the same opportunities to smoke, or drink, or take lovers. In the Village, writes Cowley, Puritanism was the great enemy, and a version of Freudian psychology the great liberator. If we are unhappy, it is because we are repressed; the solution is to remove our repressions.

It is not hard to see how the values of Greenwich Village, however fortuitously, fed into the consumption ethic. The notion of female equality, for example, had the potential to double the consumption of commodities that had previously been available only to men, such as cigarettes. The idea of living for the moment fueled credit spending, encouraging people to borrow money in order to buy a house or a car. The emphasis on self-expression encouraged consumers to buy all sorts of items that they did not really need, but which, in Veblenesque fashion, indicated who they were or wanted to be. Greenwich Village did not create the consumption ethic, of course, any more than American business set out to exploit it for the purposes of profit. But, as Cowley points out, American business and Village doctrine nourished each other in ways that neither fully realized at the time. Even as the *Saturday Evening Post* thundered against Greenwich Village, denouncing its pagan values and bohemian immorality, it was filling its pages with advertisements for cigarettes, toilet tissues, and cosmetics. Big business took Village doctrine and spread it to middle America, where, in time, "houses were furnished to look like studios" and "women smoked cigarettes on the streets of the Bronx, drank gin cocktails in Omaha and had perfectly swell parties in Seattle and Middletown."[9]

This revolution in morals after the war would have happened without Greenwich Village, admits Cowley, although it may not have happened in exactly the same way. America had been getting richer before the war, and its currents of profligacy had been held in check by hellfire Puritan preaching. During the war, however, all sorts of strict standards were relaxed. Afterward, it was hard to turn back. The war, writes Cowley, "left us with a vast unconcern for the future and an enormous appetite for pleasure."[10] Even older people who had not fought in the war were changed by it. "People of forty had been affected by the younger generation: they spent too much money, drank too much gin, made love to one another's wives, and talked about their neuroses."[11] This was the age in which the "party" flourished, understood as a social gathering where men and women drank cocktails, danced, flirted, and gossiped. Such parties had originated with the French 1830 Romantics, says Cowley, but they were introduced to America through Greenwich Village. Perhaps by 1931 the Village was dead, as the *Saturday Evening Post* declared; but if so, it was dead because its values had become the mainstream. It died of success, Cowley writes; the consumption ethic had spread to the heartland.

MOST OF WHAT are commonly called enhancement technologies today can also be described as treatments. Viagra can enhance sexuality or treat impotence; plastic surgery can enhance the body or treat disfigurements. Some technologies successfully straddle the line between the realms of enhancement and treatment, and some shift from one realm to the other. Perhaps the most familiar item of mass consumption to make the transition from treatment to enhancement during this century has been cosmetics.

Cosmetics are so ubiquitous today—so heavily advertised, so widely bought and sold, their use such a rite of passage for teenaged American girls—that it is easy to forget that the cosmetics industry is a fairly recent social development. The mass-market cosmetics industry in America dates only to the 1920s, the period where Cowley locates the birth of the consumption ethic. In fact, as Kathy Peiss reminds us in her excellent social history of cosmetics, *Hope in a Jar*, prior to the nineteenth century the preparation of cosmetics was considered part of a woman's store of ordinary household knowledge, like cooking, gardening, and caring for the sick. Women learned how to identify herbs and roots, distill their essences, and put together skin remedies.[12] Cosmetics were part of good health and hygiene, and knowledge was passed around between friends, neighbors, and family members, like recipes.[13] By the mid-nineteenth century this had changed: women were still mixing recipes, but often these mixtures called for ingredients available only at pharmacies. Some druggists mixed and sold cosmetic preparations, and even sold brand-name commercial preparations for things like cold cream and face powder. Yet it was not until the years after World War I that cosmetics were transformed into an item of mass consumption.

That transformation had a number of cultural barriers to overcome, one of which was a distinction commonly made between skin care preparations and "face-painting," such as the use of lipstick and rouge. Many women used skin care preparations, which were seen as a means of promoting a natural, healthy, authentic appearance. Face-painting, on the other hand, was seen as a kind of deception.[14] With its origins on the dramatic stage, it had an aura of theatricality and disguise. The inaugural issue of *Parents* magazine in 1926 promised to help parents cope not only with the milk-refusing baby and the college son who wants a raccoon coat, but also "the daughter in her teens who will hide her youthful bloom under cosmetics."[15] At its most extreme, face-painting was associated in the public mind with the image of an aging prostitute, painting her lips and cheeks in order to attract customers.

The stigma of face-painting was not so different from the stigma that would be attached to enhancement technologies later on, the stigma of phoniness. This is the sense that by getting cosmetic surgery for your nose, you are hiding your Jewishness; that by taking Prozac, you are hiding your true character; that by using a hair straightener, you are trying to look like a white person. The stigma is rooted in worries about fakery and passing, of trying to hide the person you really are.[16]

How did marketers overcome the aura of fakery that cosmetics carried in the 1920s? One way was exactly as Veblen might have predicted. Marketers portrayed cosmetics as a way of overcoming the restrictions of social class. Some manufacturers sought endorsements from wealthy society figures such as Mrs. Reginald Vanderbilt and Mrs. O. H. P. Belmont, portraying cosmetics as a marker of high culture. A 1924 ad for Zip depilatory shows before-and-after shots of a dark-skinned European immigrant who rids herself of excess facial hair in order to achieve social acceptance.[17] Upper-class women are not necessarily more beautiful than working-class women, these ads suggested; they just know more about the proper use of cosmetics. The appeal to status-climbing even extended to the much smaller men's cosmetics industry. An advertisement for J. B. Williams shaving cream shows an American man in a bowler next to a turbaned Indian. The copy notes that in India, a man's place is painted upon his face, while Americans judge a man's social class by how well his face is shaved. The headline reads: "We have our caste marks, too."[18]

A central value of the new consumption ethic emerging in the

1920s was that of self-expression—the idea, as Cowley describes it, that each person's "purpose in life is to express himself, to realize his full individuality through creative work and beautiful living in beautiful surroundings."[19] It was an idea beautifully suited to cosmetics marketing. At a time when cosmetics still carried an aura of theatricality, marketers countered by portraying cosmetics as a means of finding and enhancing your individuality. You are playing the part of yourself, and cosmetics are a way of playing that part more convincingly. This sales pitch skirts the common worries about disguise and deception. A disguise is not a disguise if you are dressing up as yourself; it is not deception if your public presentation more accurately reflects your inner self. The Max Factor sales staff offered individualized recommendations to consumers based on their hair and skin types, while Armand launched a marketing campaign called "Find Yourself."[20]

If all of public life is a performance, then cosmetics are not a way of hiding yourself. They are a way of expressing yourself in a world where others, even strangers, are always watching you. Cosmetics advertisements in the 1920s reminded women that they were constantly being scrutinized. Advertisers placed cameras and spectators in their magazine and newspaper ads, underscoring the notion that appearances count. A Woodbury's soap ad from 1922 showed a glamorous woman at a social affair, surrounded by men in dinner jackets and women in formal dress, and asked: "Strangers' eyes, keen and critical—can you meet them proudly—confidently—without fear?"[21] A booklet for beauty aids showed a nude woman with the caption, "Your Masterpiece—Yourself." Women, often veiled nudes, were frequently shown gazing into mirrors.[22] Seventy-five years later, the same strategy was being used to sell Rogaine, the hair growth treatment for men. Television advertisements showed a handsome, full-haired young man looking into a mirror. To his obvious dismay, a balding reflection stares back.

The thin line that cosmetics manufacturers had to walk in the early part of the twentieth century—between nature and artifice, authenticity and disguise—was much like the one walked in later years by mass producers of hair coloring. As Malcolm Gladwell has written, the selling point for Miss Clairol, the first do-it-yourself hair coloring, was that even though it would artificially color a woman's hair, the artificiality would be undetectable to the casual observer. When the ad campaign for Miss Clairol was launched in 1956, it used the tag line, "Does she or doesn't she?" followed by, "Only her hairdresser knows for sure." Just as cosmetics manufacturers thirty years earlier had portrayed cosmetics as a means of looking natural, Clairol emphasized the natural look of its new hair coloring, highlighting how difficult it was to tell if the hair had been colored artificially. For Nice 'n Easy, Clairol's shampoo-in hair color, Clairol used the slogan: "The closer he gets, the nicer you look." Clairol's advertising pitch was remarkably persuasive. From the 1950s to the 1970s, the percentage of American women coloring their hair rose from 7 percent to over 40 percent.[23]

But as Gladwell points out, it is not hard to see the downside of this kind of marketing. By playing up the notion that hair coloring is a brilliant disguise, Clairol also played up the idea that it is, in fact, a disguise—a way of hiding the person the woman actually is. Disguises can be oppressive, especially if you come to see them as obligatory. You become utterly dependent on the good opinions of others. Even if you are successful in gaining those good opinions, you never know whether the success is really yours, or if the credit belongs to your disguise. A Lady Clairol commercial in the 1960s featured a young, blonde woman by a lake who is being swung around in the air by a handsome man. The voice-over says, "Chances are she'd have gotten the young man anyhow, but you'll never convince her of that." Here is the flip side of Clairol's emphasis on passing undetected. If you succeed with the help of fakery, you will constantly wonder whether you would have succeeded without it.[24]

This helps to explain why, in the 1970s, Clairol began to lose ground to a new hair coloring, with a new kind of ad campaign: Preference, by L'Oreal. L'Oreal's advertising slogan was: "Because I'm worth it." The slogan referred to the slightly higher cost of Preference, but it also pointedly shifted emphasis from the notion of passing to that of self-expression. Where Clairol's ads had emphasized what people might say about a woman who colors her hair, the L'Oreal ads emphasized what a woman says to herself, when nobody else is around. These ads said: Forget about passing, forget about trying to fool other people; if you are going to color your hair, do it for yourself. By the 1970s, when L'Oreal took the lead, hair coloring had moved from the hair salon to the home, from the province of experts to that of a woman herself. Many more women were coloring their hair, and for that reason, hair coloring became less embarrassing: no longer did it need to be so carefully hidden. The moral background to hair coloring changed as well. The L'Oreal ads emerged at a time in which women were being encouraged to be independent and pro-gressive. Middle-class Americans were "finding themselves." "Pass-ing" had given way to pride and self-esteem. This moral shift was reflected in the L'Oreal ads, which hit upon the language of inde-pendence and liberation that has become such an important piece of advertising today.

THE WIZARDRY OF these sales pitches makes it easy to overlook the fact that they are, after all, just sales pitches, with no higher pur-pose than to sell hair coloring. In a consumer culture, though, hair coloring can be invested with magical properties. It can be seen as a genuine means of self-expression, even liberation. Just as cosmetics at the beginning of the century could be convincingly portrayed as a means of throwing off oppressive Victorian ideals of womanhood, so a new hair color in the 1970s could be convincingly portrayed as a means of throwing off the retrograde ideals of 1950s conformity. Hair coloring and cosmetics are not simply enhancements, not merely a means of self-improvement, but vehicles of liberation and self-transformation.

Veblen realized at the beginning of the century that consumer goods were coming to be seen as a way to escape being defined by the culture that surrounds you. By buying correctly, you could avoid being defined as working class. Proper consumption could liberate you. Yet Veblen was mocking the idea of consumption as social climbing even as he identified it. He tells his story of class emulation with a wink to the reader: You and I know that you cannot *really* buy your way into the upper class. Consumers may think consumption is a tool of liberation, his ironic tone suggests, but you and I are wise to the game. Thus in Veblen's world, consumption is really not so much a means of self-transformation as a kind of self-deception. You buy in order to demonstrate outwardly your high social class, but deep inside you remain the same—a poor sucker duped into thinking that money and breeding come to the same thing. Veblen, remember, lived in the same world as F. Scott Fitzgerald, whose Jay Gatsby, the former James Gatz, displays his glittering wealth and affects upper-class phrases like "old sport" in a sad attempt to transcend his humble beginnings.

The difference today, a century later, is that Veblen's story is told without the wink. The notion that you are what you buy has become so thoroughly entrenched in popular consciousness that even intellectuals can speak of it with no sense of irony or regret. Veblen's mocking tone has disappeared, or else it is used as an advertising strategy by canny ad agencies. When John Seabrook writes in *The New Yorker* that "brands are how we figure out who we are," or that "judgments about what jeans to wear are more like judgments of identity than of quality," one wonders whether Veblen would feel vindicated or horrified.[25] In his own odd way, Veblen was identifying the dawn of a new consumerist mentality and protesting against it. But these days the tone of protest has all but vanished. Americans either celebrate consumption, or they turn anti-consumption into a consumer choice itself, a mark of one's social identity as a green, pro-environmentalist, counter-cultural outsider. This is understandable: in a culture so thoroughly dominated by the market, when the consumerist mentality has so clearly won the struggle that the fact of the struggle is no longer even apparent, protest seems beside the point. If the idea that you can achieve status by what you buy becomes an article of faith among a critical mass of people, then it becomes the reality. If the culture that surrounds you sees clothes and hair as signs of liberation, then in some strange sense they are.

To make liberation an effective sales pitch, however, to make plausible the idea that by changing your hair or clothes or even the size and shape of your breasts you are liberating yourself, rather than being manipulated by the culture around you, you must portray the self as somehow independent of culture. Consumers must believe on some level that their individual attitudes, tastes, and desires are independent of the forces that surround them. They must believe that when they buy a product or a service, they are making a choice that is theirs alone. In this way, consumers can believe both that their appearance pleases other people and that the opinions of others have nothing to do with their choices. In *Modern Primitives*, a book about extreme body modification, one man explains why he has decided to cover his entire body and face with tattoos: "I definitely see it as a kind of theater for myself—people definitely perceive me totally differently than if I had no tattoos." Then he goes on to explain, with no apparent contradiction, "I've never regarded my tattoos as exhibitionistic . . . the tattoos are for myself."[26]

Susan Bordo, writing about the way women justify cosmetic surgery, points out that women often defend themselves against the claim that they are caving in to cultural pressures by saying, "I'm doing it for me." "For me" means not for their husbands and boyfriends, not as a way to please others, not in response to media images of female beauty. "In these constructions," writes Bordo, " 'me' is imagined as a pure and precious inner space, an 'authentic' and personal reference point untouched by external values and demands. A place where we live free and won't be pushed around." Thus, when a woman has a breast augmentation procedure, it is not because of the culture around her, not because others will see her as sexier, but because she herself prefers large breasts. Having larger breasts is liberating, because they give her confidence, comfort in her own body, and a sense of self-control.[27]

This particular sales pitch—buying as liberation, as self-expression, as a search for the authentic self—has been a remarkably effective one. Americans are deeply attracted to the image of the individual throwing off the oppressive limitations imposed by others, whether they be the government, the establishment, the patriarchy, the church, the rigid dictates of social class, or majority tastes. The irony of this particular sales pitch is that it uses deeply held cultural values in order to sell the idea of the individual transcending his or her culture. This is part of what Laurie Zoloth is getting at when she writes, "It is as likely that an American teenager will want to be free to do his own thing as it was that a serf would do the work of his lord."[28] It is the fact that we place such importance on values such as liberty, self-expression, and authenticity that they make such effective advertisements.

When Norman Mailer, in his 1957 manifesto "The White Negro," called upon alienated white Americans to emulate the ways and styles of black society as a mode of resistance to the conformist, work-ethic, delayed-gratification American mainstream, his call was taken up not only by the disaffected counterculture; it was also taken up by the advertising industry. Dodge, the car manufacturer, invited consumers to "Join the Dodge rebellion." Virginia Slims cigarettes told women smokers, "You've come a long way, baby," reminding them of the days when smoking by women was frowned upon. An ad for Pond's skin cream, linking women's liberation to cosmetics, featured a young woman doing mechanical work on a motorcycle, with copy that read: "You need another pale, white, virtuous hand lotion like you need another apron."[29]

As the ad agencies of the '60s realized, an advertisement can use virtually any idea to sell consumer products. It can use liberation. It can use rebellion. It can even use the idea that consumer culture is a sham. It was in the 1960s that advertisers hit on the remarkable strategy of selling consumer products by portraying consumption as an act of rebellion against consumer society. Ads became irreverent and self-mocking, poking fun at advertising itself. A magazine ad for Fisher advised readers, "How to ignore the ad man when you buy a stereo."[30] The message of 1960s advertising, writes historian Thomas Frank, was this: "Consumer culture is a gigantic fraud. It demands that you act like everyone else, that you restrain yourself, that you fit in with the crowd, when you are in fact an individual. Consumer culture lies and seeks to sell you shoddy products that will fall apart or be out of style in a few years; but you crave authenticity and are too smart to fall for that Madison Avenue stuff (your neighbors may not be)."[31] This is why you should buy our consumer products and not those of our competitors. You can buy what we are selling without selling out.

Ads like these play on a perceived gap between the self and the choices that help constitute the self. Once this gap is set into place, as sociologist Daniel Bell pointed out twenty years ago, you can simultaneously rebel in your liberated personal lifestyle while holding a comfortable job within the very system you are rebelling against. You can express your contempt with consumer culture by buying only products that are advertised with mocking disdain for consumer culture. You can demonstrate your independence from the sexist ideals of beauty purveyed by consumer culture by listening to that inner voice: "Don't get bigger breasts to please other people. Do it for yourself." Your consumer choices, unlike those of other people, liberate you from the consumer culture you profess to scorn. You are an anticonsumerist consumer.

It sounds deeply contradictory, even incoherent. Yet the idea that consumer items can liberate us from consumer culture is not limited to advertisers. Take, for example, this narrative by sociologist Grant McCracken: "There was a time when this self-invention was impossible. We were defined by others. Religion, the community, work, in-laws, husbands, children, our ethnic group, our neighbors were all happy to tell us who we were and what to do." Today, however, this has all changed. Now we are free to define who we are. "We all live lives now of active transformation," writes McCracken. "This is one of the great accomplishments of our cultural tradition and one of the great joys of our personal lives. Increasingly, transformation has become the single constant of our lives. . . . We can go from being a person who cares passionately about her social life to someone who wants nothing more than a solitary walk in the country, spaniel in tow. From someone who never misses the *Sunday Times* to someone who hardly ever reads the local paper. From someone defined by her children to someone defined by her work. From someone who lives to be married to someone who loves to be single again."[32]

Reading this enthusiastic description, you might be forgiven for assuming that McCracken was discussing the French Revolution rather than hair styling. But hair is McCracken's subject, or more precisely, the way that the hairstyles of white North American women have changed since the 1950s. McCracken's book, *Big Hair*, carries the subtitle *A Journey into the Transformation of Self*, which is a pretty good description of how McCracken sees hair. According to McCracken, women once had to tolerate rigid, oppressive hairstyles—in his memorable phrase, "preposterous bits of rococo shrubbery." In the '50s, women had to roll their hair into curlers at night, perm it, set it, even lacquer it into place with spray that made the hair seem like a synthetic substance. But with the 1960s came the great liberator, Vidal Sassoon. Sassoon made the haircut into a means of individualistic self-transformation by doing a Bauhaus, "form follows function" job on hair. After Sassoon, hair was no longer a mere ornament for the head. It became a natural part of the head itself. The work of other hair stylists needed constant maintenance. But Sassoon made women shake their hair back and forth when they got out of the salon chair. The hair was always supposed to fall naturally back into place.

The idea that a new hairstyle may be liberating is not completely absurd, of course, especially if the old hairstyle meant forcing your hair into complex positions that it resisted with equal or greater force. What is absurd is the idea that a new hairstyle can liberate you from cultural constraints. Simply because the new fashion is easier to manage than the old one does not mean that you have been liberated from the dictates of fashion. It means that fashion has changed, for better or for worse, and now you serve a new master.

Like the advertisers of the 1960s, McCracken portrays hairstyle as a way to escape being defined by other people. But changing your hair is not an escape. It is merely a transfer to another prison. Of course you can change your hair color from brown to blonde. You can even style and color it to code for one of the various cultural taxonomies of blondeness described by McCracken in a level of detail that would impress even the most obsessive Germanic mind: the sunny blonde, the bombshell blonde, the dangerous blonde, *und so weiter*. But the codes available to you are dependent on the broader culture in which you live. You can't just decide these things for yourself. You can't simply decide, for example, that Maggie Thatcher–style helmet hair codes for come-hither feminine seductiveness. The code is determined by the culture in which you are situated. The escapes from culture being sold by hair stylists and ad agencies do not leave you any less dependent on your culture, because your identity has to be negotiated with the culture. You depend on culturally agreed-upon signals for the messages you send.

The logic of consumer culture insists that you are making your own identity when you choose what to buy—your clothes, your hair, your pills, your cosmetic surgery. But identity is not merely something that anyone can simply decide upon and create, even at the outer level of hair and clothing. It is dependent on the recognition of oth-

BETTER THAN WELL ■ 117

ers. If my skin is dark and I want to pass as white, my success or failure depends on the way that the outer presentation of my identity is
read by others. The matter is not simply up to me. It depends on you
as well. And if my identity is somehow in question, how you read the
signals I send out will take on even greater significance. If I, a ninety-
pound weakling, have decided to recreate myself as a bodybuilder, it
is important to me that you recognize me as a bodybuilder. If I am an
Anglo-Canadian, living in the shadow of what Canadians wryly call
their "great neighbor to the south," it is important to me that you not
mistake me for an American. In the same way that Scots resent being
mistaken for English, Flemish for Dutch, New Zealanders for Australian, so a man who has undergone sex-reassignment surgery to
become a woman may well resent being taken for a man. When you
send out these signals, not only do you expect them to be received,
you hope against hope they are also interpreted correctly.

The meaning of these cultural signals is constantly changing, often
in ways that can be difficult for outsiders to comprehend. At the
beginning of the century, for example, suntanned skin was a mark of
a working-class background. It signified outdoor manual labor. In the
1920s, with the growth of the consumption ethic, the meaning of a
tan began to change. Tanning became associated with the leisure
class, the moneyed people whose wealth had managed to survive the
Depression. A tan signified weekends on the yacht, summers on the
Riviera. Just as Veblen would have predicted, the middle class began
to cultivate tans. The cosmetics industry began marketing tanning
lotions and artificial tanning agents. By the 1970s, the middle classes
were spending weekends oiled up in the yard or baking themselves at
the tanning parlor.

Yet the meaning of the tan continued to change. In the 1990s the
moneyed classes, newly obsessed with their health, began to stay
away from the sun for fear of skin cancer. A dark tan, like a bulging
belly, began to signify a lack of self-control. Leisure itself began to go
out of fashion. High status became associated with busyness. The
rich and powerful had no time for weekends on the yacht; they were
too busy running the world and talking on their cell phones. Once
again, Veblen would be proud of the marketing niche these changes
created: these days, in 2002, a natural tan is out, but sales of new,

artificial tanning lotions are up 40 percent over last year. Their cachet is precisely the fact that they are artificial. *New York Times* fashion reporter Gina Bellafante quotes a tanned friend: "I feel compelled to tell people it's from the bottle. I don't want anyone to think I had the time to go to the beach."[33]

A few years ago I was driving down a street in Minneapolis with my son Crawford, who was perhaps four years old at the time, and we saw a woman working in her garden wearing pajamas and a bathrobe. Crawford laughed hard when I pointed the woman out to him, being at an age when breaking the rules is one of the funniest things a person can do (coming in the house through the window rather than the door, wearing underpants on your head); but what struck me at the time was how his finding this woman funny depended on cultural knowledge that he had only recently acquired. A year earlier he would not even have known that a person is not supposed to wear pajamas and a bathrobe outdoors. Yet at four, he was conscious that wearing clothes was a rule-governed activity. He knew that a bathrobe is fine inside the house, but not outside; that it is okay to wear it in the morning and in the evening, but not in the afternoon; that you can wear it at the breakfast table with your family, but not when you have guests, and so on. You do not wear pajamas in the yard. "Why is she gardening in her pajamas?" he wanted to know. The answer "Because it is a warm spring day" would not do. He really wanted to know why she was breaking the rules— whether it was willful rule-breaking or simply ignorance. Was she aware of the signals her pajamas were sending out, even to four-year-olds? If so, did she care? Was she breaking free of convention, or simply oblivious to what convention prescribes?

If items of consumption give you liberation, then this liberation has a paradox in it. There is a sense in which you are even more dependent on the culture around you in an age of consumerist self-transformation (so-called) than you might have been in earlier times. In an age where you are defined by items of consumption—where it is *expected* that your clothes and hair and such are sending out messages about who you are—you cannot escape from the iron cage of style. You can't simply be indifferent any more. Your very indifference sends out a message: I don't care about style; I'm above that sort of thing. I will wear my pajamas in the yard. This may be the message you want to send, of course, but then again it may not be. You may not be trying to send out any message at all. You may, like me, fail even to realize that hair and clothes send messages until you begin to read academic books by fashion experts and scholars in cultural studies. Still, your very indifference sends messages to the people around you who read such things. And because your messages are read this way, whether or not you want them to be read, it takes a monumental degree of cultural insulation to escape the uncomfortable sense of self-awareness that comes with knowing how your messages are being read. As Andrew Sullivan puts it, "Even the hermit is posturing somewhere."[34]

CONSUMER CAPITALISM WORKS, at least in part, by presenting consumers with a vision of the good life. This vision of the good life suggests the ways in which a consumer's own life does not measure up, and which could be remedied by the consumer product. You could be hipper, sexier, not just liked but well-liked, if only you would buy what we are selling. To the extent that enhancement technologies have found their way into mainstream advertising, this approach has suited them quite well. Prozac will transform your gray skies into blue. Rogaine will transform your balding future into a perennially youthful one. Viagra will give you back your sexual vigor. Of the fifty drugs most heavily promoted in 1999 through direct-to-consumer advertising, thirteen were drugs that can be used for enhancement purposes: drugs for obesity (Xenical and Meridia), baldness (Propecia), wrinkle control (Renova), acne (Differin), sexual function (Viagra), contraception (Ortho tri-cyclen and Depo-Provera), social anxiety (Paxil), and menopause (Prempro, Combi-Patch, Premarin, and Cenestin). The most heavily promoted enhancement drug in 1999 was Roche's obesity drug, Xenical, which ranked at number 3 overall with $76.2 million in promotional expenditures.[35] Roche promotes Xenical on the Web with photographs of a chunky, unhappy woman and the slogan, "Inside every block of stone there is a statue."[36]

Direct-to-consumer drug advertising has grown tremendously in recent years, but it still accounts for only a very small part of pharmaceutical promotions. Most industry marketing is still aimed at doctors, who hold the keys to the pharmaceutical kingdom. Marketing to doctors takes many forms: promotional gifts, advertisements in medical journals, and so-called "seeding trials" of new drugs, among other things. The industry monitors the prescribing patterns of individual doctors with the aid of information sold by pharmacies, the federal government, and the American Medical Association. (The AMA generates $20 million in annual income by selling biographies of American doctors.)[37] The industry's most important marketing strategy is "detailing" by drug representatives. Drug representatives—or "detail men," as they used to be called—are industry salespeople who make personal visits to doctors, often with gifts and drug samples. An army of 83,000 drug representatives pitched their products directly to doctors in 1999, dispensing nearly $8 billion worth of free drug samples.[38]

Of course, there is a conceptual barrier to marketing enhancement technologies to doctors. Doctors treat "patients," not "consumers." As much as American medicine has changed in recent decades, most doctors still feel as if they are in the business of curing human illnesses rather than making people feel better about themselves. Thus, if the industry wants to sell an enhancement technology to a doctor (rather than a consumer) the technology must be transformed into a treatment. Doctors must be convinced that the problem addressed by the technology is a medical disorder. Paxil must treat social phobia rather than relieve shyness. Ritalin must treat attention-deficit disorder rather than improve concentration. Synthetic growth hormone must treat growth hormone deficiency rather than make short boys taller. The technology in question must treat a proper illness, or else there is no reason why doctors should feel obliged to provide it.

Cosmetic surgery was successfully transformed from enhancement to treatment during the early part of the twentieth century. When plastic surgery was in its infancy, mainstream surgeons were deeply suspicious of surgery performed solely to make people more beautiful. Surgeons denounced it in print. They made ethical distinctions between surgery to improve health and surgery that was purely decorative. They warned women about so-called "beauty doctors," who were widely seen as charlatans and quacks. Yet by century's end, cosmetic surgery had become a multibillion-dollar industry. It had its own professional societies, like other medical specialties. Many mainstream plastic surgeons were performing cosmetic procedures themselves.

How did this shift come about? A key turning point, writes Elizabeth Haiken in her wonderful history of cosmetic surgery, *Venus Envy*, was the notion of the "inferiority complex." The inferiority complex was a theoretical construct initially developed by psychologist Alfred Adler, who argued that a person could develop a sense of personal inferiority because of his or her physical deficiencies. As a result, these people would not have the confidence necessary to present themselves to others in a way that would ensure social and economic success. A poor appearance led to a sense of inferiority, which in turn reinforced the person's poor appearance, which in turn led to an even greater sense of inferiority.[39]

The inferiority complex provided the perfect justification for cosmetic surgery. No longer was cosmetic surgery a procedure for mere "beauty doctors." No longer was the surgery merely cosmetic. Now that it could fix self-perceived physical deficiencies, cosmetic surgery became a medical treatment. A nose job was not just a nose job anymore; it was a way of treating an inferiority complex. As Haiken puts it, cosmetic surgery became "psychiatry with a scalpel."

As odd as it might sound today, this kind of justification for cosmetic surgery was neither ad hoc nor cynical. The concept of the inferiority complex took hold in a world where the notion of self-presentation was seen as critically important. The idea that your face could really make a difference in your fate did not seem at all farfetched. America at the beginning of the century was becoming mobile, urban, and competitive.[40] This was the era that invented "the parable of the first impression," which taught the importance of physical beauty and self-presentation in job interviews. Surgeons often used the term "deformity" in medical journals to refer to prominent ears, receding chins, double chins, wrinkles around the eyes, moles on the face, and hook noses.[41] By the late '30s, the term "deformity" had come to connote any kind of physical attribute that might give rise to feelings of inferiority.

Nor was the inferiority complex mere academic jargon. It was enthusiastically taken up by the popular culture of the day. Vogue's *Book of Beauty* exhorted women to embrace new beauty products, pointing out that a woman who does not update her looks "destroys those potential personalities that psychologists tell us are lurking behind our ordinary selves."[42] Cosmetics industry spokesman Everett McDonough said that "many a neurotic case has been cured with the deft application of a lipstick."[43] In a 1939 ad for Ingram's Milkweed Cream, beauty expert France Ingram addressed a reader who had been passed over for a promotion in a Detroit department store. Ingram told her: "I believe that the dullness of your complexion may have reacted on your subconscious in such a way that your confidence in yourself has become impaired."[44] By the 1930s and 40s, writes Haiken, the notion of the inferiority complex had so pervaded American culture that *Collier's Magazine* could run a piece with the title "How's your I.C.?" assuming that readers would know what the initials meant.

In fact, the idea of using cosmetic interventions to cure psychiatric problems was taken so seriously that prison systems in California, New York, and Illinois sponsored studies where prisoners were given cosmetic surgery as a way to rehabilitate them. "The thrill of reform through face-lifting," wrote the *New York Times*, commenting on a 1927 pilot project at San Quentin in which a fifty-year-old inmate underwent a nose job, a cauliflower ear repair, and a face-lift. In New York, surgeons operated on 110 criminals selected from reform schools and prisons. The state of Illinois sponsored a similar study, which was reported in the *Journal of the International College of Surgeons* to have yielded "excellent psychologic and sociologic results."[45]

Today nobody uses the term "inferiority complex," but the idea behind it has become so widely accepted that it is now common sense. Common sense tells us that a poor self-presentation can make a person anxious, sad, self-conscious, or socially inhibited. Common sense also tells us that being anxious, sad, self-conscious, or socially inhibited makes for a poor self-presentation. Thus, a drug for your self-presentation will improve your mental state, and a drug for your mental state will improve your self-presentation. Xenical helps you lose weight and makes you more self-confident and less inhibited.

Paxil relieves your social anxiety and improves your self-presentation. The health of the self and the presentation of the self are so mutually dependent that to treat one is also to treat the other.

The pharmaceutical industry has learned this lesson well. As psychiatrist and historian David Healy points out, the industry has learned that the key to selling psychiatric drugs is to sell the illnesses they treat. Antidepressants are a case in point. Before the 1960s, clinical depression was thought to be an extremely rare problem. Drug companies stayed away from depression because there was no money to be made in antidepressants. Depression, they thought, was too uncommon. So when Merck started to produce amytriptaline, a tricyclic antidepressant, in the early 1960s, it realized that in order to sell the antidepressant it needed to sell depression. Consequently Merck bought and distributed 50,000 copies of *Recognizing the Depressed Patient*, a book by Frank Ayd that instructed general practitioners how to diagnose depression. The strategy worked. Prescriptions for amytriptaline took off, and amytriptaline was not even the first antidepressant on the market. Imipramine, another tricyclic, had been available since the mid-1950s.[46]

Forty years later, of course, it is now clear to everyone that the market for antidepressants was not a shallow one at all; that it was, in fact, a tremendously lucrative market, as the remarkable success of Prozac and its sister drugs have demonstrated. The notion of "clinical depression" has expanded tremendously to include many people who might once have been called melancholy, anxious, or alienated. Antidepressants no longer lie within the exclusive domain of psychiatry: as much as 70 percent of serotonin reuptake inhibitors are now prescribed by primary-care physicians.[47] Clinicians today use antidepressants to treat not just clinical depression but also panic disorder, social anxiety disorder, paraphilias, sexual compulsions, premenstrual dysphoric disorder, and obsessive-compulsive disorder. Like depression, obsessive-compulsive disorder (OCD) was once thought to be extremely rare. In the mid-1980s came the development of clomipramine, or Anafranil, which proved an effective treatment for OCD. Soon after clomipramine came Prozac and its sister drugs, many of which also proved effective. Today, epidemiological studies say that up to 3 percent of all people may have obsessive-compulsive disorder.[48] What has happened? At least part of what has happened is the marketing of a disease.

This does not mean that drug companies are simply making up diseases out of thin air, or that psychiatrists are being gulled into diagnosing well people as sick. No one doubts that some people genuinely suffer from, say, depression, or attention-deficit/hyperactivity disorder, or that the right medications make these disorders better. But surrounding the core of many of these disorders is a wide zone of ambiguity that can be chiseled out and expanded. Pharmaceutical companies have a powerful financial interest in expanding categories of mental disease, because it is only when a certain condition is recognized as a disease that it can be treated with the products that the companies produce. The bigger the diagnostic category, the more patients who will fit within its boundaries, and the more psychoactive drugs they will be prescribed.

Panic disorder, for example, was not even listed as a distinct psychiatric disorder in the second revision of the American Psychiatric Association's *Diagnostic and Statistical Manual of Mental Disorders* (*DSM-III*). Until the 1960s, psychiatrists generally conceptualized panic as part of anxiety. In 1964, however, Donald Klein published an article (partially funded by Geigy and Smith Kline) suggesting that panic was distinct from anxiety, and that it could be prevented with anxiolytic medication. When the APA began to develop the next version of the *Diagnostic Manual* in the 1970s, Klein was part of the task force appointed to revise it. He persuaded other members of the task force that his views on panic were correct. When the *DSM-III* was published in 1980, it included "panic disorder" as a distinct diagnosis, separate from anxiety, characterized by sweating, faintness, and the "sudden onset of intense apprehension." The Upjohn Company soon began repositioning its new anxiolytic medication, Xanax (alprazolam), as a treatment for panic disorder. Upjohn funded extensive clinical trials to demonstrate that panic disorder was an illness distinct from anxiety.[49] By 1998, panic disorder had become so widely diagnosed that the National Institutes of Mental Health was reporting that it affected 2.4 million adults between the ages of 17 and 54—1.7 percent of that age group.[50]

The genius of much of today's pharmaceutical marketing is that it does not look like marketing at all. Very often it looks like science. Take, for example, a recent supplement issue of the *Journal of Clinical Psychiatry* devoted to the topic of social phobia.[51] Published in that supplement are scientific papers by some of the foremost researchers in the field. Yet if you look at the front cover, you will see that the sponsor of that special issue was SmithKline Beecham (now GlaxoSmithKline), which, as it happens, makes Paxil, or paroxetine—to date, the only drug approved for the treatment of social phobia. Is this a conflict of interest? It is hard to see how. SmithKline Beecham appears to have had no editorial control over the issue, and the papers look balanced and fair. No conscious effort to sell Paxil is evident. The point, however, is that SmithKline does not need to sell Paxil. What they need to sell is social phobia. If an article, a journal supplement, a conference session—or even better, a best-selling book—gets the word out about social phobia, then social phobia is going to be much more widely diagnosed, and the drug that treats it is going to be more widely prescribed.

When pharmaceutical marketing does not look like science, it often looks like grass-roots patient support. When the FDA approved Paxil for the treatment of social phobia in 1999, spokesmen for SmithKline Beecham announced that they would donate substantial sums of money to patient support groups in order to promote public education about the disorder. Yet while SmithKline may have genuinely wished to educate doctors and patients about social phobia, the fact remains that money spent promoting public awareness of social phobia is money that will be multiplied and returned to SmithKline. The more people who are aware of social phobia, the greater the number of prescriptions that will be written for Paxil. Other corporations fund similar projects. National Depression Awareness Day began in 1991 and is now a national media event. In October of each year, hospitals and universities around the country offer free depression screening. People are encouraged to dial twenty-four-hour 800-numbers and take an automated depression screening test. At the end of the test, a computer analyzes the score and tells the person the severity of his or her symptoms. Who pays for the press kits, the 800-numbers, and the depression screening kits? Eli Lilly, the manfacturer of Prozac.[52]

In his history of psychopharmacology, *The Antidepressant Era*, David Healy calls this kind of seeding "the Luke Effect."[53] Healy takes the name from the parable of the sower told in the Gospel according to Luke. When a sower sows his seed, according to the parable, some of the seed falls on stony ground and withers. Some falls on a path and is eaten by birds. Some falls on fertile ground but is choked by weeds. But some of the seed falls on fertile ground and yields a good crop. For Healy, this parable is instructive because it tells us that the reception an idea gets depends not just on the idea itself, or even where it comes from, but also on the readiness of people to hear it. Ideas, like seeds in fertile soil, will bring forth fruit only if the ground is properly prepared. Anyone who is in the business of planting ideas, like a pharmaceutical company, does well to make sure that the ground is ready; otherwise the ideas will simply wither away. Scientific journals, conference sessions, post-marketing clinical trials, even donations to patient support groups are ways of fertilizing the soil for ideas like social phobia, panic disorder, or obsessive-compulsive disorder.

Many people miss this point. In 1995, many observers were outraged by the news that Ciba-Geigy, the manufacturer of Ritalin, had donated $900,000 to Children and Adults with Attention-Deficit Disorder (CHADD). CHADD had not disclosed the donation from Ciba-Geigy to the public or even to most of its own membership. Moreover, CHADD was then petitioning the Drug Enforcement Agency to loosen its controls on Ritalin, a move that would have been clearly beneficial to Ciba. Outsiders were probably right to see the donation by Ciba-Geigy in a cynical light, and they are surely right to criticize CHADD's failure to disclose the donation. But the outrage over nondisclosure misses a more important point about the contribution. Even if the support group had not been lobbying for Ciba, the $900,000 would have been money well spent, because support groups like CHADD have helped make attention-deficit disorder part of the national vocabulary.[54] CHADD has helped sell ADD.

WHEN VEBLEN PUBLISHED *The Theory of the Leisure Class* in 1899, he could plausibly describe an American consumer as motivated by status and appearances. But today's landscape looks slightly different. As early as the 1950s David Riesman was contrasting the Veblenese consumer to the "other-directed" personality type that he saw emerging. The Veblenese consumer was concerned only with appearances, wrote Riesman; the Veblenese consumer wanted to dazzle others with display. But the new, other-directed consumer wants to be *guided* by others rather than simply to impress them. The other-directed consumer worries not that he will fail to impress other people, but that he is missing out on something that they have. The concern of the other-directed consumer is to make sure that the quality of his experience matches up to that of the people he admires and envies.[55] The object of his quest is not so much status as it is self-fulfillment. He is motivated by what historian Jackson Lears calls a "fretful preoccupation with secular well-being."[56]

Today, buying has come to be seen as a legitimate, even obvious way to achieve well-being. You aim at a certain lifestyle, which is available to a certain type of person, and you buy things in order to achieve that lifestyle and that identity. When I make a choice about what to buy, the advertisers tell me, I am making a choice about what sort of person I want to be: investment banker or environmental activist, golfer or skateboarder, countercultural dreamer or pillar of the community, Malcolm X or Booker T. When an advertiser markets cosmetics or hair coloring, plastic surgery or liposuction, that advertiser is showing the consumer how to live a certain way and how to be a certain kind of person. Advertising is no longer just a means of selling goods; it is also an instrument for the transmission of values.[57] Like television and the movies, advertising teaches us how to dress, how to furnish our homes, how to eat well, and how to be cool. It also tells us what kind of people deserve respect and which deserve ridicule, what romantic love looks like and how to find it, how to lead a successful life and how to be a failure. Many Americans today learn who they want to be not by listening to a Methodist minister or a civics teacher but by watching advertisements for The Gap.

In this world, you consume in order to change the quality of your inner experience. Consumption promises that a change in outer display will bring about a change in the life underneath. Enhancement technologies become tools on the quest for self-fulfillment by ensuring that the quality of my inner experience equals that of the people

I admire and envy. They assure me that my sex life is as good as yours, that my mental life is as stimulating as yours, that my looks will bring me rewards as satisfying as those that your looks bring you. I know this because the experts tell me so—experts specializing in the problems that enhancement technologies are meant to treat. What these experts tell me is that the technologies do not merely fulfill desires; they treat psychological problems as well. Weight loss and breast augmentation and wrinkle removal are not just matters of vanity, narcissism, or frivolous self-regard; they also concern my psychological well-being, the locus of my self-fulfillment. Enhancement technologies put me in touch with my true self. Authenticity can be packaged, commodified, and put to work for capitalism.

6

THREE WAYS TO
FEEL HOMESICK

Sometimes I live in the country,
sometimes I live in town;
Sometimes I have a great notion
to jump in the river and drown.

—Leadbelly

W e've finally decided to buy our first house, Ina and I, and
we have found an open-house showing at 2:00 on Saturday. It is a three-bedroom bungalow, with a thoroughly
modern kitchen, central air, finished basement, landscaped lawn. A
fine place to raise a family. It sounded like just the thing, and now
we're out in front of the house, sitting in the car with the kids, engine
idling, just looking it over, deciding whether to go in and have a look.
It looks fine, just fine, a sensible house for a sensible family. Like us.
No reason why we couldn't be happy here, I tell myself, as I start to
sweat.

Then a curious thing happens. Another car drives up across the
street. Another family emerges from the car: husband and wife in
their mid-thirties, t-shirted and tennis-shoed, a three-year-old in
hand, a one-year-old on her father's hip, clutching like a monkey at
his shirt. All of them are smiling. They look exactly like us. As I see
this family walk up the driveway toward the house I get one of those
pan-away moments, one of those times where the camera backs
slowly away from you and the frame gets wider and wider. And there

I see myself for what I am: an Average American on the verge of buying a lovely home with a perfect lawn and a thoroughly modern kitchen; a really cute place that is infected with everydayness and despair; a contemporary American wrist-slitter. I look at Ina. She looks at me. We each let out an involuntary groan.

Ina looks away, and like Steve McQueen in *The Getaway*, she says, "Punch it, baby, punch it!" So I punch it, and off we race, gas pedal to the floor, the children momentarily terrified. We look at one another again and discover that the everydayness is gone. It has been dispelled as suddenly as it arrived, sucked out the windows as we speed away. As we drive away I begin to grasp why Americans live on houseboats on the Mississippi or deconsecrated churches in Boston; why country folk move to the city and live in abandoned warehouses while city-dwellers move to the country and live in converted barns. Maybe after the quiet desperation of American exurbs and edge cities, the relentless hipness of urban apartment dwelling, the synthetic happiness of subdivisions and gated communities, there is nothing left to do but to hole up with the survivalists in Idaho, or to set up house in a deserted gas station, or like a philosophy professor I once met in Tennessee, to move your family into an abandoned elementary school in the woods.

MUCH OF THE credit for modern anxiolytic drugs belongs to a Czech physician named Frank Berger. "Most people get nervous and irritable for no good reason," Berger once remarked. "They flair up, do not differentiate between serious problems and inconsequential ones, and somehow manage to get excited needlessly." When Berger took up a post as assistant professor of pediatrics at the University of Rochester in the late 1940s, he began to consult for a drug firm to develop a treatment for this kind of nervousness. In 1955, Wallace Laboratories introduced meprobamate, the drug treatment that Berger had developed, under the trade name Miltown. By 1956, in any given month, Miltown was being taken by one American in twenty.

Miltown was the first psychiatric drug developed to treat the anxiety and depression of everyday life. Like Prozac thirty years later, Miltown was both enormously popular during its time and the object of widespread anxiety itself. Newspaper columnists worried about the search for well-being in a pill. Intellectuals wondered why so many people needed tranquilizers to tolerate ordinary life in the most prosperous country in the world. News magazines carried headlines reading "Happiness by Prescription" and "Peace of Mind Drugs." Despite all the public hand-wringing, however, the demand for Miltown far exceeded that of any drug ever marketed in the United States.[1]

In a way, Miltown represented an ironic twist on the legacy of Freud. When psychoanalytic theory began to make its way into psychiatry in the late nineteenth century, mainstream psychiatrists were concerned almost exclusively with psychotic illness. Psychiatrists spent their time with patients who were floridly delusional, hearing voices, out of touch with reality. Psychiatry was considered a largely biological science. But Freudian analysis shifted the center of gravity for psychiatric practice. Psychoanalysts treated patients with neuroses rather than psychoses—the worried well rather than inmates of the asylum. Increasingly, they saw middle-class patients in private clinics.[2] By the 1950s, with the postwar emigration of so many European psychiatrists to America, psychoanalysis was well on its way to becoming the dominant force in American psychiatry.

Miltown reversed this trend. With Miltown, biological psychiatrists captured the terrain of psychoanalysis and made it the object of biological intervention. Anxiolytic medication gave the biological psychiatrists a treatment for the worried well, the patient on the analyst's couch. Miltown was only the first in a long series of treatments for the anxiety and melancholy of everyday life, from Valium and Ativan to Prozac and Celexa.

In an odd way, the history of anxiolytic drugs like Miltown is also bound up with the history of American suburbia. Both had their heydays in the 1950s, and both have come to represent the peculiar brand of alienation that has accompanied American prosperity. During the Miltown era of the '50s, Jack Finney was writing *The Invasion of the Body Snatchers,* a book that used alien body-snatching as a metaphor for the soul-deadening effect of suburban life. In the 1970s, when Valium had become the most prescribed drug in America, Ira Levin published *The Stepford Wives,* in which scientific

manipulation produced beautiful, eerily mechanical women, techni-
cally perfect by the standards of a conformist suburbia and happily
resigned to their places in the kitchen and the bedroom. By the time
Prozac hit its stride and *American Beauty* was winning Academy
Awards, the suburb had become America's most reliable symbol of
existential alienation, likely to send shivers down the neck of any
middle-class American born after 1960. Cartoonists who satirized
Prozac in the early 1990s inevitably drew on the imagery of 1950s
American suburbia to symbolize the psychic state to which Prozac-
users were alleged to aspire, but which the cartoon reader was supposed to dread: manicured lawns, shiny cars, mom in an apron, dad
in a suit and hat. For better or worse, suburbia has come to stand for
something that can be survived only with minor tranquilizers.

This is probably not an accident. If it is true that suburban alienation has become a cliché, it is also true that every cliché contains a
sliver of truth. American cartoonists can use suburbia as a stand-in
for anomie precisely because they know that American readers will
get the joke. What is harder to put a finger on is the precise characteristic of suburbia alleged to produce the kind of depression and
anxiety that psychoactive medication is needed to cure. Loneliness?
Social conformity? A thoroughly modern kitchen? Whatever the
problem of suburbia is, it is related to the problem of feeling homeless at the very place where you should feel most at home. House,
kids, husband, job: what could be wrong with that? Everything, you
think, as your heart sinks. "Show me that Norman Rockwell picture
of the American family at Thanksgiving dinner," writes Walker Percy,
"and I'll show you the first faint outlines of the death's-head."[3]

Susan Sontag has written that most "serious thought in our time
struggles with the feeling of homelessness."[4] Homelessness is a
metaphor Sontag uses for good reason. It stands in for questions of
meaning—or maybe better, questions of meaninglessness. Why do I
feel homeless at the very place where I am supposed to be at home?
Why am I not as happy as the other Phi Delts, the other new mothers, the other eager-to-please go-getters at the office? We are apt to
ask these questions when we take a step backward out of our lives
and start looking at them in a moment of cool detachment; when we
get that flash of insight and see ourselves as others see us: a tubby,

middle-aged mother pushing a stroller through the mall, an anxious young man in a business suit riding a commuter train to nowhere, a distracted father sitting in the audience at the school play with a laptop on his knees. These are the times when we are apt to look up, blinking, and think: Good God, is this how it's going to be? Is this really what it's all about?

Homelessness can stand in for meaninglessness precisely because home, at least for late-modern Westerners, is where the meaning is. Existential questions like these would have looked very different, say, to a medieval Christian. A medieval Christian would have worried about his relationship to God, about the state of his soul. But we don't worry about these things anymore, not even Christians. What we worry about (even when we worry about God) is ordinary life— the life of home and work and family. Should I get married? What should I do for a living? Should I have children? Where should I live? It is no wonder that the home has become a symbol of such anxiety: home is where it all happens. The home is the locus of meaning for the late modern life. If you feel homeless at the very place where you are supposed to feel most at home, if you question the point of the very things that are supposed to give your life its point, it's no wonder you might start thinking about psychoactive medication. Nor is it any wonder that home is ground zero for three of the most perceptive critics of postwar American life: Richard Ford, Richard Yates, and Walker Percy.

FRANK BASCOMBE, THE narrator of Richard Ford's novel *Independence Day*, is an ex-fiction writer living in the "Presidents Streets" section of Haddam, New Jersey. He makes his living by selling real estate. His wife, Ann, has divorced him, married an architect named Charley O'Dell, and moved to Deep River, Connecticut with their kids. Frank lives in Ann's former house. The series of events that have led him to this point in his life are not exactly happy ones—a failed career, the death of a young son, adultery, exile, and divorce. But neither are they especially unusual for a middle-aged American. Not unless your point of comparison is a white paper about the "ideal American family" put out by some right wing think tank, as Frank puts it: "propaganda for a mode of life that no one could live without access to the very impulse-suppressing, nostalgia-provoking drugs they don't want you to have."[5] Frank is just getting by. He calls this time of his life the Existence Period.

A successful practice of the Existence Period, Frank writes, is to ignore things he doesn't like or that strike him as worrisome. They usually go away eventually. When he first came to Haddam, he had thought differently. At that time he had thought that since he had "paid handsome dues to the brotherhood of consolidated mistake-makers," everything ought to go perfectly for him. Having survived his mistakes and personal tragedies, he deserved to be happy, very happy, all the time. These days he has more or less given up on that. He has resigned himself to smaller expectations, not a life of high drama, not a life of passion and abandon, but a life of detached reflection and careful insulation. "A high-wire act of normalcy," as he calls it. More than anything, the Existence Period means a willingness to let life take him where it might, in the hope that worries and contingencies will vanish along the way. He does not count on good things waiting for him at the end of the line. "Where's the good mystery?" his girlfriend, Sally Caldwell, asks him. Frank replies, "The good mystery's how long anything can go on the way it is. That's good enough for me. The Existence Period par excellence." (Then he adds: "Sally and Ann are united in their distaste for this view.")[6]

Frank himself has some doubts now and then, lying on the bed at Sally's beach house, reading a paperback copy of *Democracy in America*. At one point in his life, he would have thought that this is the best feeling on God's earth, the very state that the word "life" was invented to describe: floating toward sleep in an air-conditioned house, awaiting the arrival of an eager and sympathetic woman. But now? Nothing. Not a thing, even though the stage is set and all the props are in place. Real life is gone. "Left only is some ether of its presence and a hungrified wonder about where it might be and will it ever come back. Nullity, in other words." He lies back and listens to the voices on the beach. He starts to muse on the Existence Period. "Possibly this is just one more version of 'disappearing into your life,' " the way career telephone company bigwigs, overdutiful parents and owners of wholesale lumber companies are said to do and never know it. You simply reach a point where everything looks the same but nothing matters much. There's no evidence you're dead, but you act that way."[7]

Yet there are times when the Existence Period and its tenets serve him very well: selling real estate, for example, which he sees as its ideal occupation, and to which he brings a meditative reverence. Frank realizes that selling real estate is not simply about selling people a house. It is about selling them a life. What he finds especially congenial about the real estate business is its blend of intimacy and detachment, of existential hope and the hard bare facts of a market economy. The one gnostic truth of real estate, says Frank, is that nobody gets the house they want. A market economy has nothing remotely to do with getting what you want. It has everything to do with making yourself feel good about what is available. There is absolutely nothing wrong with this, and the sooner you realize it the better off you will be.

Frank is patiently trying to find a house for Joe and Phyllis Markham, who are moving to Haddam from Vermont. Joe Markham is an ex-trigonometry teacher from Aliquippa who used to play nose guard for his high school football team, while Phyllis is a plump, frog-eyed ex-DC housewife. Back in the '60s, when both were married to other people, Joe and Phyllis had each decided to give up their old lives, pack it all up in a trailer, and give Vermont a try. And so they did: moved to Island Pond, Vermont, got mixed up with all the other flatlanders who had moved to Vermont for the same reasons, started taking classes, setting out on new degrees, trying out new partners and new lives. Eventually Joe and Phyllis split with their spouses and wound up with each other. Joe, working for the Department of Social Services and not obviously a creative type, found he had a knack for pottery; Phyllis, a gift for design and papermaking. Soon, to their surprise, they were winning prizes in craft shows and selling their wares to upscale department stores all over the country. They built a new house with cathedral ceilings and a hand-laid hearth, hidden at the back of an apple orchard. They started giving free studio classes to college students and eventually had a child together. But neither of them saw the "Vermont life" as their final destination, both having strong opinions about dropouts and social nonproducers. Joe says, "I didn't want to wake up one morning and

be a fifty-five-year-old asshole with a bandana and a goddamn earring and nothing to talk about but how Vermont's all fucked-up since
a lot of people just like me showed up."[8]

They say they are moving to Haddam for the schools. The Vermont schools didn't work out too well for their other kids (one married a Hell's Commando, another is serving time for armed robbery)
and so they want something better for Sonja. Haddam is also close
enough to New York for Joe's work, and so they're looking for something modest, a little three-bedroom place with hardwood floors and
crown moldings, a Cape or converted saltbox set back on a stream or
a cornfield. The problem is that those houses do not exist anymore,
at least not for the kind of money the Markhams are able to pay.
What they can pay will get them a builder-designed colonial in a
development with a name like Mallard's Landing. There are no
streams or cornfields in Mallard's Landing, just a fiberglass-bottomed
"pond." This brute fact has sunk them deep into brooding depression
(Phyllis) and righteous anger (Joe). After months of searching for
houses, of driving down from Vermont every weekend and seeing
their savings sucked away by motel bills, they are still no closer to
finding a house. Often they will not even get out of the car to look at
the houses Frank has set up appointments for them to see. They are
fighting with each other, snapping at Frank, sinking deeper and
deeper into a funk. Joe accuses Frank of showing them only places he
hasn't been able to unload on anyone else. "I don't want to live in
that particular shithole," Joe fumes, and on they drive to the next
house, in the rain.

The Markhams are stuck. They have given up on a life in Vermont,
sold their house, quit their day jobs, made the decision to move, and
now it is all coming undone because they can't decide on a house. A
new house is a new life, and the Markhams cannot bear the thought
of making a new life in a suburban housing development or a dank
two-bedroom place in the Haddam village. They can't even make
peace with the idea of the unknown, of taking a step that may have
unforeseen consequences. Every house they see has something wrong
with it: too small, too dark, bad plumbing, a shared driveway. They
have started to brood about all their past mistakes, the wrong turns
they have made, how things could have been otherwise. "As regret

goes, theirs, of course, is not unusual in kind," says Frank. "Though finally the worst thing about regret is that it makes you duck the chance of suffering new regret just as you get a glimmer that nothing's worth doing unless it has the potential to fuck up your whole life."[9]

Joe and Phyllis Markham have what Frank calls the "realty dreads," which are not about the fear of losing money, or even about house-buying itself, which could be one of life's most hopeful experiences. The realty dreads are about that "cold, unwelcome built-in-America realization that we're just like the other schmo, wishing his wishes, lusting his stunted lusts, quaking over his idiot frights and fantasies, all of us popped from the same unchinkable mold." The realty dreads are about facing up to the cold hard fact that our lives are no more extraordinary than those of anyone else, despite what we are told by the sitcoms and magazine ads and children's books. So when the deal's almost closed and the papers signed and the real estate agency is sending us generic housewarming gifts and notes of "congratulations," what we feel, as often as not, is panic. Good schools? Fire protection? A fine place to raise a family? It is enough to make anybody want to bolt. Because what we sense, as Frank says, is that "we're being tucked even deeper, more anonymously, into the weave of culture, and it's even less likely we'll make it to Kitzbuehel."[10]

WHAT FRANK BASCOMBE realizes (and the Markhams fear) is that an American house is no longer just a home. A house is an expression of who you are. It says something not just about the place where you have come from, your family roots, or even your social status; it is also an expression of your identity *as an individual*. The reason the Markhams can't stand the thought of moving into a suburban development is that they can't stand the thought of *themselves* as the kind of people who would live in a place with a fiberglass-bottom "pond." Suburban housing developments have become the most reliable symbol of this sort of existential dissonance, but by no means do they exhaust all its possibilities. Other people have a hard time imagining themselves as the kind of people who would live in a commune or a gated community or a small town in Indiana. And when they do decide to move to such a place, as the Markhams did when they decided to give the "Vermont experience" a shot, more often than not it is because they want to see themselves as different people. They want to change their lives, of course; that goes without saying. But a changed life means a changed person, and if a house is part of who you are, then it is crucial to the change you want to make. In fact, the change may well be little else.

Identity has become fused with lifestyle, with one of the most obvious parts of lifestyle being the place where it is lived: student flat, artist's loft, executive apartment, beachcomber's cottage, religious commune, gay quarter, retirement community. Not just the house itself, but how it is designed, where it sits, and how it is decorated. Today it is expected that you will be able to look at a dwelling and tell something important about the person who lives there: what sort of books are on the shelves, what is hanging on the walls, the furniture in its rooms, the neighborhood in which it is situated. This sociological current is related to what Robert Bellah and his *Habits of the Heart* coauthors call "expressive individualism." By expressive individualism, which they trace to the eighteenth- and nineteenth-century Romantics, they mean the idea that each person has a core of feeling and intuition unique to themselves, the expression of which is necessary for that person to realize his or her individuality.[11] It is also a key part of a consumption culture. Once a life is detached from a socially and historically rooted narrative, it becomes possible to *construct* an identity to an extent far greater than before. Identity is not who your parents are, where you grew up, what church you grew up in, not the narrative of a nation or a family, but something that you mold through your conscious choices. Where you live, whom you live with, what you do for a living, how you spend your free time, and what you buy with your discretionary income can be seen as expressions of individual identity.

The word "individual" is important here. Words like self-love, self-confidence, self-command, self-esteem, self-knowledge, and self-pity appeared in English or French only two or three hundred years ago.[12] The same goes for other words that describe the interior life, like conscience, disposition, character, ego, egoism, sensible, sentimental, melancholy, apathy, agitation, and embarrassment. It is no coincidence, suggests historian John Lukacs, that the interiors of homes also began to change during this same period. Before the seventeenth century, even the wealthiest and most aristocratic houses had no rooms for specific purposes. Furniture was portable and often collapsible, even beds. People ate, slept, danced, worked, and entertained visitors in the same rooms. "As the self-consciousness of medieval people was spare," writes Lukacs, "the interiors of their houses were bare, including the halls of nobles and of kings. The interior furniture of houses appeared together with the interior furniture of minds."[13] You can see something of this shift in paintings by Vermeer and Rembrandt, which mark a new attention to the interior life, both in their psychological complexity and their physical setting. This inward turn, the growing self-consciousness of a vocabulary describing the life of the mind, was mirrored in the way people lived. As Lionel Trilling put it, "It is when he becomes an individual that a man lives more and more in private rooms."[14]

But privacy is only one part of individualism, a part that has been with us for centuries. Expressive individualism is more recent. It is when a person becomes an "expressive individual" that he lives more and more in private rooms located in converted grain warehouses, dwellings perched over waterfalls, or houses whose walls are made entirely of glass. The antidote to life in an anonymous suburb is to live in a dwelling absolutely unique to yourself. This is the impulse that motivates clients of high-style architecture, and leads people to make houses out of old fire towers, cabooses, or missile silos. Who else lives in a converted missile silo? Nobody. Or at least that's what you hope; a subdivision of missile silos laid out in neat blocks will not have that same glow. What is important here is style, for which you are willing to trade comfort and convenience. The style in which you live marks you as different.[15]

Yet it is not all about being different. Here is where the appeal of the makeshift dwelling differs from that of high-style architecture. "Like Robinson Crusoe," architect Witold Rybczynski says, "the builder (of makeshift dwellings) makes do with whatever is at hand."[16] This analogy with Crusoe hits the mark square on, because the real appeal of makeshift dwellings is the way they can dispel the everydayness of day-to-day existence. Rybczynski thinks this has something to do with childhood memories, of turning a refrigerator carton into a bungalow or building a treehouse. I doubt it. The appeal is not just that of building something. Building a missile silo, then living in it, would strike most people as silly. But converting a silo into a house has a certain undeniable enchantment. It is the same sort of enchantment that, on a more humdrum scale, leads people to make lamps out of canary cages and coffee tables out of ventilator duct grills. Ordinary houses, like ordinary lamps, coffee tables, and cabooses, have been drained of life and rendered invisible.[17] Reshaping the things of ordinary life transforms them and thus makes them visible again. The walls of a former fire tower, a Baptist church, or a caboose quiver with a life not their own: not the ordinary dreary life of pot roast in the kitchen and Oprah on the tube, but an extraordinary life of fire-jumpers, shouted sermons, and life lived on the rails.

What worries Bellah and his colleagues about expressive individualism is not so much that Americans live in private rooms, or even that the rooms are located in missile silos or perched over waterfalls, but that they live in private rooms and never come out. The worry of expressive individualism is a worry about the loneliness and spiritual impoverishment that come when people make decisions solely to satisfy some vision of themselves. In *Habits of the Heart*, they describe the development of "lifestyle enclaves," such as retirement communities, at the expense of more traditional communities. The ties of lifestyle enclaves are the ties of expressive individualism. What links members of a lifestyle enclave to one another are not shared moral or civic visions, but aspects of private life, mainly leisure and consumption. Retirement communities, for example, are made up of people whose only shared characteristic is that they are older and do not work for a living anymore. Retired people often share some leisure interests, such as golf or bridge, but they do not share common religious convictions, an ethnic identity, or a political vision. They do not share a past—nor do they share any vision of a future together. (Nor, for that matter, do some suburbanites, who are often tied together only by a convenient commuting distance to work.) Lifestyle enclaves are groups whose boundaries are marked primarily by individual choice.

Perhaps this is the best we can do in a radically individualistic society, where meaning is increasingly found in private rather than public life. Maybe groups organized around lifestyle—like bridge clubs, retirement communities, self-help groups, or as Frank Bascombe describes in *Independence Day*, the Divorced Men's Club—are the contemporary equivalent of the "associations" Tocqueville thought were the counterpoint to America's individualism. "Religious, moral, futile, serious, very general and very limited, immensely large and very minute," is how Tocqueville describes them. "Americans of all ages, all stations in life, and all types of dispositions are forever forming associations."[18] The problem with lifestyle enclaves is the absence of any moral character or civic commitment to these associations, which a person joins only because he shares some aspect of private life with its members (devotion to wine tasting or needlepoint, the loss of a spouse, a fondness for jogging, or a substance abuse problem) and which, like the Divorced Men's Club, a person may even be expected to leave once he finds a new partner. Even marriage can become a lifestyle enclave if it is simply a means for encouraging individual self-development, with no moral character apart from the mutual fulfillment of its contractees.[19]

The language of therapy is as useful for describing this kind of fulfillment as it is for justifying enhancement technologies. The therapeutic worldview offers a moral vision of the good life, but it describes that life in a language that pretends to be free of moral judgment. The point of life is to achieve a lifestyle that works. A lifestyle that works is one that is financially affordable and psychologically tolerable. The locus of meaning is the self, not any higher commitments outside the self. Just as enhancement technologies ("lifestyle drugs") are often justified using the vocabulary of therapy—self-fulfillment, liberation from the expectations of others, promotion of psychic well-being—so are decisions about where and how to live. Both are decisions about a lifestyle. The "genius" of the vocabulary of therapy, write Bellah and his colleagues, is that "it enables the individual to think of commitments—from marriage to work to political and religious involvement—as enhancements of the sense of individual well-being rather than as moral imperatives."[20]

Therapeutic relationships are ideally suited to Frank Bascombe's Existence Period, particularly their peculiar combination of intimacy and distance. In therapy, one person talks; the other listens. One person explores her interior life; the other helps her do it. One person pays; the other is paid. The therapeutic relationship is designed to give people a safe space to examine themselves, a space for full and open communication, yet it is circumscribed by strict rules (no sex, no gifts, fixed time limits on sessions, etc.). It is not too different from Frank Bascombe's brand of real estate sales, which is why Frank sees real estate as the ideal occupation for the Existence Period. Standing in the presence of strangers, listening to the stories of their lives, selling them a house, then disappearing forever with the slam of a car door. AIt is one of the themes of the Existence Period that interest can mingle successfully with uninterest in this way, intimacy with transience, caring with the obdurate uncaring."[21]

And what about community? What about those involuntary ties, that civic spirit, that sense of past and future that is supposed to bind people to one another in towns like Haddam? This is Frank's problem, indeed the central problem of the Existence Period, not to mention the problem of expressive individualism: these ties seem to have disappeared. What used to be thought of as the involuntary ties of "community" have been replaced with the voluntary ties of expressive individualism. As Joel Garreau writes in his book *Edge Cities*, "If you don't like the ties that bind you to others—for even the most ephemeral or transitory or stupid reasons—you can and may leave."[22] The late Eudora Welty may have been the last person in America to live her entire life in the house where she was born. The idea of home may still tug at many of us, but so do the ideas of independence, convenience, and a better "lifestyle." Garreau writes, "Americans will leave behind houses that were the most emotion-filled places of their lives to move to a 'retirement community.' When asked why, they tell interviewers it was because they got tired of mowing the lawn."[23]

In THE OPENING pages of Richard Yates's 1961 novel *Revolutionary Road*, April Wheeler is performing the lead in the inaugural production of a new community theater group, The Laurel Players. The whole town has come to see the opening, including April's husband, Frank. The actors are all very nervous, but the director has assured them that things have finally come together. At the dress rehearsal the night before he told them, "Well, listen. Maybe this sounds corny, but something happened up here tonight. Sitting out there tonight I suddenly knew, deep down, that you were all putting your hearts into your work for the first time."[24] As it happens, the director is dead wrong. The performance that evening is a disaster. The leading man gets the flu and the director has to stand in for him. Old and balding, he is spectacularly ill-suited for the young man's part. He constantly flubs his lines. April, a former student of a leading New York drama school, is so thrown that her performance is even worse than the rest. She is absolutely humiliated. So is everyone else. The audience murmurs embarrassed congratulations to the actors as they file out of the theater.

As we are led to expect, life in *Revolutionary Road* follows art. The fakery and petty humiliations of this amateur stage production are nothing compared to the hypocrisies and betrayals of the Wheelers' suburban life. If Richard Ford's *Independence Day* is about contingency and the fragility of independence, *Revolutionary Road* is about fakery and the illusions of authenticity. It is as if Holden Caulfield has grown up, moved to the suburbs, and become one of the very people he called a phony back when he was fourteen.

Frank and April Wheeler are acting out a charade not just for the benefit of others, but also for the benefit of themselves. Frank works at a job meant for automaton, commuting to a corporation where all he has to do is turn up, wear a suit, and pretend he is doing something. April plays the part of loyal mother and wife. They live in the suburbs but pretend they are not real suburbanites, have sexual affairs while pretending they are in love, make fun of their shallow neighbors as if they are somehow different. Everyone in the novel is a fake, from the chirpy real estate dealer, who makes happy small talk about the weather while her schizophrenic son hurls abuse at everyone within hearing distance, to the husky he-man, Shep, genteelly pampered throughout his childhood and consequently determined to prove he is a man's man by studying mechanical engineering at State Tech instead of going to Princeton or Williams. The only person who is not self-deceived is the asylum inmate, John Givings, who, in a state of agitation, points out to the people around him the lies that they are living. We are given to believe that John Givings is the only one who has faced up to the truth, to the meaninglessness and hope-lessness of this upbeat American life, and the experience has driven him insane.

Like its spiritual cousin, *The Catcher in the Rye*, the tone of *Revolutionary Road* is suffused with a kind of knowing sarcasm. *Revolutionary Road* scorns every idea and institution it treats, from marriage to childbearing to work. It reserves its most bitter sneers for Frank and April's snobbishness about suburban life, their feeling that they are different, their idea that they are rebels. (Revolutionary Road is the name of the anonymous suburban street where they live.) Frank thinks of himself as a "decent but disillusioned young family man, sadly and bravely at war with his environment."[25] April pictures herself as "the girl who could have been The Actress if she hadn't got-ten married too young."[26] Both of them survive life in the suburbs by telling themselves that they are different, that they are special, that they, unlike all their neighbors, are aware of the absurdity of subur-ban life. They believe they are living suburban lives ironically, while their neighbors are living them out in earnest. Watching April and the rest of the Laurel Players humiliate themselves on stage, Frank tells himself with apparent sincerity that a failed play is not worth getting upset about. "Intelligent, thinking people could take things like this in their stride, just as they took the larger absurdities of deadly dull jobs in the city and deadly dull homes in the suburbs," Frank thinks. "The important thing, always, was to remember who you were."[27]

But "remembering who you are," in the world *of Revolutionary Road*, is the biggest charade of all. *Revolutionary Road* is not a great novel, and its themes were pretty worn even by the late '50s. But what puts it a notch above the stacks of novels and plays about suburban dysfunction published at midcentury is its willingness to suggest that even the search for authenticity is a charade. Most critiques of subur-ban conformity suggest that the problem of the suburban life is paying too much attention to the opinions of others. The remedy is to be true to yourself, because only then can you achieve self-fulfillment. But in *Revolutionary Road*, even being true to yourself is an exercise in pre-tence and self-deception. The only time Frank and April feel truly alive to themselves is when they start to plan their escape from suburbia. They will move to Paris and let Frank find himself, discover what he really wants to do with his life. He is a bright young man, a promising young man, as April tells him in the first flush of their romance, "the most interesting person I have ever met." Paris is April's idea. She thinks that Frank needs to discover who he really is, work at a job that is truly meaningful. "I don't care if you decide after five years that what you really want is to be a bricklayer or a mechanic or a merchant seaman," April tells him. "Don't you see what I'm saying? It's got nothing to do with definite, measurable talents—it's your very *essence* that's being stifled here. It's what you *are* that's being denied and denied and denied in this kind of life."[28]

Of course, the Wheelers' plan for self-fulfillment falls through. April suggests that it makes more sense for them to go to Paris rather than, say, Greece or Italy because, after all, in Paris Frank could speak the language. This gives Frank a shock. Had he really pretended to April that he could speak French? Again Frank has to bluff his way out of a charade, chuckling that after all this time he has probably forgotten most of his French anyway. The character he has been performing for her, the worldly disillusioned intellectual, speaks French and knows the streets of Paris. But in reality, most of what Frank knows about Paris geography he picked up from *The Sun Also Rises.*

While all the inhabitants of this sad suburb are performing their lives, Frank Wheeler is the actor whose performance goes deepest: he performs when no one else is around. April eventually realizes that her pose of being an aspiring actress was really just a pose. She even realizes that the life she and Frank have made for themselves, playing the role of sophisticated intellectuals temporarily exiled into suburbia, is really no more than complex role-playing. But Frank never gives up the pose. Even when he is railing against the fakery of suburban life he is faking. He pretends he is going to Paris when he really does not want to go. He has an affair with a secretary then tells himself it is a mark of his new self-confidence. He even talks April out of an abortion only to realize that he himself wants the child less than she does. Everything he does is calculated, everything is a show for others, when the real point is to serve his own narrow, narcissistic interests. His is the shallowness of performance all the way down.

In the hands of a pseudointellectual poser like Frank, discovering yourself and finding a true vocation are just poses to be used instrumentally, a means to make yourself look a certain way in the eyes of other people. For Yates, this mirrors the problem of American suburban life. It is not really American life in itself that is objectionable, or even suburban life in particular; what is alienating is the pretence that these things (or anything, for that matter) are something different from what they are. The America in *Revolutionary Road* is insufferable precisely because it is built on appearances, like the Emerald City in Baum's *The Wizard of Oz*, where everything glitters emerald green because you must wear green-tinted glasses to get in. The whole game of suburb-husband-wife-kids-train-job is a massive exercise in self-deception. You pretend to be working and raising a family; I pretend to believe you; we all pretend that the entire exercise is not really about money, status, and competition.

This is an old complaint about American life, of course, and one that has motivated some of the best and worst of American fiction. This fiction suggests that Americans profess to seek rewards that they are not actually seeking, and even if they were actually seeking them, those rewards are not as valuable as Americans often pretend. It is hardly an original observation, yet each generation of Americans apparently needs to hear it. In a country built on the idea that worldly success is within the grasp of every citizen, the novel of alienation provides a crucial social function. It tells the reader: Even if you fail in the world of kitchen-and-kids or cubicle-and-computer, don't worry. This kind of life isn't all it is cracked up to be anyway. If you fail, at least you are not doomed to work at a job you hate, acquire material objects you don't care about, and pretend to be happy when you are not. The world out there is not necessarily what it seems to be, and the point of living there is not as unquestionably valuable as many people think. You can opt out of it if you choose.[29]

THE DISCOVERY THAT you can opt out of a worldview can feel tremendously liberating, of course. This is part of the reason novels of alienation are so popular among adolescents and young adults. It is reassuring to discover that the rules that govern life in the adult world are not as iron-cast and inflexible as they initially appear. But this discovery can also be profoundly disorienting. With no bedrock of certainty about what counts as a successful life, any choice about how to live a life may come to seem arbitrary. No framework of meaning looks absolutely secure, because any framework is subject to challenge. The result is often uncertainty, or what Charles Taylor calls "vertigo"—a sense of imbalance, because not only don't you know what kind of life to live, you don't know what, if anything, can tell you.

A characteristic modern response to this sense of vertigo has been technological. Faced with a nagging sense of dissatisfaction about the way we are living our lives, we look to technology to fix that dissatisfaction, even when something very different may be called for. We like competitive sports, but we also want to win the competition, so we take a performance-enhancing drug that will assure us of victory. We want others to like and admire us, and this requires a beautiful body, so we take steroids or get cosmetic surgery. We want to feel happy in our work and satisfied in our homes, and if we do not feel what we think we should feel we look to Valium or Prozac. But we give up the joy of the game when we focus entirely on winning; we lose sight of the human relationships that matter when we focus entirely on the body; and we may fail to recognize the deeper source of our spiritual malaise when we focus entirely on brain states.

The problem-oriented thinking that leads us to embrace technological solutions is connected to what Taylor calls "instrumental rationality." By instrument rationality, Taylor has in mind the kind of reasoning that focuses solely on means rather than ends, and measures success by the most economical use of means to a given end. Instrumental rationality is quite familiar to medicine, of course, where critics have complained for a century that a mechanistic approach to illness is eliminating the kind of attention to the whole person required by humane medical practice. But it is also familiar to Frank Bascombe and Jack Wheeler, who struggle to see home, family, and friends as something more than mere instruments for achieving a fulfilling lifestyle.

Of course, it can be tremendously exciting to see the world as an instrument for the achievement of our interests. This is part of the promise of American life. If the world is not given but made, then it can also be remade to suit our plans and designs. But instrumental rationality also runs the risk of what Max Weber called "disenchantment." This is the sense that the world, by being bent to accommodate human designs, has been stripped of the very things that once gave it richness and meaning. The world no longer has value in itself, but rather has value only insofar as it serves human interests and needs.

People who complain that suburbs are convenient but soul-deadening are getting at this aspect of instrumental rationality. Rather than being places of engagement with the world, suburban houses often seem designed to satisfy certain human needs and desires: sleeping, eating, safety, entertainment. The house is located in a "bedroom community," the point of which is a convenient commute to work. It is as if suburban houses are designed to make their inhabitants more comfortable and their lives more efficient, and so various items are constantly being added, all for the point of increasing comfort and efficiency: central heat, electric garage-door opener, heated garage, dishwasher, garbage disposal, riding mower, leaf blower, cordless phone, and answering machine (not to mention the acronym accoutrements: TV, VCR, DVD, SUV). The appeal of such devices is obvious. This is why we buy them. But in the end they help transform the house, in Corbusier's famous phrase, into a "machine for living."

Technology has transformed the suburban house from a "thing," to use the philosopher Albert Borgmann's rather obscure terms, to a "device." In Borgmann's terminology, things are different from devices. A thing, whether it is a house, a stove, or a baseball, is inseparable from its context. And so our engagement with the thing is also an engagement with the thing's context. Our engagement with a basketball is an engagement with the game in which it is used: the rules, the rims, the style and swagger of the game, a blacktop court pounded by thousands of players in high-tops. But a device is the product of instrumental rationality. A device presupposes a distinction between the purpose of a given practice and the means of reaching that purpose.[30] With a device, only the purpose is important. To engage with a device is merely to engage with the purpose of the device, the end result. A basketball is a thing, but a home exercise machine is a device.

Things are often replaced by devices. Borgmann's favorite example of the transformation from thing to device is the way we have come to heat our houses. In former times, Americans used a hearth to heat their houses—a wood-burning stove or a fireplace. But a hearth provided more than just physical warmth. It was a central focus of the household. Life revolved around it, both work and leisure. The mother built the fire, the children were responsible for keeping the firebox filled, the father cut the firewood. The day started with the stove cold, and the rhythm of the day moved with it. But gradually this all changed. Fireplaces and stoves were replaced by the coal-fired central plant, and then by natural gas or oil, and then forced air heating, until gradually the "thing" (the fireplace or stove) was replaced by a "device" (central heating). Only the purpose, or end, of the hearth has been preserved, which is to heat the house in the most efficient way possible.

The result is a house designed like the one in South Carolina where I grew up. That house, built in the late '60s, has a big living room with easy chairs and sofas. At the center of the room is a brick fireplace. It is a very comfortable room, yet when my brothers and I go back there with our families, nobody really spends any time in the living room, unless they are reading alone or watching television. The room to which everyone seems drawn, as if by some invisible force, is the kitchen. We loiter in the kitchen even when there is no available space there. We sit on the counters, next to the stove, on the floor, drinking beer, playing with the kids. It is logical that life would revolve around the kitchen, where the cooking is done, but the house itself is designed as if life revolves around the hearth, the fireplace in the living room. The original purpose of the hearth, heating and cooking, has been replaced by more efficient means of heating and cooking, so all that remains for the hearth is a kind of ceremonial place in the house. A few years ago, in fact, my parents simply gave up, closed off the chimney, and replaced the fireplace with artificial logs and a gas burner.

In many ways, the story of technology in America is the story of this kind of transformation. We embrace fast food because it is an efficient means of satisfying hunger, then find that the life of the table has been replaced by plastic forks and anonymous service providers. We embrace the car because it is an efficient means of getting from one place to another, but in return we get a landscape of asphalt parking lots and strip malls. In the South, we have embraced air-conditioning because it makes the house so much more comfortable for six months of the year, but as a result we have lost the culture of the porch. Once a fabled place of meandering conversations, the Southern porch in the age of air-conditioning has been largely reduced to a functionless attachment where Christmas decorations can be hung.

Devices, almost by their very nature, are replaceable. Not because they are poorly built, but because the psychological appeal of a device wears out so quickly. A device is designed to accomplish its purpose with a minimum of skill and effort. If we see our house as a device designed to achieve comfort and entertainment in the most efficient way possible, it is predictable that we will find ourselves drawn to ever more elaborate means of achieving those ends—leaf-blowers, big-screen televisions, and automatic sprinklers. But devices often demand so little of us, so little engagement and so little skill. After the novelty wears off, the device naturally becomes boring, and it must be replaced by another device.

Devices also have more insidious psychological effects. Treating something as a device flattens it out. It reduces it to surfaces. When we think of a fireplace as a heating device rather than as a hearth, we lose the context that gives the thing its meaning, and think of it only in terms of its instrumental value. When we think of the wilderness as a device, we treat it as something to look at or admire, rather than to experience. Animals become meat production devices (this is part of the philosophical critique of factory farms), while women, in the eyes of men, become sexual devices (this is part of the philosophical critique of pornography). Part of what lies behind the force of these critiques is the idea that this transformation from thing to device takes place insidiously or even subconsciously, that these images or values or ways of interpretation come to us almost without our realizing it. We do not consciously intend to see a thing as a device, and often do not even realize when we have begun to see it that way. All we feel is a gap, what historian Jackson Lears calls a sense of "weightlessness," a vague sense of longing for what has been lost. Once we see our homes not as an end in themselves, but as a means to achieve self-fulfillment, then it is natural that any home will soon wear out, that we will always be looking for the next house, the one that has not been worn out yet, like Joe and Phyllis Markhams, leaving their "Vermont experience" behind in search of something else. We will long for something more authentic, closer to nature or God or our inner selves, a life that expresses our individuality or puts us in touch with our callings. Like Jack and April Wheeler, we may decide to move to Paris and write novels so that our true selves can emerge.

A FEW YEARS AGO I was one of several people teaching a one-week bioethics course to academics and health care workers. At the beginning of each day, the moderator asked us all to introduce ourselves and answer a single question, as a means of getting a discussion started. The question varied from day to day. One day the question was, "What did your parents do for a living?" The question drew some interesting answers. Many people were the children of doctors or teachers. Some were the children of domestic workers. One man was the son of an exterminator. But while just about everyone had a father who had worked at an identifiable job, many had mothers who had not worked outside the home. The answers these people gave were the most interesting of all. To a person, they said things like, "My mother raised six children and put all of them through college even though she had never been to college herself," or, "My mother was a full-time mom who nevertheless found time to be president of the Woman's Club, sing for thirty years in the church choir, and work as a volunteer for the Girl Scouts." It was not possible to say simply, "My mother kept house and raised the children," or, "My mother did not have a career." A curriculum vitae had to be invented. It was as if human life was being conceptualized as a project, and the only possible measure of success was accomplishment. The more items on the CV, the more successful the project.

The unstated pressure that led people to answer this way is related to what Charles Taylor calls the "affirmation of ordinary life."[31] By ordinary life, Taylor means the life of work and householding. The affirmation of ordinary life is one of the most powerful ideas of the modern age. Participation in the life of work and householding is what gives contemporary men and women their dignity. You command the respect or contempt of other people by virtue of your work, or by raising and providing for a family. When you succeed, you can count your life successful. But when you fail, you lose your dignity. The prospect of losing dignity is what leads a middle-aged man to continue to dress in a business suit, pack a briefcase, and pretend to commute to work for years after he has unexpectedly lost his job, solely to keep up appearances in the eyes of his wife and neighbors. It is also what leads middle-aged academics to feel the need to invent CVs for their mothers. What was sufficient to give an American woman's life dignity fifty years ago—raising children and managing the affairs of the home—is not sufficient to give it dignity today. A life of dignity requires a career. A life without one requires an apology, or at the very least, an explanation.

The affirmation of ordinary life, the moral importance of which we often take for granted, is in many ways a uniquely modern phenomenon. In Aristotle's Greece, for example, ordinary life is merely the background to what has significance, which is the life of contemplation and activity as a citizen. With the aristocratic European ethic, what is important is honor and glory. But with the Reformation, Taylor argues, we began to get a Christian-inspired sense that ordinary life *is* the good life. The critical issue became whether a person leads his or her life "worshipfully and in the fear of God." People were expected to live out a God-fearing life in their marriages and in their callings.[32] With this change came a certain social leveling. So-called higher lives of honor and glory, inaccessible to ordinary people, were knocked off their pedestal, and so were the elites who led these higher lives. There was no longer any great ship, as Taylor puts it; all people rowed their own boats.[33]

This transformed the meaning of work. The key figure in this transformation was Luther. For Luther, the way to please God was not to renounce the world for a life of monastic asceticism, but to immerse yourself in the worldly life and fulfill the duties that the world imposes on you. This was your calling. As Max Weber wrote in *The Protestant Ethic and the Spirit of Capitalism*, a calling "is an obligation which the individual is supposed to feel and does feel toward the content of his professional activity, no matter in what it consists."[34] The notion of a calling gave ordinary life a heightened moral significance. Ordinary life became crucially important to salvation. What struck Weber, for example, was not just that so many people worked hard to get more money, or that they worked for fame or glory, but that work had taken on this specifically *moral* character. Work had become a moral ideal. It had become morally important for Americans in particular, thought Weber, with Benjamin Franklin as a case in point. In Franklin's writings, to lose money or waste time is not just bad business or even foolishness; it is also a moral failing.

It is hard to listen to middle-class Americans talk about work today without hearing echoes of Franklin. Not just the way so many Americans apologize for taking time off from work, the way we pretend to be busy even when we are not, the frenzied, work-like nature of our vacations, but the way that we have begun to see a role in our work for psychopharmacology: beta-blockers or Paxil to take the edge off business presentations, Ritalin to improve our attention and concentration, Prozac to give us the confidence to apply for a promotion. For Americans, work is not merely a means of making money, but also a way to achieve dignity and fulfillment. To succeed at work is to succeed at life, and to fail at work is a sin.

When Luther wrote of work as a calling, he anticipated the crucial role that work would later come to play in the notion of self-fulfillment. For Luther, your calling came from God. For contemporary middle-class Americans, a calling comes from *within*. You discover your calling by looking inward to discover your own particular talents, values, and desires, and you fulfill your calling by following these things wherever they lead you. A meaningful life is a fulfilling life, and fulfillment is something to be found through the life of work and householding. Success at work, inside or outside the home, becomes a crucial element of self-fulfillment, and thus a crucial element of a meaningful life.

With an ethic of self-fulfillment, however, comes the sense that some lives are *un*fulfilling. This is part of what lay behind the early feminist critiques of keeping house and raising children (that this life is not as fulfilling as the life of work available to men), and it also lay behind the intellectual critiques of suburban American affluence that began to emerge in the 1950s and '60s. For many critics of suburbia, the problem of the suburbs was that many Americans were simply pretending at their lives, just going through the motions of work and householding. Suburbanites were slaves to the opinions of others. They were responding not to that still, small voice within them, but to the voices of their suburban neighbors. "[I]t's your very *essence* that's being stifled here," as April tells Frank in *Revolutionary Road*. "It's what you *are* that's being denied and denied and denied in this kind of life."

Yet once we take on the idea that a life can be less meaningful, even a failure, if it is not fulfilling, then we open another door for the use of psychoactive drugs. Work is not just as a means to make money, and taking care of children is no longer just an obligation to the children themselves. These activities must be fulfilling. They must be *enjoyed*. If you fail to enjoy them, your life is incomplete. You are missing out on something important that life has to offer. If a psychoactive drug can help you enjoy your work, enjoy keeping house, enjoy taking care of children, then it is not just an instrument for the relief of boredom. It is a way to achieve a meaningful life.

Dr. Tom More, the hero and narrator of Walker Percy's 1971 satire *Love in the Ruins*, is a resident of Paradise Estates. Paradise Estates is an exurb in Feliciana Parish, Louisiana, located between a golf course and a swamp. *Love in the Ruins* is set at some time in the unknown future, when the United States is on the verge of another civil war: left against right, white against black, believers against non-believers. Wolves prowl the streets of Cleveland. Vines sprout in New York City. Minnesota and Oregon have established consulates in Sweden, while some southern states have established diplomatic ties with Rhodesia. Dr. More himself is an alcoholic psychiatrist, a lapsed Catholic, and the inventor of the More Qualitative-Quantitative Ontological Lapsometer. The Ontological Lapsometer is an existential medical tool that promises to bridge the gap between body and mind. It is a "caliper of the human soul," as More puts it, an instrument with which he can diagnose and treat ailments of the spirit. Lapsometer in hand, More can take readings of a patient's "pineal selfhood" or "red nucleus activity" or "vagal rage," pinpointing the precise brain abnormalities that lead a person to become socially anxious, sexually repressed, or spiritually alienated.

Love in the Ruins was published fifteen years prior to the development of antidepressants like Prozac. Yet many of Tom More's patients share the same complaints as today's antidepressant users, and the Ontological Lapsometer works in much the same way. When More uses the language of neurochemistry to describe the spiritual ailments of the late modern age, he sounds very much like the biological psychiatrists who inhabit contemporary university medical centers. Where More speaks of pineal selfhood and red nucleus activity, biological psychiatrists speak of dopamine and serotonin transmission. Where More talks about measuring "perturbations of the soul" through electronic microcircuitry, biological psychiatrists talk about measuring depression and anxiety with standardized interviews and diagnostic instruments. Where More speaks of a pineal massage with the Ontological Lapsometer, psychiatrists speak of a six-week course of SSRIs. All of which work, at least on occasion. Put a shy, anxious woman on Paxil and she becomes outgoing and confident. Put a sexually obsessed man on Celexa and his obsessions disappear. Give More's alienated patients a pineal massage with the Lapsometer and soon they are back to work, healthy and happy and fulfilled.

With the Ontological Lapsometer, More can do more than simply treat his patients' anxiety, depression, or sexual inadequacy. He can give them a meaningful life. Like the psychiatrists who prescribed Miltown for anxious organization men in the '50s and Valium for bored suburban housewives in the '60s, Dr. More helps his patients *enjoy* playing bridge and shopping at the mall. He can help them take real pleasure in watching the Christian baton-twirlers of Valley Forge Academy. No longer must they face the death-in-life of Paradise Estates. No longer must old people simply endure endless days of shuffleboard and Papa Putt-Putt at the Senior Centers to which they have been exiled. Their alienation can be treated. When the ex-golf pro Charley Parker takes to wearing high-stomached shorts, looking at himself in the mirror and saying, "Charley, who the hell are you? What the hell does it all mean?" More can give him a pineal massage with the Lapsometer and his life has meaning again.

The Ontological Lapsometer sounds a lot like Prozac, and it sounds even more like some of the mechanical interventions currently being investigated for the treatment of depression, such as transcranial magnetic stimulation and deep-brain stimulation.[35] If such interventions sound like parodies of the scientific worldview—a worldview so powerful that it can even encompass spiritual alienation—this is exactly Percy's point. Percy is poking fun at a view that treats human beings as biological organisms whose well-being depends solely on the satisfaction of biological and psychological needs. This is the joke behind the pretensions of the Lapsometer, which reduces spiritual ailments to ailments of the brain, and it is also the joke behind the Love Clinic, where sex researchers monitor dials and screens at the vaginal console while Lonesome Lil, their star subject, masturbates herself to orgasm. For Percy, it is absurd to see human beings solely as objects of scientific study, absurd to buy into a scientific worldview that sees sex, death, and even prayer as "behavioral responses." The scientific worldview says that a human being will flourish if she can satisfy her various needs. But Percy is struck by the fact that a person can satisfy all her needs and still find her life unbearable. "One has only to let the mental health savants set forth their own ideal of sane living," writes Percy, "the composite reader who reads their books seriously and devotes every ounce of his strength to the pursuit of the goals erected: emotional maturity, inclusiveness, productivity, creativity, belongingness—there will emerge, far more faithfully than I could portray him, the candidate for suicide."[36]

When the psychiatrist looks at the unhappy man or woman in the suburbs, she sees someone in need of treatment. She sees a shy, introverted, socially anxious woman who could function better on Paxil; an underachieving, inattentive, socially anxious teenager who could function better on Ritalin; a sorrowful, melancholy, socially anxious man who could function better on Prozac. And she might well be right. If you see your job as helping people to *function* better—not as making them dumb and happy, as the critics of psychiatry often unfairly suggest, but helping them to do their jobs and keep their friends and make their cautious, troubled way through the hazard zones of ordinary life—then you will quite reasonably see psychoactive medication as a useful tool in your black bag.

But when Percy looks at the unhappy man or woman in the suburbs, he sees something very different. He does not see a patient with
a problem, but a person in a predicament. And part of that predicament is that the person has come to see herself in just the same way
that the psychiatrist sees her: as a person in need of treatment. She
has come to see herself as an organism whose well-being can be measured in terms of her mental health, her sexual happiness, the state of
her body, the way she "functions" at work and at home. She has
stepped onto the bathroom scale of psychological well-being and is
horrified by what she sees. But her real predicament, at least in Percy's
view, the predicament that she may not even realize she is in, is
something far deeper and more profound. It is not a medical problem, but an existential problem. It is not the predicament of an
organism in an environment, but that of a wayfarer who has lost her
way.

Percy asks, "Given two men living in Short Hills, New Jersey, each
having satisfied his needs, working at rewarding jobs, participating in
meaningful relationships with other people, etc., etc.: one feels good,
the other feels bad; one feels at home, the other homeless. Which one
is sick? Which one is better off?"[37] For the psychiatrist measuring
depression with a standardized diagnostic instrument, there can be
no question which man is better off. It is better to feel good than to
feel bad, better to feel at home than to feel homeless. It is reasonable
for the man who feels bad and feels homeless to want a medication
that will make him feel better and at home. "Isn't it better to feel
good than bad?" Art Immelman asks Tom More in Love in the
Ruins. "Isn't the purpose of life in a democratic society to develop
your potential to the fullest?" For Percy, however, the answer is not
so clear. Sometimes it is not unequivocally better to feel bad than to
feel good. Some situations call for depression or alienation or anxiety. Some things call for fear and trembling.

Percy is not challenging the effectiveness of psychoactive drugs or
even the existence of the problems they treat. He is challenging a
framework of understanding that presents our mental states as scientific problems defined by the language and techniques of psychiatry,
rather than as existential problems defined by our predicament as
mortal beings who must die. Within this framework, suffering

becomes a problem of brain chemistry. A drug that fixes the chemistry solves the problem of suffering. Death, loss, grief, fear, anxiety, sexual inadequacy become medical problems to be addressed by experts with prescription pads. Thus do the existential interests of a mortal being harmonize perfectly, in a way that perhaps only Adam Smith could appreciate, with the financial interests of the pharmaceutical industry.

For doctors, the body and the mind are objects of control. Therapeutic control is arguably the very point of modern medicine. But once we see human beings as objects of therapeutic control, a human life becomes a project that can be tweaked and reworked and adjusted in accordance with a person's own private wishes and desires. The fantasy here is not just about adjusting the body to suit the demands of the world; it is also about adjusting the soul. This is a powerful fantasy, yet for Percy it is not the only possible moral framework that our cultural resources have made available to us. Whatever the moral value of exerting control over a life—whatever the genuine value of self-reinvention, of taking charge of a life and wrenching every last drop of meaning from it—it does not exhaust all moral possibilities. We are not locked into seeing our lives as projects and our selves as instruments for self-fulfillment. We can still opt out.

Percy hints at this possibility at the end of *Love in the Ruins*. Five years after the dread latter days, five years after the Mephistopheles-like drug rep Art Immelman has taken More's Ontological Lapsometer off to Denmark and oil has been discovered in the Louisiana swamp, making millionaires of black squatters and turning the white residents of Paradise Estates into paupers, More and his Presbyterian wife, Ellen, have settled into small quarters down on the bayou with their kids. Times are different now, says More. He is poorer, but happier. He is still a bad Catholic, but he has learned a few things. Back in the old days, he says, "We planned projects and cast ahead of ourselves. We set out to 'reach goals.' We listened to the minutes of the previous meeting. Between times, we took vacations." These days you still work, More says. You hoe collards and run trotlines for catfish. You still work, but there is a difference. "Now while you work, you also watch and listen and wait."[38]

What Percy is describing here is something close to what philosopher James Edwards is getting at when he suggests an alternative to a life of *order*.[39] Technology does not simply serve our needs, Edwards points out. Technology orders our world for us, so that it is available for us to use with maximum efficiency and minimal effort. We see the world through the frame imposed on it by our technology, and through that frame we see the world as an instrument for our own designs. By virtue of the way we live, the way our world is put together, we come to see the things of the world as instruments, standing in reserve for our own use. A computer, a car, a house, or a box of Prozac capsules—all are tools with which we can take control of our lives and put them in order.

Yet there is an alternative to this way of seeing the world. The alternative is not a life of passivity (not any more than the kind of life that Thoreau describes in *Walden* is a life of passivity) but it is a kind of surrender, writes Edwards, a "surrender of oneself into a kind of activity that aims not at order but at full acknowledgement."[40] This kind of surrender suggests a willingness to court disorder. It suggests a willingness to forget about planning projects and reaching goals and listening to the minutes of the previous meeting. As Edwards puts it, it suggests a person who does not care much about training for the race that most of us are running.

It is no simple thing to opt out, of course. It is not easy to imagine how to lead a life so radically at odds with the values and structures of the dominant culture. It is not even clear that a life at odds with the values and structures of the dominant culture would be a *better* life. Edwards does not argue that we *ought* to opt out of this aspiration to technological order, only that we *can*. Opting out is a live possibility. As Edwards puts it, we can nurture a sensibility that aspires less to control than to clarity, less to working furiously on the project of a life than to understanding what gives that mysterious project its pathos.

Can Miltown, Valium, or Prozac help the sad and anxious suburbanite "function" better? Probably. Thoreau would probably function better out on Walden Pond. Tom More would hoe his collards faster and more efficiently, and he would catch more catfish. Medicated, we might well feel better about all those thousands of hours in front of the television. We would spend happier evenings at the health club, climbing the Stairmaster to heaven. On Prozac, Sisyphus might well push the boulder back up the mountain with more enthusiasm and more creativity. I do not want to deny the benefits of psychoactive medication. I just want to point out that Sisyphus is not a patient with a mental health problem. To see him as a patient with a mental health problem is to ignore certain larger aspects of his predicament connected to boulders, mountains, and eternity.[41]

7

PILGRIMS AND STRANGERS

I am a pilgrim, and a stranger
Traveling through this wearisome land
I have a home in
That yonder city, oh Lord
And it's not
Not made by hand.

—Traditional

One of my favorite passages in Walker Percy's 1966 novel, *The Last Gentleman*, begins when Will Barrett, a young southerner temporarily exiled in the North, is hitchhiking south from New York. Sitting patiently on the side of the road for an hour and a half, Barrett is almost ready to give up when a bottle-green Chevrolet pulls over. The driver is a well-dressed Negro in a brown suit. Barrett takes him for a preacher, or possibly a teacher. His name is Isham Washington. A bit of good fortune, thinks Barrett. This is the sort of colored man who will converse on all manner of high-minded subjects. Barrett stows his gear in the back seat and climbs in.

But there is something odd about the man. Barrett can't quite put his finger on it. This man talks about Einstein. He carries on about air-conditioning, and landscaping, and how they upset the balance of nature. "There is the cause of your violence!" he all but shouts. This is not the way an educated colored man talks, thinks Barrett. An educated colored man does not cry "Capital!" and "Marvelous!" in a nervous, reedy voice.

As they drive, the man leans over to Barrett and says, "I have a lit-

tle confession to make to you." "Certainly," Barrett replies. The colored man continues. "I am not what you think I am." He pushes up
his coat sleeve and shows Barrett a light patch of skin on his arm. He
is not really a Negro, he tells Barrett. Nor is his name Isham Washington. His real name is Forney Aiken, and he is a photojournalist on
an investigative trip to the South—"below the cotton curtain," as
Aiken explains it. He is doing a journalistic series on the "behind-the-
scenes life of the Negro." And what better way to do such a series
than to become a Negro himself? Aiken tells Barrett that he persuaded a dermatologist friend up North to administer an alkaloid to
turn his skin dark, and that it can be reversed with a skin-lightening
cream. He then acquired the personal papers of a black man called
Isham Washington, an agent for a burial insurance firm in Pittsburgh.
Aiken has just begun his journey south in disguise, and Barrett is his
first test. Aiken has a hidden camera in his necktie.[1]

Americans who came of age in the 1960s and '70s will recognize
Aiken as a fictional stand-in for John Howard Griffin, the best-
selling author of *Black Like Me*.[2] Griffin was a novelist and journalist who, like Aiken, underwent dermatological treatment to
darken his skin in 1959, and then spent six weeks disguised as a black
man in the deep South. His account of his experiences was serialized
in the magazine *Sepia*, and then published in book form in 1961.
Black Like Me turned Griffin into a minor celebrity and a spokesman
on civil rights. Many white Americans found themselves deeply
moved by Griffin's account of the racial prejudice he experienced as
a black man. But others vilified him. In his hometown, Griffin was
hung in effigy.

Black Like Me has had a curious legacy. On one level it was hugely
successful. It became an international bestseller and a standard text
in many school classrooms. Once a minor novelist, Griffin became a
well-known media figure. Even today, *Black Like Me* is included on
the syllabus of many African-American Studies courses. For white
Americans in particular, Griffin's experiment seems to have an enduring appeal. In 1964, *Black Like Me* was turned into a Hollywood
movie with James Whitmore. Four years later Grace Halsell, a White
House aide in the Johnson administration, repeated Griffin's experiment, living as a black woman in the South and in Harlem. She pub-

lished a book about her experience called *Soul Sister*.[3] As recently as 1994, Joshua Solomon, then a student at the University of Maryland, undertook his own Griffin-inspired experiment and wrote about it for *The Washington Post*.[4]

Yet there has always been an undercurrent of discomfort with Griffin's experiment. Many black readers were uneasy with the preposterous idea that it took a white man's testimony to verify racial prejudice in the South, and as the 1960s came to a close, Griffin found himself marginalized within the Civil Rights movement—a development he admits with bitterness in his later writings, yet never quite seems able to understand. Griffin also became an easy mark for satire. In *The Last Gentleman*, Percy turns him into a clownish Yankee who hangs out with Hollywood actors intent on staging a "morality play" in Alabama. Percy refers to him as "the Pseudo-Negro."

What accounts for the lasting appeal of Griffin's experiment? At least part of it, I suspect, comes from the actual intervention itself, the concrete, physical act of darkening your skin. This is not posturing, or at least not in any simple way; nor is it merely an act of imagination—the body actually changes color. And what American cannot identify with the existential thrill of taking on the identity of another person, of becoming a stranger in your own body? Ethnic impersonation has a long history in American life, from blackface minstrels and the Oriental princesses in Wild West medicine shows to the strange public career of Asa Carter, an ex-Klansman and speechwriter for George Wallace who, under the pseudonym Forrest Carter, posed as a Cherokee Indian and faked a best-selling autobiography called *The Education of Little Tree*.[5] Griffin meant well, but many of us still cringe involuntarily at the thought of what he did. Self-transformation has its dangers, and one is the danger of fakery, to yourself as well as to others. This is part of what Percy is hinting at with the figure of Forney Aiken, who is less an investigative journalist than a voyeuristic thrill-seeker. One danger of the way we live now lies not just in the way that our selves are packaged and given to us by others, but also in the promise of liberation through self-transformation. These days, self-transformation is part of the package too.

O NE ETHICAL WORRY about enhancement technologies is the way they can play into racist ideals of beauty. The demand for many kinds of cosmetic surgery has long been tied to a desire to efface ethnicity, to get rid of the so-called "Jewish" nose, say, or "Asian" eyes. The cosmetics industry itself has a long history of selling skin-lighteners and hair straighteners to African-Americans. Critics of these products argue that by undergoing a procedure to change or efface your ethnicity, you may be reinforcing the racist ideals of beauty that led to your desire for the procedure in the first place.

Black Like Me turns all these concerns on their heads. It describes not a skin-lightener, but a skin-darkener, undertaken not for a black man to pass as white, but for a white man to pass as black. What should a right-thinking, race-conscious liberal make of *this* kind of medical intervention? Griffin claimed to be undergoing the procedure in order to investigate racism in the South, which is surely a worthy goal, but in fact, by 1959 nobody really had any doubts that racism existed in the South. Besides, why should it take a white man to tell people what it is like to be black? Plenty of black writers were able to do that, and do it much better than Griffin could. Whatever the reason for the popularity of *Black Like Me*, it seems to go beyond the ordinary appetite for investigative journalism.

In some ways, reading *Black Like Me* is like reading the memoir of a spy, or a plainclothes detective. As you, the reader, accompany Griffin on his journey in disguise, it is as if you travel with him into another world, where his (and thus your) identity is hidden from sight. The effect is like watching Jimmy Stewart look through his binoculars in *Rear Window*, or reading about Huck going ashore at Goshen dressed as a girl: you can see but you cannot be seen, or at least seen for what you really are. I suspect that even a black southern reader might get this vicarious thrill, and might even have gotten it in 1961 when the book was first published. Not because a black southern reader would need Griffin to tell him what conditions were like in the South in 1961, but because this kind of knowledge is secondary to the book's main appeal, which is the appeal of hiding, of passing, of looking at things undetected.

Yet the unspoken premise of *Black Like Me* is that Griffin can, in some deep sense, become a black man—that he is not just posing, but has taken on a new identity, an identity otherwise foreign to him, and is looking at the world from this new vantage point. Seen this way, Griffin's experiment looks weirdly like that of Civil War reenactors thirty years later, men who dress in period uniforms and stage mock reproductions of battles at Shiloh or Gettysburg. In his book *Confederates in the Attic*, Tony Horwitz describes the time he spent with a group of "hardcores" called the Southern Guardsmen who marched barefoot, ate hardtack and salt pork, spoke in the style and accents of the 1860s, and dressed in the filthy, frayed uniforms of Confederate or Union soldiers. ("Look at these buttons," one hardcore tells Horwitz. "I soaked them overnight in a saucer filled with urine.") Especially prized is the gaunt, hollow-eyed look that comes from months of near-starvation diets. One hardcore named Robert Lee Hodge specializes in "bloating," whereby he impersonates a swollen corpse: his belly distended, his mouth contorted, his hands curled up like a dead soldier at Antietem. Done properly, the hardcores tell Horwitz, this obsessive loyalty to the 1860s will produce a transformational thrill, or what they call a "period rush."[6]

Many enhancement technologies hold just this sort of draw. Their appeal lies in the way they transform experience. Some operate directly on consciousness itself, altering the way you see the world. Ritalin allows you to concentrate your attention; Prozac makes the world look brighter and more vivid. They change the way you perceive the world and the way you act in it. Other enhancement technologies work to change the way you are perceived. Larger breasts, greater height, straighter hair, Gentile nose: you feel different, but you feel different because of the way other people perceive you. In both cases there is a feedback loop between the way you see the world and the way the world sees you: you look and behave differently, so you are treated differently; you are treated differently, so you look and behave differently. When Joshua Solomon, John Griffith's 1994 imitator, disguised himself as black, he found himself being excessively polite to white people. He did it, he says, as a means of getting the respect that was denied him because of his black skin.

When W. E. B. Du Bois used the term "double consciousness" to describe the experience of being black in America, he was getting at this sort of feedback effect, this "sense of always looking at one's self through the eyes of others." Double-consciousness can describe both the danger and the appeal of using enhancement technologies as a strategy for transforming experience. The danger comes when you buy wholeheartedly into a standard of value against which you will inevitably fail to measure up. Given a set of aesthetic standards according to which light skin is superior to dark skin, straight hair superior to curly, and European features superior to African, black Americans run the danger of constantly seeking an ideal of beauty that they will never quite reach. By virtue of the cultural norms that shape and sustain their desires, Du Bois worried, black folks in America might well find themselves doomed to self-loathing or futile striving.

Yet the very appeal of these technologies (as John Griffin seems to have realized, however vaguely) is that of seeing yourself through the eyes of another. What is it like to travel not just as another person, but another person whom others will treat very differently than they ordinarily treat you? Will you come to see yourself differently if others see you differently? You will, of course. This is a lesson familiar not just to drag queens, bodybuilders, and undercover cops, but also to expatriates of the more conventional sort. You discover how American you are by living in Berlin, how southern you are by living in Boston. Your accent changes, your vocabulary, your dress, your manner; you start to behave in ways that would be unrecognizable to the folks back home. (You hide your southernness and talk like Ted Kennedy, or you exaggerate it and talk like Strom Thurmond.) Your identity shifts depending on how you are seen by others. Sometimes, in fact, your identity shifts so much that it is no longer clear to you just who you are—which is exactly what is disturbing about Griffin's experiment.

"For years the idea had haunted me, and that night it returned more insistently than ever. If a white man became a Negro in the Deep South, what adjustments would he have to make? What is it like to experience discrimination based on skin color, something over which one has no control?"[7]

Griffin set out to answer these questions, which open *Black Like Me*, by changing the color of his skin. After acquiring sponsorship from the black-owned magazine *Sepia* and informing the FBI of his plans, Griffin traveled to New Orleans to see medical specialists, with the hope that medical treatment could transform him into a Negro.

His request was fulfilled by the first dermatologist he saw. The dermatologist gave him oxsoralen, a medication ordinarily used to treat a skin condition called vitiligo, and which he thought would darken Griffin's skin. Griffin spent hours under a sun lamp, shaved his head, and stained his skin with vegetable dye. Looking at himself in the mirror four days later, he saw a stranger, "a fierce, bald, very dark Negro." He writes: "The transformation was total and shocking. I had expected to see myself disguised, but this was something else. I was imprisoned in the flesh of an utter stranger, an unsympathetic one with whom I felt no kinship. All traces of the John Griffin I had been were wiped from existence."[8] Thus humbled, Griffin set out into another world to which he was a complete stranger, the segregated world of black southerners in Louisiana, Alabama, Georgia, and Mississippi. He traveled on foot and by bus, looking unsuccessfully for work, living in segregated boarding houses and hotels and eating in segregated restaurants. His story is one of cruelty and hate stares from whites, and good-natured kindness from blacks, with whom he finds a welcome solidarity in a racist South. Griffin stayed on the road for six weeks before he returned home.

But there is something a little odd about *Black Like Me*, something that may be more apparent now than when it was published. As you, the reader, try to imagine yourself in Griffin's place, you can hardly help but ask, "How is Griffin going to pull this off?" It is no small thing for a white man to pass as black. It is no small thing, in fact, to impersonate anyone whose way of life is unfamiliar to you, to notice and make your own the sensibility of people of another culture. Yet Griffin appears to have been oddly confident. Initially, he is very anxious about his *physical* appearance. One black man in whom Griffin confides points out that Griffin might be given away by the white hairs on his arm, and this possibility worries Griffin a lot. But once he shaves his arm hairs and spends a few days undetected as a black man, his anxiety seems to dissipate. Even as he takes painstaking care with his physical disguise, shaving his head and dying his skin, he pays no attention at all to anything else —nothing about his manner, his speech, his voice, his way of carrying himself. He does not give any thought to the way black folks in the South talk, or what they talk about, the way they laugh or make jokes. He does not seem to know anything about their music, or churches, or really anything at all about their lives apart from the fact of racial oppression.

Yet it is not hard to see why Griffin was so preoccupied with skin color. The white South itself was obsessed with it, of course, and it was crucial to Griffin's moral purpose to show that this obsession was absurd. Griffin wanted to hammer home the point that deep down, regardless of skin color, human beings are all the same. In America we profess to judge people as individuals, he writes, not as types. Yet if this were true, then "my life as a black John Howard Griffin would not be greatly changed, since I was that same human individual, altered only in appearance."[9] His life *did* change, of course, and this is the point of the book. He was insulted, patronized, threatened, blocked from using public facilities reserved only for whites—all because his skin had been darkened. Hence his obsession with skin color. To concede that black southerners really *are* different in significant ways other than skin color would have been to give in to the segregationists. It would have undermined the moral force of Griffin's experience.

But Griffin does not stop at convincing the reader that black and white Americans are no different from one another. He seems to have also convinced himself. The most unnerving element of Griffin's book is the way he seems genuinely to convince himself that during the time he was wearing his disguise he *actually changed races*. He constantly refers to himself as a Negro, and when he mentions white people, he refers to them unself-consciously as "they" and "them" (rather than "we" and "us"), who live in a world utterly apart from the world that "we Negroes" inhabit. It is as if Griffin really believes he is black.

After Griffin eats a humble supper with a black family in Alabama, he writes, "I felt more profoundly than ever the totality of *my* Negroness, the immensity of its isolating effects."[10] Commenting on white customers whose shoes he is shining, he writes, "All of them [whites] showed *us* how they felt about the Negro, the idea that *we* were people of such low morality that nothing could offend *us*."[11] As he eats beans and rice in a segregated restaurant he wonders: "The distance between them [whites] and me was far more than the miles that physically separated us. It was an area of unknowing. I wondered if it could really be bridged."[12] And as he sits in the home of the Alabama family on whose floor he spent a night, thinking of his children in Texas, Griffin writes, "They slept now in clean beds in a warm house while their father, a bald-headed old Negro, sat in the swamps and wept, holding it in so that he would not awaken the Negro children."[13]

Of course, it might be that the experience of being treated like a black man really did transform Griffin's consciousness; that when he wrote these words he truly did feel like a black man, and not merely like a disguised white man. Some confusion is understandable. Occasionally Griffin even slips between identities, forgetting which race "we" refers to. Writing on one particularly dreadful night in Hattiesburg, Mississippi, Griffin describes "the onrush of revulsion, the momentary flash of blind hatred against the whites who were somehow responsible for all this, the old bewilderment of wondering, "Why do they do it? Why do they keep us like this? What are they gaining? What evil has taken them?" "They" in this passage means white people. Yet only a few sentences later in the very same paragraph, "they" becomes "we" and Griffin is white again: "My revulsion turned to grief that *my own people* could give the hate stare, could shrivel men's souls, could deprive humans of rights they unhesitatingly accord their livestock."[14]

Even if Griffin honestly felt like a black man while he was disguised as black in 1959, it would take no small amount of self-deception to do the same thing eighteen years later when he was writing a new epilogue to his book. In that 1977 epilogue, Griffin writes as if he had been an actual victim of racial segregation twenty years earlier. Look, for example, at this passage, in which Griffin describes the more subtle kind of racial prejudice that pervaded southern life: "[W]e did not see WHITE ONLY signs on the doors of libraries (where *we* could find learning and books) but *we* knew that we had better not try to enter one. We saw no WHITE ONLY signs on the doors of schools or universities, but we knew it was suicidal to try to enter one."[15] "We," for Griffin, still refers to "we Negroes." Thus does a white, southern, university-educated novelist on a pilgrimage through the South speak of his oppression at the hands of people just like him. Whether this was the result of a self-conscious rhetorical style or an unconscious identification with others, Griffin seems to have forgotten that he was never really black.

To DESCRIBE GRIFFIN as a pilgrim does not require much of a stretch. In fact, the metaphor of the pilgrimage as an interior, spiritual journey has become so firmly entrenched in popular consciousness that it is now a cliché, a staple of self-help literature and Disney cartoons. The metaphor has become so worn that it is sometimes easy to forget that it is, after all, still a metaphor—that a pilgrimage is, first and foremost, a journey to a real place. (A *New Yorker* cartoon has Queen Isabella asking Columbus: "I don't want to hear about your self-discovery. Tell me about the new continent.") The pilgrim does not merely travel in search of another state of inner, spiritual well-being; she travels physically to Jerusalem or Mecca or Lourdes. For some religions, like Islam, a pilgrimage is strictly required of all believers. For others it is not required, yet may be undertaken to strengthen a believer's spiritual faith. Pilgrimages are ancient in origin, but by no means are they dying out. Often they arise spontaneously. Where once a Christian pilgrim may have journeyed on foot to Jerusalem, now he is more likely to travel in an RV to Conyers, Georgia, where the Virgin Mary has appeared in a cow pasture.

What ancient pilgrimages held in common was travel to a holy place, a place where miracles had happened or might happen again. The contemporary pilgrimage, in contrast, is a journey not to a holy place, a place made sacred by external frameworks of meaning, but an interior journey in search of identity. The self is what is sacred now. In America, we are told, who you are is not a matter of what external standards of meaning say you are, but rather what you make of yourself and what you discover yourself to be. The point of life is to discover, articulate, and follow the markers of your own identity. Your physical journey mirrors this interior journey. As Eddy Harris describes it in *Native Stranger*, a memoir of his journey through Africa, "To paraphrase Harry James Cargas, we each have a certain destiny and the real adventure in life is to discover it; to discover how we may fully develop into who we are."[16]

In Griffin's case, we see a convergence not just between spiritual and physical pilgrimages, but also between the ancient pilgrimage and the contemporary. The contemporary pilgrim leaves home to discover who she really is. By leaving home you see yourself through the eyes of others. What is interesting about Griffin's journey in *Black Like Me* is that it turns this trope about journeys on its head. He is traveling, but he is not really leaving home: he is a southerner traveling through the South. He is constantly being made aware of his identity in a way that he has never had to before, but of course, it is not really *his* identity: he is in disguise. And while he does not explicitly set out to discover anything about himself—on the contrary, the whole point of his journey is to investigate the experience of the black man—he winds up discovering things about himself that make him rather uncomfortable. When he sees himself in the mirror, he is shocked not just at what stares back at him ("a fierce, bald Negro") but also by his own negative reaction to what he sees. He does not much like his reflection, and he does not much like himself for not liking it.[17]

If the contemporary pilgrimage sounds rather self-obsessed and inward-looking, this is exactly the point. The purpose of the contemporary pilgrimage is not to discover something about the world, but to discover something about the self. What was true in 1959 is doubly true today. To see how far we have come, compare Griffin's journey to the journey of Joshua Solomon, Griffin's imitator forty years later. Like Griffin, Solomon does not profess any worries about his ability to pass convincingly as a black person. But unlike Griffin, Solomon does not spend any time with black people. His only extended contacts on his journey are with white people, who are uniformly rude, patronizing, distant, or downright hostile. As an argument that racism is alive and kicking, the article makes a forceful point, but as an investigation into the experience of black people it is oddly self-centered, like an ethnography of a foreign culture that records the feelings of the ethnographer and fails to mention the natives. The question it asks is not, "How does it feel to be black in America?" but "How would it feel for *me* to be black in America?" And the subtext to that question, in turn, is "How does it differ from the way I ordinarily feel?" Here, perhaps, is the real appeal of this kind of enhancement: not so much a passport into another existence as a tool for self-exploration. This is part of what Walker Percy was poking fun at with the figure of Forney Aiken in *The Last Gentleman*, who is not only a Pseudo-Negro, but also a Pseudo-Pilgrim.

The classic pilgrimage tale for Americans, of course, is *The Wizard of Oz*, which combines spiritual odyssey, consumerist fantasy, and self-help propaganda.[18] Like *The Last Gentleman*, *The Wizard of Oz* is about a quest—for brains, for a heart, for courage, for home—and like many quests, it ends up exactly where it started. Dorothy, carried by a tornado into Oz, must follow the Yellow Brick Road to the Emerald City, where she will ask the Wizard to help her get back to Kansas. On her way to the Emerald City, Dorothy is joined by three companions: the Scarecrow, the Tin Woodman, and the Lion. Yet when they all finally reach the Wizard, they discover that the very things they are looking for they have had in their possession all along. The Scarecrow, who asks for brains, is already the most intelligent of the lot; the Tin Woodman, who asks for a heart, is the most compassionate; and the Cowardly Lion, who asks for courage, is the bravest. Their problems lie not in who they are, but in who they *think* they are. The Wizard is not really selling brains, or heart, or courage. He is selling self-esteem.

Like today's drug marketers, *The Wizard of Oz* teaches that unhappiness can be remedied by what you buy. The Wizard himself is the very prototype of an American consumer capitalist. When Dorothy and her companions come to him for help, he agrees to grant their requests, but only at a price. ("In this country," he says in Baum's original book, "everyone must pay for everything he gets.")[19] The price the Wizard demands is the broomstick of the Wicked Witch of the West. He fully expects Dorothy and her companions to fail, of course. He does not think they can really destroy the Witch. But he also knows full well that if they succeed, he won't be able to fulfill his end of the bargain except by fakery. So when Dorothy kills the Witch and comes back to the Emerald City expecting him to fulfill his end of the bargain, the Wizard is exposed as a fraud. He is just an ordinary carnival huckster from Kansas. "You are a very bad man!" Dorothy tells him angrily. "No, my dear," he replies, "I'm a good man. I'm just a very bad wizard." In fact, though, just the opposite is true. He is a bad man, but a very good wizard. Which is to say: he is a very good businessman. His virtues are those of American salesmanship, the ability to persuade others to do what he wants them to do, even command their respect, by way of smooth talk. The Wizard is a cross between a therapist and a con artist. He has power, but it is not the power of the military or of Big Brother. It is the power of Hollywood and Madison Avenue. It is the ability to carefully manage his image.

The message of *The Wizard of Oz* is no different from the message of the self-help books on the shelves at Borders. Both teach that unhappiness comes from self-doubt and a lack of self-confidence. As the Wizard knows, the secret to selling enhancement technologies is to take advantage of a person's perceived inadequacies. The Cowardly Lion needs self-confidence. He feels like a fraud because he is supposed to be King of the Forest, yet deep inside he feels like a coward. The Wizard cures him by pinning a medal on him. By doing this, the Wizard sells the Lion two ideas. First, he convinces the Lion that, despite his doubts and fears, he really is a lion of genuine courage. Second, he persuades him that the medal will allow his true, courageous self to emerge. This is the genius behind the Wizard's methods. Not only does he sell the Lion a vision of himself that is at odds with what the Lion fears himself to be; he also convinces him that this is the way he really is, deep inside.

Here is a key to understanding the place of enhancement technologies in contemporary America. The Scarecrow, the Tin Man, and the Lion do not go to the Wizard because they want to be "enhanced." They go because they want to be *themselves*. In *The Wizard of Oz*, as in contemporary America, the search for the good life is an inward search for authenticity. As Dorothy says, "If I ever go looking for my heart's desire again, I won't look any further than my own backyard. If I don't find it there, I never really lost it to begin with." Cliché aside, this is a very powerful idea. The quest for the good life will differ from one person to the next, the story tells us. Dorothy and her friends are each searching for different things. *The Wizard of Oz* says that we must all look inward to discover our own particular talents and desires and needs, then choose a path that allows us to develop and fulfill them. To point out that this notion has become a staple of twentieth-century self-help literature is not to belittle it. Just the opposite: it is a sign of its power. The fact that so many of us are moved by this kind of language, that we find the metaphors persuasive, should tell us something about how deeply rooted in our culture this idea is.

At the end of *The Wizard of Oz*, when the balloon floats off to Kansas without Dorothy in it and she is left standing on the platform in her ruby slippers, Glinda the good witch tells her that she has always had the power to go back to Kansas. An extraordinary remark, when you think about it. Dorothy has risked her life and the lives of her friends trying to steal a broomstick when she could have gone home at any time. She has been tricked, utterly deceived; yet when Glinda reveals this to her, we are not outraged. Neither is Dorothy. The notion of self-discovery is so deeply ingrained that instead we think, with Glinda, "Yes, she had to learn it for herself." This is how you learn life's lessons. You have to find your own way. You must discover for yourself what is valuable in life, and you discover it by looking inside yourself.

IN *THE LAST GENTLEMAN*, Percy places Aiken side by side with another traveler, Will Barrett, the lost young southern hitchhiker who hops into Aiken's bottle-green Chevrolet. But Barrett is no ordinary traveler. The epigraph for *The Last Gentleman* is a remark by Kierkegaard: "If a man cannot forget, he will never amount to much." Forgetting, however, is exactly what Barrett does, involuntarily and in spectacular fashion: he forgets who he is and then he wanders the country. Barrett is subject to fugue states, episodes of amnesic wandering where he will disappear for weeks on end and come to himself miles from the site of his last memory. During these fugue states Barrett is haunted by vague feelings of déjà vu and nostalgia for the South. "Most of this young man's life was a gap," we are told. "The summer before, he had fallen into a fugue state and wandered around northern Virginia for three weeks, where he sat sunk in thought on old battlegrounds, hardly aware of his own name."[20] Barrett calls it a "nervous condition."

Barrett's "nervous condition" is not a mere product of Percy's literary imagination. As Ian Hacking has written in his extraordinary book *Mad Travelers*, the fugue state, or "dissociative fugue," was a real condition that flourished for a brief twenty years or so in Europe, particularly France, then disappeared.[21] Like, say, anorexia nervosa, or multiple personality disorder, the fugue state was a product of a particular time and place, a confluence of cultural forces that somehow came together to produce episodes of forgetful wandering. Men in fugue states would disappear for weeks or months at a time and travel far from home, then suddenly come to themselves, with no memory of the time during which they wandered. The most famous case of fugue, that of Jean-Albert Dadas, was reported by a medical student, Philippe Tissie, in late-nineteenth-century Bordeaux, a region that would become the focus of a minor fugue epidemic. As Hacking persuasively argues, the sudden emergence and later disappearance of the fugue state as a psychiatric entity reveals something important about the cultural and historical conditions of nineteenth-century France. But, as Percy realizes, the fugue state also represents something about the appeal of travel and its peculiar relationship to identity.[22]

As Hacking relates the tale, Jean-Albert Dadas was a Bordeaux gas-fitter who was twenty-six years old in 1886 when he first came to the attention of a medical student in the Saint-Andre' Hospital, Philippe Tissie. The story Dadas told was extraordinary. He generally lived a quiet, uneventful life, working for a gas company. For several days before lapsing into a fugue he would become anxious. He would lose sleep, suffer from headaches, masturbate five or six times a night. And then off he would go. He would travel obsessively, on foot, and when he eventually came to, often months later in Prague or Vienna, he would have no memory of his travels. (Unless, that is, he was under hypnosis; then he could give details of the places he had traveled and the events that took place during his amnesia.) Sometimes he was picked up by the police, destitute, or arrested for vagrancy; sometimes he would report to the French consul, who would arrange for his travel back home. Occasionally he would find temporary work and come home on his own. His first fugue came when he was only twelve years old and working as an apprentice to a manufacturer of gas equipment. One day he simply disappeared. Later he was found in a nearby town helping a traveling umbrella salesman. When his brother tapped him on the shoulder, Dadas woke up, groggy and disoriented, astonished to find himself where he was.

Once he heard the name of a place, Dadas would be compelled to take to the road and find it. Usually he would travel on foot—in the words of Tissie, deserting "family, work and daily life to walk as fast as he could, straight ahead, sometimes doing 70 kilometers a day."[23] On one occasion he traveled by ship to Algeria, was eventually advised to return home, and upon his return was arrested for having no identity papers. He did a month's forced labor as punishment. His most spectacular journey came when he was in the army, working as a cook. He took his uniform to the police station in Mons, turned it in, and headed east, eventually winding up in Moscow. There he was mistakenly arrested as a nihilist following the assassination of the czar. He spent three months in a Russian prison, then was forcibly marched to Turkey by Cossack guards. He eventually made his way back to France, where he was arrested as a deserter from the army and sent back to Algeria for three years of hard labor.

When Tissie, the medical student, published this tale in his doctoral dissertation in 1887, he set off an epidemic of fugue states. Within a year the famous French neurologist, Jean-Martin Charcot, had presented a similar case that he termed *automatisme ambulatoire*. Almost immediately the fugue state became a recognized mental disorder. Germans wrote of *Wandertrieb*; the English, of "dromomania." It became a topic of learned debate at academic meetings and in scholarly publications. Not that its status was not fiercely debated: some thought these cases were epilepsy, some hysteria. Nowadays clinicians engaging in the misguided enterprise of retrospective diagnosis might conclude that, in contemporary terms, many of these patients had posttraumatic stress disorder, or that their difficulties arose from early head injuries. (Dadas had a concussion at age eight.) Whatever its causes, the disorder became much more widely diagnosed. Was the fugue state a "real" disorder? Or more to the point: what would it mean to say that it was real? While Dadas, like others, was deeply upset by his fugue states and his consequent inability to live a normal life, it is hard to avoid concluding that his travels also satisfied some very deep needs.

What exactly brought about this fugue epidemic? One important thing to remember is the financial and social circumstance of those who suffered from fugues. As Hacking points out, the vast majority of *fugueurs* were working, urban poor: shopkeepers, artisans, deliverymen, and the like.[24] They did not come from the middle and upper classes, whose financial means gave them the opportunity to travel. Nor were they peasant farmers, tramps, or vagrants—and it is important to recall that this was a time when many French people saw vagrancy as a worrying social problem. Vagrancy signified racial degeneracy, and France passed strict antivagrancy laws in 1885. The class of people for whom the fugue state appealed were neither vagrants nor aristocrats, but those for whom travel was a way to escape a life of dull provincialism. Even the fugueurs who deserted the army were typically not wartime deserters. As Hacking puts it, "Fugue was a medical entity of peace, boredom and dull regimentation."[25]

Fugue states were never widely diagnosed in the United States, or even in Britain. In the United States, a person did not need to go into a fugue state to be able to travel. As Hacking puts it, "Go west, young man: the *fugueur* never came back."[26] The same went for the British, says Hacking, who could travel or even emigrate to the colonies in a way that never seemed quite as acceptable for the French. Perhaps just as importantly, neither the United States nor Britain had a system of forced military conscription during this period. Many of the young French and German men who suffered fugue states were those drafted into the army. In France, the authorities required that all citizens carry passports if they left their home region to travel to another one. Hence anyone who looked suspicious, especially young men of draft age, could be stopped by the police and asked to present identity papers. If a traveler was a deserter or a vagrant or a fugueur, his identity could be easily discovered. But in Britain or America, travelers of all sorts could move undetected.

Of all the cultural factors that formed the cultural niche into which the fugue state fit, perhaps the most striking is this: the latter half of the nineteenth century ushered in the age of mass tourism. In the earlier part of the nineteenth century tourism had been generally restricted to the wealthy or aristocratic classes. But by the late nineteenth century, travel was growing popular with the bourgeoisie. This was the age of Thomas Cook and Sons, the still-popular British travel agency that began sending British tourists to the continent on organized tours by the thousands. It was the age of the Baedeker tourist guides, of the travel narratives of Robert Louis Stevenson and Mark Twain, of the fantasies of Jules Verne. It was also the age in which bohemianism was born, with its romantic imagery of itinerant artists and idlers, liberated from the ties of family and daily habit. The bohemian ethic allowed a man like Paul Gauguin to abandon his wife, children, and workaday routine as a stockbroker to sail to the South Pacific and paint masterpieces. The fugue state fit neatly between moneyed tourism, vagrancy, and bohemian artistry. It provided a release for people who were not wealthy enough to be tourists, whose social class barred them from bourgeois bohemia, and whose morals were not sufficiently loose to permit them entry into the underworld associated with vagrancy.

By the early years of the twentieth century, however, the fugue state as a medical diagnosis had all but disappeared. Today it remains on the books in name only, as "dissociative fugue." It is rarely if ever diagnosed, rating hardly more than a historical footnote in most courses of psychiatric training. Why the fugue state disappeared is a matter for historical speculation. Perhaps where psychiatrists once saw fugue states they began to see other conditions, such as temporal lobe epilepsy. Perhaps the romantic appeal of travel eventually dissipated in the flood of mass tourism. But perhaps the dawn of the consumerist economy in the early twentieth century simply made the fugue state redundant. As identity hitched itself to consumer goods, becoming less a matter of the interior life and more a matter of self-presentation, the cultural niche for the fugue state disappeared. Once you are able to buy a new identity, losing your old one in a fugue state is no longer necessary.

Unless you are a man like Will Barrett. It makes sense that Barrett would lose his identity through fugue states: he is not sure what his identity is supposed to be. Barrett is Percy's "last gentleman," a relic of a time and an age that have all but disappeared. He is a southern gentleman in a South that has been transformed into a landscape of golf courses and auto dealerships. According to the moral map he has been given by his forebears, Barrett ought to go back home, revive the plantation, and live as an honorable man. But the structures of meaning that would make such a life possible have disappeared. The old South has given way to the businessman's South, a formidably cheerful place where happiness conquers and destroys everything in its path. Will is the last of the Barrett line, a relic of an age that has slipped imperceptibly away: an age where honor was honor and sin was sin and a gentleman knew who he was and what he was to do. When Barrett was a boy he used to think what a wonderful thing it would be to grow up and be a man and know how to live. But then he had grown up and still he did not know.

For a man caught between an age that has passed and a future that looks inexplicably hard to bear, the possibility of losing that identity through travel can be very attractive. Barrett is constantly taking to the road. When he was a child, his parents once put him in a summer camp while they vacationed in Europe. He had no use for the camp whatsoever. One evening when the campers were gathered around the fire listening to stories, the director asked everyone to stand up and make a decision for Jesus Christ as their personal savior. Barrett crept out of the circle, lit out down the road to Asheville and bought a bus ticket home. He spent the rest of the summer with a black friend, reading comic books in a tree house. Years later he repeated himself at Princeton. He joined a good club, did well in his studies, made the boxing team, but nonetheless was overtaken by an immense melancholy. He envied the janitors. How much better to go home to a cozy cottage along the railroad tracks than to be sharing quarters with young Republicans from Bronxville and Shaker Heights. "Walking around in New Jersey was like walking on Saturn, where the force of gravity is eight times that of earth."[27] These are supposed to be the best of times, Barrett told himself. What is the matter with me? On the afternoon of the Harvard-Princeton game, he looked in the mirror, let out a groan, and two hours later he was leaving Princeton on a bus.

Travel is deeply attractive to a man in search of who he is, yet, as Percy realized, the contemporary pilgrim can no longer travel in the conventional way. Mass tourism has made that impossible. Tourism has become so thoroughly packaged and routinized that it rarely brings about self-discovery. It rarely even measures up to the expectations of the tourist. Traveling in disguise like John Howard Griffin is one way to escape the routine, though Percy clearly has no patience for Griffin's muddy-headed intentions. A far better way is forgetfulness: if you have forgotten who you are and where you are going, like Jean-Albert Dadas, then you will never be disappointed in your travels. The fugue is Barrett's unconscious solution. He wanders the country in a state of partial amnesia, waking after weeks on the road to find himself working at a bakery in Cincinnati or clutching a tombstone at Gettysburg. "Like the sole survivor of a bombed building, he had no secondhand opinions and could see things afresh."[28] Barrett's fugue states, like Forney Aiken's disguise, are methods of transcending the ordinary.

PEOPLE WHO USE enhancement technologies often compare their experiences to journeys. A makeup artist boasts that "creative make-up will be the guide during the pilgrimage to the Holy Land of personality."[29] "Gender crossing is a good deal like foreign travel," writes Deidre McCloskey, a transsexual economist.[30] Historian Susan Stryker agrees, suggesting that people who stay the same gender all their lives are like people who never leave their hometown.[31] And of course, the central metaphor for the psychedelic experience has always been "the trip." Aldous Huxley, one of the early psychedelic evangelists, described mescaline as a vessel to "cross a dividing ocean into the world of the personal unconscious." "Wafting across it on the wings of mescaline," wrote Huxley, "we reach what might be called the Antipodes of the mind. In this psychological equivalent of Australia we discover the psychological equivalent of kangaroos, wallabies, and duck-billed platypuses."[32]

The comparison is not hard to understand. As I write these words, I am sitting cross-legged on a *bale* next to my cottage in Nyuh Kuning, a small village outside Ubud on the island of Bali. My family and I have been here for a month. In front of me stretch green rice terraces, acres and acres of them, ringed by palms and banana trees. Behind me is a shrine covered with a bright yellow cloth, to which the neighborhood women bring offerings every day. Sitting here under a clear blue sky, the pungent scent of incense and mosquito coils in the air, it is easy to understand the existential exhilaration that lay behind the wanderings of Will Barrett, John Howard Griffin, or Jean-Albert Dadas. Some Americans come here and never go back.

When Bali enjoyed its first vogue as a traveler's destination in the 1920s and '30s, Europeans and Americans made the long journey by ship because they saw Bali as somehow a more genuine or "authentic" place than Europe or America. The early travel books, such as Hickman Powell's *The Last Paradise* or Colin McPhee's *A House in Bali*, communicate the sense that American and European life had become encrusted with fakery and superficial things, and that travelers could somehow find a deeper, more genuine way of living in Bali. Even today, after decades of mass tourism in Bali, many travelers still think that Bali is different. Ubud, for example, is supposed to be closer to the "real" Bali than, say, the surfer-hippie-Aussie mecca of Kuta Beach, or the decaying hotels of Sanur, which has the look of a 1960s Elvis movie and the feel of an abandoned shopping mall. In fact, however, Ubud is not so much closer to the real Bali (whatever that might mean) as it is closer to the heart of international backpacker culture. A haven for leather-skinned ex-hippies and grad school dropouts, Ubud is the kind of place where travelers idle for months reading, meditating, learning how to play the gamelan or cook Balinese. Some people wander like this for years, living cheap, carrying worn paperbacks in their packs, working in Australia or Europe just long enough to keep going for a while longer.

It is not hard to see why this kind of travel has become so closely associated with self-discovery. Travel brings out the contingent features of your life and throws them into relief. The rhythm and shape of life in another place can be so different that you naturally begin to wonder just how it is that you came to be living the way you do. Why one God, rather than many? Why deodorizer and meatloaf rather than frangipani and jackfruit? The traveler can hardly help but see himself as alien, his own life calling for some kind of justification. Life in a new place takes on an intensity that it did not have at home: motorbikes buzzing past like horseflies, *bemo* drivers careening crazily along roads without stoplights, gamecocks lined up outside houses in wooden cages, statues of dancing frogs and Ganesha, the elephant boy. To get to Ubud we must pass through a forest inhabited by aggressive macaque monkeys who survive on bananas fed to them by tourists. Walking through the forest, I find myself treating these monkeys like panhandlers in Chicago. Don't make eye contact, I tell myself, otherwise they may turn nasty.

The marvel is that it does not last. After only a month in Nyuh Kuning, even the exoticism of Balinese life is starting to seem ordinary. I am getting used to barong masks, mosquito nets, and shrines to unfamiliar gods. I am becoming accustomed to the theater of Balinese life, the rituals and flowers and sticks of incense nestled in banana leaves. It seems normal to lie on my back and watch the gekkos on the ceiling. I have even settled into a work routine: get up at dawn, work under the shade of the *bale* while it is cool, drinking boiled coffee, then ride with Crawford into town on the bicycle to hang out at the English library or the *Tutmak Kopi Warung*. How quickly life becomes ordinary. The everydayness is not here yet, but a few months more and it will surely arrive.

It is a phenomenon that Walker Percy would have recognized. For Percy, ever the student of Kierkegaard, the great problem of contemporary life is boredom. Emptiness, alienation, and loneliness, yes; but from one day to the next the problem is boredom. Your work is boring. Your hometown is boring. Your vacations are boring. Even sex becomes boring, if you do it the right way. Kierkegaard said that most of us simply bore other people, but if you are really gifted at boredom, you even bore yourself. When your boredom reaches its zenith, he wrote, either you die of boredom, or you shoot yourself out of curiosity.[33] Hence the marriage of the existential and the mundane, the problem of meaning and the problem of boredom. Ask not what you should do with your life, but what you should do after lunch.

Experience is not merely there for the taking anymore. It must be *recovered*. And this is what the pilgrimage promises to do. You are bored and suffocated with malaise, your life does not feel the way the experts have told you it should, yet you can recover it all by traveling. Set out for parts unknown, where the landscape looks different. You can hitchhike to New Mexico, hop a plane to Bali, ride a bicycle to British Columbia. ("Home may be where the heart is," says

Percy, "but it's no place to spend a Wednesday afternoon.")[34] A similar strategy is disguise. Don the persona of someone else entirely. Take on his behavior and his costume: hell-raising, southern-boy poet, bearded Left Bank intellectual, Ivy League preppie in an L.L. Bean windbreaker. Stain your skin black and become a Pseudo-Negro. Or best of all, like John Howard Griffin, do both: take to the road in disguise. You will see the world differently, and the world will see you differently too.

Whether these are anything more than temporary solutions to the malaise, of course, is a matter for debate. Certainly Percy and Kierkegaard thought not. Both travel and enhancement technologies run out eventually: you can only change yourself so often before even that becomes habit and routine. Stay in Bali long enough and even trances and elephant Gods will start to seem ordinary. Kirkegaard writes, "One tires of living in the country, and moves to the city; one tires of one's native land, and travels abroad; one is *europamuede*, and goes to America, and so on; finally one indulges in a sentimental hope of endless journeyings from star to star."[35] But for Kirkegaard this sort of exercise can go on indefinitely, and it is ultimately futile. One can only search for diversion from boredom for so long. Better to stay home like me, says Kierkegaard, and become a genius of solitary inventiveness.

But for the contemporary pilgrim, as Percy realized, the problem is even more complicated. Travel does not solve the problem of boredom, and this is not just because the novelty of travel runs out. It is because travel itself has been packaged so thoroughly that even the first trip is not a novelty anymore. The Caribbean cruise, the adventure tour to Alaska, the *Wanderjahr* through Europe, the family trip to Disneyland or the Grand Canyon or Hilton Head: all have been so thoroughly described, photographed, documented in travel books and brochures and even academic ethnographies that they cannot be experienced for themselves anymore. Tahiti can never really match up to your expectations, and Switzerland will never be the way it looks in the movies. After Griffin's book, in fact, even a white person's pilgrimage through the South disguised as a black person cannot be experienced for itself. To try was Joshua Solomon's mistake, and perhaps the reason why his pilgrimage lasted only a day. Merely to impersonate a black person among white people in the South is no way to dispatch the malaise anymore. The only real way to salvage a journey that has been so thoroughly documented, photographed, filmed, and theorized is to get lost, or have your bus break down, or chance upon a black person who has lightened his skin in order to pass as white.

For those of us who persist, there remains only the favorite strategy of intellectuals, the strategy Percy calls "The Familiar Revisited." After a lifetime of avoiding guided tours, you take the most thoroughly conventional tour you can imagine. Then you step back and watch the watchers. You look at your fellow tourists busily taking their photographs. You look sidelong at the fellow on the mule next to you and try to see the Grand Canyon through his eyes. This is often a strategy of last resort, a strategy for the person who has seen it all. For him, leaving the beaten path has become a beaten path itself, the most worn-out strategy possible. He has to see the world from the shoulders of other people.

Yet even this strategy may not work anymore. For intellectuals, ironic detachment has become too familiar a stance. You take the mule tour of the Grand Canyon with a knowing wink and write about it for *Harper's*. You go to Disneyland not as a person intending to experience it directly, but as an ironic observer of American ritual. Had Joshua Solomon taken this stance, he would have not simply repeated Griffin's experiment, but repeated it and written about it with a wink to the reader: isn't this amusing? We are both in on this game.

Like all strategies, though, this one is running its course; even the detached ironic stance has become packaged. You know all the steps by heart. You have read too many articles in *Harper's*, taken too many cultural studies courses in college. So you have to take another step back. It will no longer do to watch the watchers; now you must watch the people who are watching the watchers. You go to Indonesia not to see the Bali of Mead, Bateson, and Geertz, but to watch the cultural anthropologists following in the footsteps of Mead, Bateson, and Geertz. You go to the South Seas not to see the Tahiti of Gauguin, but to watch the art historians tracking the path of Gauguin.

You go to the Grand Canyon and take the mule tour, but you go with a professor of cultural studies. Instead of watching the Iowans on the mule tour, you watch your fellow professor watch the Iowans. And so you keep stepping back, and back, and back, until you step backward into the canyon itself.

8

RESIDENT ALIENS

If you're white, you're all right
If you're brown, stick around
But if you're black, whoa brother:
Get back, get back, get back

—Big Bill Broonzy

"Negro Announces Remarkable Discovery: Can Change Black to White in Three Days" reads a newspaper headline at the start of the African American writer George Schuyler's 1931 novel, *Black No More*. The "Negro" of the headline is Dr. Junius Crookman, a physician-businessman who has invented a revolutionary medical technique for changing black people into white. Crookman's technique can lighten skin color, straighten hair, even change facial features. All this in only three days, as long as the proper fee is paid. For Dr. Crookman is more than a brilliant, German-trained black physician. He is also a canny entrepreneur and a "race man," whose dedication to the advancement of the Negro people is exceeded only by his dedication to the advancement of his bank account. When Crookman announces that he has developed a method to turn black people white, his Black No More clinic is besieged by thousands of black people willing to pay heavily for the privilege. As he explains to the press, there are only three ways for the Negro to solve the race problem in America: "To either get out, get white, or get along."[1]

Getting white, as it turns out, is not the unqualified success Crookman imagines. As black Americans rush to Black No More Incorporated, they abandon black social structures and businesses. Black banks collapse. So does the segregated housing market. Black civil rights organizations panic and black-owned businesses go belly-up. Meanwhile, white people become obsessed with finding out which whites were born white and which ones have undergone the Black No More procedure. This distinction is important. Changes brought about by Black No More are not hereditary: converted whites will still have black children. (Though, as Crookman notes, Black No More Inc. can change a black child to white in only twenty-four hours.) Max Disher, the book's converted black-to-white hero, must hide his racial origins when he marries a young woman whose father is the Imperial Grand Wizard of the Knights of Nordica. Schuyler dedicated *Black No More* to "all Caucasians in the great republic who can trace their ancestry back ten generations and confidently assert that there are no Black leaves, twigs, limbs or branches on their family tree."

Schuyler's book is more than science fiction or even social satire. It is a political novel that takes on controversial issues of beauty and racial identity. For ethnic minorities in a consumption culture, apparently simple matters of hairstyle or skin cosmetics have a much larger political significance. If you are a black person in a culture whose standards of beauty are determined by the white majority and reinforced by media images and advertising, then even a simple decision to have your hair straightened risks the charge of self-hatred or ethnic betrayal. And if you are a woman, the problem is even more complex, since the very identity of American women has often been bound up with their physical beauty. Both women and ethnic minorities are often made to feel ashamed and inadequate if their appearance deviates from accepted cultural standards.

From an ethical standpoint, the issue is complicated by the fact that Americans tend to think of every moral issue as a matter of personal choice and individual rights. American bioethicists generally frame dilemmas in terms of the autonomy of patients. Thus the bioethics literature is filled with patients who want life-sustaining treatment pitted against doctors who don't want to give it to them, doctors who want to get expensive treatments for their patients versus managed care organizations that keep turning them down, women who want abortions versus religious zealots who want to stop them. Even in the debate over health care reform in the early '90s, Americans turned the debate into a choice between systems that allow patients to *choose* their doctors versus mythical Canadian-style systems that do not. American bioethicists generally presume that unless strong reasons to the contrary are produced, patients should get what they want.

But with cosmetic surgery the problem is different. The problem here is not whether people should get what they want, but why they want what they want, and what happens when they get it. Americans have a hard time resisting anything that can be phrased in terms of self-determination. Autonomy, liberty, freedom: these are among our most powerful words. When they run up against terms like community and solidarity, there is little question which ones will win out. What Schuyler realized, however, was how tightly solidarity and community are bound up with identity. He portrays the black American's dilemma brilliantly by putting autonomy and self-determination at the service of self-betrayal. You can get exactly what you want, says *Black No More*, but the cost will be all the things that have made you what you are. When you lose your appearance, you will also lose your family, your friends, your neighborhoods, and your culture.

Framing moral dilemmas as a matter of resisting oppression is easy when you can identify an individual oppressor: P. W. Botha grinning like a crocodile, Lester Maddox standing in the doorway of his chicken restaurant, stroking his axe handle. But when the oppression is more diffuse, enforced by no laws or regulations, it is harder for resistance to get any purchase. How do you resist aesthetic values that exist nowhere but in people's minds? It is one thing to resist oppressive ideals of beauty when they are championed by the enemy. It is quite another when you are convinced that they are *your* ideals, a part of *your* authentic self; that remaking yourself by the light of these ideals marks the pathway from shame to happiness. How do you resist the oppressor when he has taken up residence in your own head?

IF YOU WERE to look solely at the numbers, you might well conclude that Americans are wildly enthusiastic about cosmetic surgery. Cosmetic surgery is more popular now than at any point in American history. According to the American Society for Aesthetic Plastic Surgery, Americans underwent 4.6 million cosmetic procedures in 1999, a 66 percent increase over the previous year. Part of this steep increase is due to the growing popularity of cosmetic dermatological procedures, such as chemical peels, Botox injections, and laser hair removal. But major surgical procedures are on the rise as well. A study by the American Academy of Cosmetic Surgery found that breast augmentation procedures increased over fourfold during the 1990s, with 255,254 women undergoing breast augmentation in America during 1999. The most popular procedure in 2000 was liposuction, with over 670,000 procedures performed, a tenfold increase from 1990. Another professional society, the American Society of Plastic Surgeons, found that breast augmentations were up 413 percent since 1992, liposuction procedures rose 389 percent, and eyelid surgeries increased 139 percent. These newly modified Americans are apparently very pleased with their new bodies. According to one survey, 82 percent of women and 72 percent of men say they would not be embarrassed if people outside their family knew that they had undergone cosmetic surgery. Another recent headline reads: "Ninety-Seven Percent of Breast Augmentation Patients Happy with Results."[2]

Beneath all this apparent happiness, however, runs an undercurrent of apprehension. Why are so many Americans unhappy with the way they look? Many of these procedures are invasive and painful. Some are quite expensive. Face-lifts, nose jobs, and full-body liposuctions can each cost upward of $8,000. If Americans are willing to risk this much money and discomfort for a better body or face, there must be some powerful reasons behind the choice, and this is precisely what worries many critics of cosmetic surgery. People may not be getting cosmetic surgery for its advantages, but because they desperately dread the alternative: a body or a face of which they are deeply ashamed. For women and ethnic minorities, this shame may come from failing to meet the sexist and racist standards of beauty as defined by the dominant culture. Cosmetic surgery may remedy their shame, but it also reinforces the very racist or sexist standards that fueled the desire for surgery in the first place.

Philosopher Margaret Olivia Little nicely captures the problem of enhancement technologies like cosmetic surgery with the phrase "cultural complicity." The handicaps that enhancement technologies are meant to fix—social inadequacy, stigmatization, shame, problems finding a partner or a job—are the result of social values and attitudes that ought to be changed. Yet not only do enhancement technologies do nothing to improve those attitudes, they may also make them worse. The more breast augmentations that are performed, the more entrenched the preference for large breasts. The more nasal surgeries that are done, the more entrenched the preference for Gentile noses. The more skin lightener and hair straightener that are sold, the more entrenched the preference for white skin and hair. This is why Little uses the word "complicity." These procedures may relieve individual suffering, but in so doing they make the social problem even worse.

The first Americans to seek out cosmetic surgery in significant numbers were Jews who were unhappy with their noses.[3] American surgeons had begun to experiment with nasal cosmetic surgery late in the nineteenth century, and the surgery became popular during the early part of the twentieth century, when America underwent its first wave of immigration from eastern and southern European countries such as Italy, Poland, and Russia. These immigrants wanted to fit in, and fitting in meant effacing the features that were most often caricatured. For Jews, this meant hiding the so-called Jewish nose, a term that had found its way into popular currency by the 1920s. The wish not to look Jewish was not limited to Jews, however. Italians, Greeks, Armenians, Iranians, and Lebanese all feared that a nose of a certain shape would lead to their being mistaken for Jews or another undesirable ethnic minority.[4] The popularity of nasal surgery grew most rapidly during the 1940s, when the dangers of being seen as Jewish were at their peak. Even through the 1960s, over half of all clients seeking nasal surgery were first- or second-generation American Jews.[5]

Not that clients of surgery themselves always saw their choices this way. Most people undergoing nasal surgery simply said they wanted a nose that looked more attractive. Unattractive noses were not always described as "Jewish." Often they were said to be "over-large" or "humped." Plastic surgeons, aware of the racist implications of this kind of surgery, insisted that they were simply doing as their patients asked. They claimed to want nothing more than to help their patients become happier and more attractive.[6] Yet most Americans were aware of the social handicaps that came with looking like an ethnic minority. When actress Fanny Brice had her nose altered in 1923, she claimed that looking Jewish had nothing to do with her decision. But Dorothy Parker said out loud what many Americans secretly thought when she said that Brice "cut off her nose to spite her race."[7] By 1936, Vilbray Blair, a Washington University surgeon and a founder of the American Board of Plastic Surgery, could endorse cosmetic surgery to minimize markers of ethnicity: "Change in the shape of the pronounced Jewish nose may be sought for either social or business reasons."[8]

Asian Americans have undergone similar experiences with surgery for their eyes. Beginning in the mid-twentieth century, Asians began to seek out "blepharoplasty" (cosmetic eye surgery) in order to make their eyes look more like those of Europeans. One of the most popular remedies has been the "double eyelid" procedure, which creates the superior palpebral fold that is naturally present over the eyes of Caucasians, but which is absent from the eyes of many Asians. The double eyelid procedure became popular in Japan after World War II, when the Allied occupation exposed Japanese citizens to Western images of beauty. The military conflicts in Korea and Vietnam had similar effects in those countries. Today, even the People's Republic of China supports a lively cosmetic surgery industry. In America, the double eyelid procedure is the most popular form of cosmetic surgery for Asian Americans, yet surgeons (and many patients) often deny that it is a way of westernizing Asian eyes. Typically, they will say that it is a way of making the eyes look less tired, or the face more open and friendly.[9]

African Americans, on the other hand, have traditionally been less likely than members of other ethnic minorities to seek cosmetic surgery. This may be partly because dark skin is more likely to develop

keloid scars after surgery. It may also be because no amount of surgery will hide dark skin. Historically, the real debate for African
Americans has not been about cosmetic surgery, but about cosmetics.
When George Schuyler wrote *Black No More* in 1931, the cosmetics
industry was a focus of intense political debate within the black community. "Black No More" was, in fact, the name of a skin bleach of
the period.[10] In the preface to his book, Schuyler refers to a popular
hair straightener called "Kink No More," a preparation for the
"immediate and unfailing straightening of the most stubborn Negro
hair."[11] (The name was not entirely accurate, Schuyler points out,
since users of Kink-No-More had to renew the treatment every two
weeks.) Schuyler's criticism was echoed thirty years later in a famous
passage in *The Autobiography of Malcolm X,* where Malcolm
recounts his first and last "conk," a painful procedure that used lye
to straighten black people's hair. "This was my first really big step
toward self-degradation," writes Malcolm, "when I endured all of
that pain, literally burning my flesh to have it look like a white man's
hair."[12]

For many black intellectuals of Schuyler's day, the sale of skin
whiteners, face powders, and hair straighteners represented the worst
form of exploitation. Not only did these products reinforce white
ideals of beauty, they did it by taking money from the black person's
pocketbook. One of the less admirable characters in Schuyler's book
is Madame Sisseretta Blandish, the operator of an ornate hair-
straightening shop. Blandish has been elected vice-president of the
American Race Pride League for the fourth consecutive time,
"because of her prominence as the proprietor of a successful enterprise engaged in making Negroes appear as much like white folks as
possible."[13] Readers in the 1930s would have recognized Blandish as
a thinly disguised caricature of Madam C. J. Walker, the wealthy
founder of a cosmetics empire that sold hair care products to black
Americans. "Look your best," said Madame Walker's ads. "You owe
it to your race."[14] Yet Walker was far from the worst exploiter of
white ideals of beauty. She refused to sell skin bleach, and she emphasized hair care rather than hair straightening.[15] Other firms, many of
them owned by whites, were far less discreet. The white-owned
Plough Chemical Company used explicit, up-from-slavery imagery in

selling its skin bleach. "Bleach Your Dark Skin; Race Men and Women Protect Your Future," said its advertisements. "Be attractive! Throw off the chains that have held you back from the prosperity and happiness that belong to you."[16]

There were good reasons behind the success of these cosmetics, of course: American society gave concrete rewards for light skin and features that looked more "white." Yet it was also true that black society enforced color hierarchies of its own, favoring light skin over dark. Schuyler pokes fun at these hierarchies repeatedly in *Black No More*, especially the black man's preference for light-skinned women. At one point Schuyler's narrator says of two characters: "Both swore there were three things necessary for the happiness of a colored gentleman: yellow money, yellow women and yellow taxis."[17] His caustic remark captures the issue that faced many black Americans of the time, and with which many still struggle today. That issue was not simply staying loyal and resisting white standards of beauty, but also the fact that they had internalized white standards. The oppressor was not just walking the corridors of power in political and corporate America. He had also set up shop in their homes. A person can try to create new ideals of beauty, of course, yet she can only go so far in changing her own preferences, much less those of others. Even progressive blacks of the time who called for new ideals of beauty to counter those of the white majority often seemed unable to imagine what those new ideals might be. When the 1904 issue of the magazine *Voice of the Negro* published a drawing of the "New Negro Woman," notes the historian Kathy Peiss, the woman looked exactly like a white Victorian woman, only with slightly darker skin.[18]

Every society has its own somewhat arbitrary fashions, tastes, and preferences. It is hard to imagine life without them. How do we tell the difference between these ordinary tastes and those that are (as Little puts it) "morally suspect?" Of course, it is not hard to see the difference between social attitudes that say skin looks better without warts and pimples and attitudes that say white skin looks better than dark. But after the obvious examples, matters become more complicated. Is the American preference for women with thin waists and large breasts a suspect standard, or is that just an ordinary standard of beauty? What about the preference for blonde hair or straight teeth? If the culture tells men they look better with big biceps, a washboard stomach, and a hairless back, is this too a sign of cultural oppression?

We can't expect a society to regard everyone as equally attractive, or even equally likely to succeed economically. As Little points out, men who are seven feet tall have opportunities for fame and wealth in America that are unavailable to men who are five feet tall, simply because they live in a country that is crazy about basketball and not about horse racing. Too bad for the short guys, but that is the way the cards fall. The same goes for beauty. Some people, in the eyes of their fellow Americans, look better than others. The less attractive people may be less fortunate, but society can't be blamed for their misfortune. No one would argue that society should be held culpable.

Yet racist standards seem different. One important difference between racist standards and ordinary standards of beauty is the *content* of the standards. A society can make any standard feel oppressive if its members humiliate those poor souls who fail to meet it. But racist standards seem disgraceful and unfair quite apart from the severity with which they are enforced. Racist standards seem more objectionable than the others not because they cause more suffering (the actual suffering they cause may even be less) but because of what they say. For Little, a standard that says dark skin is less attractive than light is worse *in itself* than a standard that says, say, ears look better if they lie flat against your head, or buck teeth are funny-looking, or a pot belly is better kept hidden. Racist standards are offensive because their very content is offensive.

Like many feminist theorists, however, Little goes one step further: when it comes to women, *all* standards of beauty are oppressive. These standards are oppressive not because they are enforced with special brutality, not because women who fail to meet them are singled out for special humiliation, but because these standards are part of a broader sexist ideology. Women, unlike men, have traditionally been defined in terms of their physical appearance. Women's bodies have traditionally counted for more than their minds, and the beauty of that body has been a significant part of female identity. For this reason, Little believes that extensive surgery to bring a woman's body in line with prevailing standards of female beauty—liposuction, cheekbone surgery, rib extraction, breast augmentation—is on a moral par with surgery to make a black person resemble a white one. She writes that for women, "Norms of appearance turn out to be, then, not norms of a *good-looking woman*, but norms of a *good woman*, full stop." This makes them different from norms of attractiveness for men. According to Little, "a man who fails in this category has failed in something that is only incidental to his nature; a woman has sinned against one of her deepest charges."[19]

I am not so sure. Women may have been traditionally defined by their physical appearance, but that does not make standards of women's beauty similar to racist standards. It is not the *content* of these standards that is suspect (the content of the standards of women's beauty have, in fact, changed over the years), but the place held by *any* standard regarding women in the larger social system. Is it the fact that American society has a standard that prefers large breasts to small ones that is the problem, or is it the fact that *any* standard is made so important?

Critical to Little's argument is a distinction between misfortune and injustice, or what is unfortunate and what is unfair. As she puts it in the case of racist standards, "It is no *accident* that the standard of beauty prevalent in the West favors white European features over black African ones. It reflects a long-standing tradition in which being black is devalued and being white in valorised."[20] The key word here is *accident*. The distinction between misfortune and injustice draws on a perceived distinction between accident and conscious human intention. It is unfortunate if you lose your house in a hurricane; it is unjust if I take it from you. It is unfortunate if you lose your shirt in the stock market; it is unjust if I cheat you out of it in a poker game. Bad events can be unjust only if they are the product of conscious intentions. God can be unjust, but the results of nature are merely unfortunate.

But this distinction between unfairness and misfortune becomes much more complicated once we start blaming an entire society rather than a single person. Clearly we are blaming *something*, in the sense of holding it culpable. To say that society should be blamed and held culpable for propping up a suspect standard is to say that the standard is unfair rather than unfortunate. It is to say that being a victim of the standard is more like losing your house to a con man than like losing it to a hurricane. Blame implies agency rather than accident. It suggests that some*one* has acted unjustly.

But who or what, exactly, are we blaming when we blame the society? We are not blaming any single person. We are not even blaming a group of people for acting in a conscious, intentional way. To say that a society's standards of beauty are racist is not like saying that George Wallace and Ross Barnett were racists. It is to say that these racist standards are so entrenched that even the *victims* of oppressive standards have internalized them, often without even realizing it. It is to say that these racist standards are buried deep within other social attitudes and permeate the structure of a society. Of course, many people in a racist society will have acted in an intentionally racist way, but often they are long dead; it is their thought, their ideology, and their institutions that have endured. This account, surely, has some truth to it, but it also blurs the line Little wants to sharpen between misfortune and injustice. If society is to blame, then no one (or everyone) is culpable for the injustice. To blame society is a little like blaming God. You have the satisfaction of pinning the crime on somebody, but you know He is not really going to take the rap.

In practical terms, the problem with blaming society is that idiosyncratic aesthetic preference can almost always be easily redescribed as oppressive ideology. Little named ideologies involving African Americans and women. But she could have also named the poor, the elderly, Jews, American Indians, Asian Americans, Latinos, Arab Americans, gays and lesbians, the transgendered, the intersexed, the disabled, and the Deaf. The class of Americans described as oppressed by an unjust system is constantly expanding. For many, it is very hard to dispute this redescription. The poor *are* victims of an American free market capitalist system in a way that they are not in many other industrialized countries. American Jews *have been* victims of systematic racist violence. In the 1990s Americans such as James L. Byrd, Matthew Shepherd, and Teena Brandon were murdered for their ethnic or sexual identities. Yet it is also true that even privileged Americans can easily call up some aspect of social discrimination with which they can identify—stigmatization of people who are fat, short, shy, or clumsy, who speak with the wrong sort of accent, have the wrong sort of name, or come from the wrong side of the tracks. I never fail to be taken aback by the number of Americans who remember being picked last for sports teams when they were children.

Let me emphasize that I find quite a number of these redescriptions persuasive. I don't want to ally myself with conservative critics who see the victimization mentality as a sign of American moral decay; I just want to point out how many people find these descriptions compelling. For many contemporary Americans, this story of unjust suffering strikes a rich and resonant chord. Stories of oppression or marginalization, of the suffering a people have undergone, of being humiliated or made to feel small—these narratives capture something deeply significant about the way contemporary Americans experience their lives. If there is any single group of Americans that the rest of the country sees as *not* oppressed, as the very opposite of oppressed, it is the group of which I myself am a member—white southern men. Yet if you ever find yourself in South Carolina, just mention the name William Tecumsah Sherman to a white man of a certain age and you may well hear a sermon about the evil visited upon the South when Sherman's army marched through the state over 140 years ago. Stories of injustice and oppression are among the most authoritative narratives of our times.

To see this, try to come up with a case of social suffering in America that *cannot* be redescribed as ideological oppression. It is not easy to do. Little's own case was an imaginary one in the form of a joke: a single-chinned man in a society that admires double chins. An imaginary joke case has the advantage of defusing, in advance, the potential objections that could be raised to a real case by people who see their own suffering mirrored there. The other example that Little mentions in passing is our society's preference for tall men over short men, pointing out that opportunities for fame and wealth are available to very tall men in a way that they are not available for short men. This preference might seem a likely candidate for the kind of idiosyncratic aesthetic preference that a society can legitimately have. Yet when growth hormone for short children was being debated in the mid-1980s, partisans were quick to point out that greater height for men is identified with greater social status, increased physical attractiveness, sexual desirability, business success, and political electability. Short boys face brutal teasing by their peers; short men have more trouble finding wives and partners. Business school graduates over 6 feet tall, it was pointed out, get starting salaries 12.4 percent higher than shorter graduates; college-educated men taller than 6 feet 2 inches have incomes 10 percent higher than those under 6 feet; and when salary differences between men and women are adjusted for height, they disappear. Some commentators noted that the taller candidate had won 80 percent of U.S. presidential elections this century. Of all U.S. presidents, only five have been below average height. Even our language, it was argued, reflects a bias towards height. (When we admire people, we look up to them; when we want to humble them we make them feel small; Heaven is above us, Hell is below; and so on.)[21]

If stigma is a form of oppression, then in America no group has a monopoly on oppression. Some groups are more stigmatized than others, but very few Americans escape it entirely. Sociologist Erving Goffman, for example, thought that almost everyone experienced stigma in some form or another, if only because of the fact that so many people experience the stigma of growing old. Stigma is not a tightly circumscribed condition unique to small groups of marginalized people. "[I]n an important sense," Goffman wrote, "there is only one complete unblushing male in America: a young, married, white, urban, northern, heterosexual Protestant father of college education, fully employed, of good complexion, weight and height, and a recent record in sports."[22]

Being part of an oppressed group has undeniable advantages, of course—you get the sympathy of others and you get the moral high ground.[23] This may be why some people who have not personally experienced oppression are nonetheless tempted to describe themselves as oppressed, attaching themselves to an oppressed group by virtue of shared ethnicity, history, or ancestry. Yet once oppression is connected to markers of identity rather than to direct personal experience of oppression, the number of oppressed people is certain to grow. I am oppressed because my people have been oppressed. I am a victim because other people like me have been victimized. I have a grievance against the North because I am a South Carolinian, a descendant of South Carolinians whose farms were burned and looted by Sherman's troops in 1865. In these narratives of oppression, any connection to a group that can be identified as the oppressor, rather than the oppressed, is conveniently forgotten. Thus southerners like me are apt to describe themselves as victims of northern aggression, not as descendants of white slaveholders.

It is sometimes said that Americans are obsessed with the question of identity, but this is only partly true: Americans worry very little about their national identity *as* Americans (nothing approaching the degree of worry or division apparent in, say, Scotland or Quebec). Yet at the same time, we see individual Americans attaching tremendous importance to their identities *within* various American subgroups, such as ethnic minorities (African Americans, Native Americans, Latinos, Jews), communities centered around sexual identity and orientation (gays, lesbians, the transgendered, the intersexed), groups organized around biology and illness (the Deaf community, disabled rights groups, AIDS and breast cancer activist organizations), and membership in various subcultures (Goths, punks, hackers, skateboarders, surfers, Deadheads, bikers, bodybuilders, etc.). What is notable about these identities is that, unlike an identity *as* an American, most are closely linked to marginalization or oppression. As citizens of one of the wealthiest and most powerful countries in the world, Americans struggle to tell a plausible narrative of oppression *as* Americans. But within a particular American subgroup, that narrative often rings very true.

Some social critics suggest that identity has become so closely bound up with oppression because of the absence of more solid, genuine markers of identity, especially in immigrant countries. As a society assimilates immigrants and minorities it becomes more homogeneous, and the identity of those minorities begins to feel shallower and more superficial. The more assimilated a particular cultural group becomes, and the more social equality that its members attain, the more that group looks like the mainstream. But the more a group looks like the mainstream, the more tenaciously it clings to what makes it different. The pairing of identity and suffering, it is suggested, is part of a larger attempt to climb back out of the melting pot. To reclaim suffering is to connect oneself to a time when identity looked more substantial, to what Kwame Anthony Appiah calls the "rich, old kitchen comforts of ethnicity."[24]

This explanation may fit some ethnic minorities, but it does not explain why other groups embrace narratives of suffering and oppression. It is not only national and ethnic groups who link identity to oppression; it is also a part of gay, lesbian, and transgender identity, of disability rights activism, of the women's movement, of survivor groups, of activist movements of all stripes. The aim of these movements is often not to remember a forgotten identity but to create a new one. If a marker of identity has been regarded as humiliating, limiting, or shameful—being gay, being a woman, being intersexed—then the task is to create an identity in which the marker is seen in a more positive way. These groups may make oppression essential to their identities, but the reason behind the effort seems less a way of connecting with history than a way of connecting with others. It is a way of creating solidarity with those with whom you might otherwise have little in common.

In contrast to the Jim Crow South or apartheid South Africa, much of what is called oppression today is not the threat of actual physical harm or legal injustice, but social stigma. Stigma is largely a matter of shame and embarrassment, of feeling humiliated for some aspect of one's identity. Yet we all have things that we are ashamed of, and a lot of these things are not our fault. Some shameful things we are simply born with, and others we acquire through no effort of our own. We can describe the fact of our shame as a matter of oppressive ideology, and in the sense that society holds certain characteristics (for which we are not responsible) to be shameful, that description will be correct. But when so many shameful characteristics can be redescribed as oppression—when so much misfortune can be transformed into injustice—it is time to start looking into the deeper social structures and attitudes that make these redescriptions plausible.

AT A MEETING a few years ago in Minneapolis, a research group discussing enhancement technologies found itself split over the hypothetical case of an aging woman who is considering a face-lift. As Hilde Lindemann Nelson presented the case, a woman with many years of service to a company is worried that she will be forced out of her job because of her age. The company wants to present a young, energetic face to the world, and this woman is worried that her own aging face will be a handicap. Her job may be at stake. Nelson argued that if this woman were to get a face-lift, she would not necessarily be selling out. A plausible case could be made for the face-lift as an empowering act. By getting the face-lift, she is acting positively rather than allowing others to act upon her. She has taken charge of her situation and used the prevailing norms of beauty for her own ends. The story of caving in to oppression is not the only story that can be told here, argued Nelson; the woman may tell a counterstory of her own.[25]

Of course, many people around the table resisted this spin on the case, especially the women. For them, getting a face-lift was to submit to patriarchal, media-driven ideas of female beauty. It was to give in to an unjust ideology. There followed a spirited back-and-forth about whether a face-lift was an act of moral surrender or a canny manipulation of cultural norms. In the middle of this discussion, all but one of whose participants were white North Americans, came a question from the single non–North American at the table, Jing-Bao Nie, a scholar from China. Nie's question was: What if your new appearance would bother other people? We expect people to take the feelings of others into account when they decide what clothes to wear to work, for example. Doesn't this woman have a duty to consider the feelings of her coworkers?

An embarrassing silence ensued. The group was speechless. The notion that you might be obligated to consult other people before getting a face-lift, particularly your coworkers, was so bizarre to Americans and Canadians that no one knew how to respond. Finally, someone said that the idea of a social system where one had to take into account the feelings of others in such a way struck them as deeply oppressive and morally objectionable.

Many Americans would probably agree. What struck me about Nie's remark, however, was just how dependent on American cultural norms our discussion until that point had been. For the people on one side of the debate, the issue was power and status. If women are going to make any kinds of social gains, this side argued, they must

202 ■ CARL ELLIOTT

take advantage of existing cultural norms. Go for the surgery, they urged. Get what you can, while you can. If this means taking advantage of unjust standards, then so be it: these standards will never be changed until women get more power. For the people on the other side of the table, the issue was about rebellion and nonconformity. Women need to undermine existing cultural standards if they are going to have any chance of succeeding in North American society. To conform to existing cultural standards is to cave in. It is to collude with an unjust system. What we all agreed upon, however—at least until Nie's remark—was our particular way of conceptualizing the debate: losing status versus selling out.

Yet the values on which this conceptualization rests are themselves open to question. If we sympathize with a woman who needs cosmetic surgery to get ahead in life, at least part of the reason we sympathize is because we can imagine feeling the same desire ourselves. And not just the desire to get ahead, but also to get ahead in a particular way; it is revealing that Nelson puts the case in terms of a woman who needed a face-lift for her *job*. I can hardly see the professional women around the table nodding in agreement if the case had been a woman who wanted a face-lift to please her husband. For sheer rhetorical power, even the particular job Nelson describes is well-chosen. The case would probably not have been as persuasive to many feminists if, instead of a face-lift to get ahead at the office, the woman had wanted breast augmentation to boost her career as a stripper.

On the other hand, when we criticize "caving in" to oppressive mainstream ideals of beauty, we are situating that criticism within standards that say social conformity is a form of weakness. According to these standards, to act in conformity with the mainstream is to give up. It is to subordinate yourself to the desires of others. Self-fulfillment comes not by simply accepting the values of the majority, but also by discovering and creating your own. The notion that standards of beauty are oppressive, then, is itself parasitic on other standards of self-reliance and independence. These standards are in turn part of a larger worldview in which rebellion wins out over conformity, independence over self-sacrifice, self-fulfillment over social solidarity.

Take a step back, though, and it is hard to avoid the suspicion that the values on which this critique of oppressive standards rests—independence, self-sufficiency, self-fulfillment—are part of a larger Western ethos that is alien (though perhaps growing more familiar) to a large proportion of the world's population. In Japan, writes Ruth Benedict, conformity is seen as a sign of strength. The weak person gives in to his own wishes and desires, while the strong person is able to resist them in order to fulfill his obligations. "Strength of character," she writes, "is shown in conforming, not rebelling."[26] Calls to resist the mainstream may well be persuasive to me, but like other people born and raised in the United States, I have been primed from an early age to celebrate resistance.

The larger point here is that the problem with cosmetic surgery is not just racism or sexism, not just a matter of unjust ideology; it is also an ethos in which the opinions of other people—especially their opinions about an individual's bodily appearance—have taken on such enormous significance. The irony of our group's reaction to Nie's remark is the form it took: that a social system that required a person to pay attention to the feelings of his or her coworkers would be deeply oppressive. It is ironic because in some important ways this is the system we have in America. We may resent being told that we *ought* to consult with coworkers or friends or even family before getting cosmetic surgery, but in fact, it is our obsessive attention to the opinions of others that pushes us into cosmetic surgery in the first place. We don't feel the need to consult the opinions of others as a moral requirement; rather, we feel their opinions are a barrier to our own personal happiness.

In America the solution to oppressive opinion is to rebel against it, and American protest movements inevitably develop public emblems of rebellion against the strictures enforced by the mainstream. For the women's movement it was foregoing bras and shaved legs; for punks, it was spiked Mohawks and safety pins through the nose; for African Americans, it was the Afro. In his memoir, *Colored People*, Henry Louis Gates Jr. writes, "This people who had spent a couple of hundred years ironing, frying, greasing and burning their hair, doing everything but pulling it out by its roots in an attempt to make it unkinky, had all of a sudden become converts to a new religion, the

Holy Order of the Natural Kink." For them, writes Gates, "An Afro looked like a crown of cultural glory on the right head."[27] Natural hair and dark skin became symbols of racial pride, as well as rebellion against the white mainstream.

Sometimes, of course, the protest works. By the mid-eighties, cosmetic surgeons were reporting that an "ethnic" look was becoming fashionable.[28] So perhaps it should not be all that surprising to hear feminist philosophers such as Kathryn Morgan argue that women should fight against oppressive standards of beauty by enlisting the help of cosmetic surgery itself. In a call for women to "revalorize" ugliness, Morgan suggests that women should have their breasts pulled down, bleach their hair gray, and ask surgeons to induce wrinkles into their faces, all as a way of protesting oppressive standards of beauty. Morgan writes that women can "constitute themselves as culturally liberated subjects through public participation in Ms. Ugly Canada/America/Universe/Cosmos *and use the technology of cosmetic surgery to do so.*"[29]

As a protest strategy, of course, Morgan's suggestion is a little problematic. (Wouldn't cosmetic surgery to promote ugliness be just another way to funnel women's money into the pockets of cosmetic surgeons? Would "revalorized" ugliness still be ugliness, or just another kind of beauty?) This strategy depends not just on the idea of rebellion as liberation (women who bleach their hair gray rather than blonde are "culturally liberated"), but also on the idea that social protest is crucially bound up with self-expression. This idea has become familiar: you express something about yourself, in accordance with the aims and standards of the protest movement, with the expectation that you will be affirmed, if not by the world, then at least by the movement. The difficulty is that this kind of self-expression often becomes subject to the same kind of problems that produced the need for it in the first place. You are still expected to express yourself in accordance with given social standards—not those of the world the movement is rebelling against, but the standards of the movement itself. And of course, these standards can be just as conformist as the ones that they are intended to undermine. Gay men who moved to the Castro in San Francisco in the '70s were, by the end of the decade, complaining of the rigid dress code: Levis, leather vests, boots, short hair, and clipped mustaches, with absolutely no room for deviation. One Castro resident says, "During the 1970s the gay movement here created an almost totalitarian society in the name of sexual freedom."[30]

Goffman noted the psychic costs of this kind of protest, especially the way a new self-presentation may eventually come to feel just as false and stifling as the one it has replaced. As he points out, the stigmatized person who acts and behaves in accordance with the standards of the stigmatized group "will have accepted a self for himself; but this self is, as it necessarily must be, a resident alien, a voice of the group that speaks for and through him."[31] The resident alien manages the oppression of mainstream society by submitting to the rules of the protest movement, yet even as he does so, he surrenders something of his own individual identity.

ASKED TO COMMENT on the social forces that were leading so many women to use tranquilizers in the early 1960s, writer Marya Mannes wrote, "Every woman is deluged daily with urges to attain this impossible state, to buy this, to do that, in order to keep a man and be forever happy. The girl with small breasts is tortured by the fear that men will not love her because of them. Women quail at the first wrinkle, the first grey hair, the thickening of the waist, because they are daily told that these signal the end of attraction."[32] Such anxieties have not gone away in the forty years since Mannes wrote these words, and they will be familiar, in one form or another, to anyone whose appearance fails to measure up to the aesthetic standards current in American culture. The mistake is to assume that this is simply a problem of sexism or racism. The problem is not just that certain people's looks don't meet the standards of the culture, but also that the underlying set of social structures demand so much of self-presentation. In America, your social status is tied to your self-presentation, and if your self-presentation fails, then your status drops. If your status drops, then so does your self-respect. Without self-respect, you cannot be truly fulfilled. If you are not fulfilled, you are not living a truly meaningful life. This is the cruel logic of our particular moral system.

In *The Triumph of the Therapeutic*, Philip Rieff famously argued that the typical American has come to think of himself less as a citizen than as a kind of patient, whose life purpose is to develop, sustain, and fine-tune his psychological well-being. For Rieff, this therapeutic turn is a logical consequence of civic and spiritual decline. Somehow our sense of the purpose of living has slipped out of joint from the social conditions that once sustained it. We are no longer at home with ourselves, never quite comfortable with our place in the world. Instead, we are like castaways on a strange island, unfamiliar with local conditions, unable to rely on the old ways of going on. Perhaps something about the way we live now produces this distance from one another, or perhaps we distance ourselves from one another and live the way we do as a result. Either way, we have become more narcissistic, but narcissistic in a way that is peculiarly dependent on things outside ourselves: that is to say, what other people are saying and thinking about us. Rieff puts it this way, "When so little can be taken for granted, when the meaningfulness of social existence no longer grants an inner life at peace with itself, every man must become something of a genius about himself."[33]

If there is something a little sad about Rieff's diagnosis, there is also something sad about thousands of Americans so unhappy with the way they look that they seek out cosmetic surgery to fix it— aging women going to suburban Botox parties, sixteen-year-old girls getting surgical birthday presents, Michael Jackson's slow morph into a white man. It is the sadness of the stumbling actor, wearing the wrong costume or struggling to play a role for which he is not suited. When we become geniuses about ourselves, the world is important, but it is important mainly in the way that an audience is important: for the way that it reacts to the performer. The audience must applaud at the right times, with an extraordinary degree of enthusiasm; it must laugh at our jokes and feel our pain. It must approve of our performance. When it does not, we are crushed with disappointment.

As long as we live in a society in which a person's own happiness is so dependent on the opinions of others, we will always have the problem of people feeling oppressed by cultural standards. We may be able to detach the problem from racism, so that beauty snobbery is racially egalitarian. We may be able to detach it from sexism, so that men are just as obsessed and fretful about their bodies as women are. We may be able to detach it from social biases against the short, the able-bodied, the gray-haired, and the wrinkled. But the problem will not go away. Like a particularly enthusiastic leech, it will find some other place to attach itself, and the deeper problem will remain untouched. That deeper problem is not simply the problem of racism or sexism (although those are problems too), but the fragility of selves that depend so intimately on the good opinions of others for their survival.

9

AMPUTEES BY CHOICE

I get glimpses of the horror of normalcy.
—Arturo Binewski in *Geek Love*

In January 2000 British newspapers began running articles about Robert Smith, a surgeon at Falkirk and District Royal Infirmary, in Scotland. Smith had amputated the legs of two patients at their request, and he was planning to carry out a third amputation when the trust that runs his hospital stopped him. These patients were not physically sick. Their legs did not need to be amputated for any medical reason. Nor were they incompetent, according to the psychiatrists who examined them. They simply wanted to have their legs cut off. In fact, both the men whose limbs Smith amputated have declared in public interviews how much happier they are, now that they have finally had their legs removed.[1]

Healthy people seeking amputations are not nearly as rare as one might think. In May 1998 a seventy-nine-year-old man from New York traveled to Mexico and paid $10,000 for a black-market leg amputation; he died of gangrene in a motel. In October 1999 a mentally competent man in Milwaukee severed his arm with a homemade guillotine, and then threatened to sever it again if surgeons reattached it. That same month a legal investigator for the California state bar, after being refused a hospital amputation, tied off her legs with tourniquets and began to pack them in ice, hoping that gangrene would set in, necessitating an amputation. She passed out and ultimately gave up. Now she says she will probably have to lie under a train, or shoot her legs off with a shotgun.[2]

For the first time that I am aware of, we are seeing clusters of people seeking voluntary amputations of healthy limbs and performing amputations on themselves. The cases I have identified are merely those that have made the newspapers. On the Internet there are enough people interested in becoming amputees to support a minor industry. One discussion listserv has over 3,200 subscribers.

"It was the most satisfying operation I have ever performed," Smith told a news conference in February 2000. "I have no doubt that what I was doing was the correct thing for those patients."[3] Although it took him eighteen months to work up the courage to do the first amputation, Smith eventually decided that there was no humane alternative. Psychotherapy "doesn't make a scrap of difference in these people," psychiatrist Russell Reid, of Hillingdon Hospital in London, said in a BBC documentary on the subject, called "Complete Obsession."[4] "You can talk till the cows come home; it doesn't make any difference. They're still going to want their amputation, and I know that for a fact." Both Smith and Reid pointed out that these people may unintentionally harm or even kill themselves trying to amputate their own limbs. As retired psychiatrist Richard Fox observed in the BBC program, "Let's face it, this is a potentially fatal condition."

Yet the psychiatrists and the surgeon were all baffled by the desire for amputation. Why would anyone want an arm or a leg cut off? Where does this sort of desire come from? Smith has said that the request initially struck him as "absolutely, utterly weird." "It seemed very strange," Reid told the BBC interviewer. "To be honest, I couldn't quite understand it."

IN 1977, MENTAL health professionals published the first modern case histories of what Johns Hopkins University psychologist John Money termed "apotemnophilia"—an attraction to the idea of being an amputee.[5] Money distinguished apotemnophilia from "acrotomophilia," a sexual attraction to amputees. The suffix -*philia* is important here. It places these conditions in the group of psychosexual disorders called paraphilias, often referred to outside medicine as perversions. Fetishes are fairly common sorts of paraphilias. In the same way that some people are turned on by, say, shoes or animals, others are turned on by amputees. Not by blood or mutilation—pain is not usually what they are looking for. The apotemnophile's desire is to be an amputee, whereas the acrotomophile's desire is turned toward those who happen to be amputees. In the *Bulletin of the Menninger Clinic* that same year, another group of researchers described a patient who would have qualified as both an apotemnophile and an acrotomophile: a twenty-eight-year-old man who was sexually attracted to female amputees, and who intensely wished to be handicapped himself.[6]

I found John Money's papers on amputee attraction at the University of Otago, in Dunedin, New Zealand, shortly after the Falkirk story made the news. Money is an expatriate New Zealander, and he has deposited his collected manuscripts in the Otago medical library. I had gone to Dunedin to work at the university's Bioethics Centre, where I had worked as a postdoctoral fellow in the early 1990s. I had never heard of apotemnophilia or acrotomophilia before the Falkirk story broke. I wondered: Was this a legitimate psychiatric disorder? Was there any chance that it might spread? Like Josephine Johnston, a lawyer from Dunedin who was writing a graduate thesis on the legality of these amputations (and who first brought the Falkirk case to my attention), I also wondered about the ethical and legal status of surgery as a solution. Should amputation be treated like cosmetic surgery, or like invasive psychiatric treatment, or like a risky research procedure?

Reviewing the medical literature, it is easy to conclude that apotemnophilia and acrotomophilia are extremely rare. Fewer than half a dozen articles have been published on apotemnophilia, most of them in arcane journals.[7] Most psychiatrists and psychologists I have spoken with—even those who specialize in paraphilias—have never heard of apotemnophilia. On the Internet, however, it is an entirely different story. Acrotomophiles are known on the Web as "devotees," and apotemnophiles are known as "wannabes." "Pretenders" are people who are not disabled but use crutches, wheelchairs, or braces, often in public, in order to feel disabled. Various Web sites sell photographs and videos of amputees, display stories and memoirs, recommend books and movies, and provide chat rooms, meeting points, and electronic bulletin boards. Much of this material caters to devotees, who seem to be far greater in number than wannabes. It is unclear just how many people out there actually want to become amputees, but there exist numerous wannabe and devotee listservs and Web sites.

Like Robert Smith, I have been struck by the way wannabes use the language of identity and selfhood in describing their desire to lose a limb. "I have always felt I should be an amputee." "I felt, this is who I was." "It is a desire to see myself, be myself, as I 'know' or 'feel' myself to be." This kind of language has persuaded many clinicians that apotemnophilia has been misnamed—that it is not a problem of sexual desire, as the -philia suggests, but a problem of body image. What true apotemnophiles share, Smith said in the BBC documentary, is the feeling "that their body is incomplete with their normal complement of four limbs." Smith has elsewhere speculated that apotemnophilia is not a psychiatric disorder but a neuropsychological one, with biological roots.[8] Perhaps it has less to do with desire than with being stuck in the wrong body.

Yet what exactly does it mean to be stuck in the wrong body? Even people who use more conventional enhancement technologies often use the language of self and identity to explain why they want these interventions: a woman who says she is "not herself" unless she is on Prozac; a bodybuilder who says he took anabolic steroids because he wants to look on the outside the way he feels on the inside; a transsexual who describes her experience as "being trapped in the wrong body." The image is striking, and more than a little odd. In each case the true self is the one produced by medical science.

Some people are inclined to think of this language as a literal description. Maybe some people really do feel as if they have found their true selves on Prozac. Maybe they really did feel incomplete without cosmetic surgery. Yet it may be better to think of these descriptions not as literally true but as expressions of an ambivalent moral ideal—a struggle between the impulse toward self-improvement and the impulse to be true to oneself. Not that I can see no difference between a middle-aged man rubbing Rogaine on his head every morning and a man whose discomfort in his own body is so all-consuming that he begins to think of suicide. But we shouldn't be surprised when any of these people, healthy or sick, use phrases like "becoming myself" and "I was incomplete" and "the way I really am" to describe what they feel, because the language of identity and selfhood surrounds us. This is simply the language we use now to describe the way we live.

P ERHAPS THE QUESTION to be answered is not only why people who want to be amputees use the language of identity to describe what they feel, but also what exactly they are using it to describe. One point of contention among clinicians is whether apotemnophilia is, as John Money thought, really a paraphilia. "I think that John Money confused the apotemnophiles and the acrotomophiles," Robert Smith wrote to me from Scotland. "The devotees I think are paraphilic, but not the apotemnophiles." The question here is whether we should view apotemnophilia as a problem of sexual desire—a variety of the same genre of conditions that includes pedophilia, voyeurism, and exhibitionism. Smith, in agreement with many of the wannabes I have spoken with, believes that apotemnophilia is closer to gender-identity disorder, the diagnosis given to people who wish to live as the opposite sex. Like these people, who are uncomfortable with their identities and want to change sex, apotemnophiles are uncomfortable with their identities and want to be amputees.

But deciding what counts as apotemnophilia is part of the problem in explaining it. Some wannabes are also devotees. Others who identify themselves as wannabes are drawn to extreme body modification. There seems to be some overlap between people who want finger and toe amputations and those who seek piercing, scarring, branding, genital mutilation, and such. Some wannabes, Robert Smith suggests, want amputation as a way to gain sympathy from others. And finally, there are "true" apotemnophiles, whose desire for amputation is less about sex than about identity. "My left foot was not part of me," says one amputee, who had wished for amputation since the age of eight. "I didn't understand why, but I knew I didn't want my leg."[9] Another says, "My body image has always been as a woman who has lost both her legs."[10] A woman in her early forties wrote to me, "I will never feel truly whole with legs." Her view of herself has always been as a double amputee, with stumps of five or six inches.

Many devotees and wannabes describe what Lee Nattress, an adjunct professor of social work at Loma Linda University, in California, calls a "life-changing" experience with an amputee as a child. "When I was three years old, I met a young man who was completely missing all four of his fingers on his right hand," writes a twenty-one-year-old woman who says she is planning to have both her arms amputated. "Ever since that time, I have been fascinated by all amputees, especially women amputees who were missing parts of their arms and wore hook prostheses."[11] Hers is not an unusual story. Most wannabes trace their desire to become amputees back to before the age of six or seven, and some will say that they cannot remember a time when they didn't have the desire. Nattress, who surveyed fifty people with acrotomophilia (he prefers the term "amelotasis") for a 1996 doctoral dissertation, says that much the same is true for devotees. Three quarters of the devotees he surveyed were aware of their attraction by the age of fifteen, and about a quarter wanted to become amputees themselves.[12]

Many of the news reports about the case at the Falkirk and District Royal Infirmary identified Smith's patients as having extreme cases of body dysmorphic disorder. Like people with anorexia nervosa, who believe themselves to be overweight even as they become emaciated, people with body dysmorphic disorder are preoccupied with what they see as a physical defect: thinning hair, nose shape, facial asymmetry, the size of their breasts or buttocks. They are often anxious and obsessive, constantly checking themselves in mirrors and shop windows, or trying to disguise or hide the defect. They are often convinced that others find them ugly. Sometimes they seek out cosmetic surgery, but frequently they are unhappy with the results and ask for more surgery. Sometimes they redirect their obsession to another part of the body.[13] But none of this really describes most of the people who are looking for amputations—who, typically, are not convinced they are ugly, do not imagine that other people see them as defective, and are usually focused exclusively on amputation (rather than on, say, a receding hairline or bad skin). Amputee wannabes more often see their limbs as normal, but as a kind of surplus. Their desires frequently come with chillingly precise specifications: for instance, an above-the-knee amputation of the right leg.

Like many conditions, it is not clear whether the desire to be an amputee is new, or whether it is merely taking a new shape in response to changing cultural conditions. The psychiatrist Douglas Price has unearthed and translated a 1785 text by the French surgeon and anatomist Jean-Joseph Sue that describes an Englishman who may have been both a wannabe and a devotee. The Englishman was in love with a woman who was an amputee, and wanted to become an amputee himself. He offered 100 guineas to a French surgeon to amputate his healthy leg. The surgeon refused, protesting that he did not have the proper equipment. But he changed his mind when the Englishman produced a gun, and then he proceeded to amputate the Englishman's leg under threat of death. Later he received a letter in the mail, along with payment for the amputation. "You have made me the happiest of all men," explained the Englishman, "by taking away from me a limb which put an invincible obstacle to my happiness."[14]

When John Money designated apotemnophilia a "paraphilia," he placed it in a long and distinguished lineage of psychosexual disorders. The grand old man of psychosexual pathology, Richard von Krafft-Ebing, cataloged an astonishing range of paraphilias in his 1906 classic *Psychopathia Sexualis*, from necrophilia and bestiality to fetishes for aprons, handkerchiefs, and kid gloves. Some of his cases involve an attraction to what he called "bodily defects." One was a twenty-eight-year-old engineer who had been excited by the sight of women's disfigured feet since the age of seventeen. Another had pretended to be lame since early childhood, limping around on two brooms instead of crutches. The philosopher René Descartes, Krafft-Ebing noted, was partial to cross-eyed women.[15]

Yet the term "sexual fetish" could be a misleading way to describe the fantasies of wannabes and devotees, if what is on the Web is any indication (and, of course, it might well not be). Many of these fantasies seem almost presexual. This is not to suggest that there is any shortage of amputee pornography on the Internet. *Penthouse* has published in its letters section many of what it terms "monopede mania" letters, purportedly from devotees, and *Hustler* has published an article on amputee fetishism. But many other amputee Web sites have an air of thoroughly wholesome middle-American hero worship, and perhaps for precisely that reason they are especially disconcerting, like a funeral parlor in a shopping mall. Some show disabled men and women attempting nearly impossible feats—running marathons, climbing mountains, creating art with prostheses. It is as if the fantasy of being an amputee is inseparable from the idea of achievement—or, as one of my correspondents put it, from an "attraction to amputees as role models." "I've summed it up this way," John Money said, a little cruelly, in a 1975 interview: "Look, Ma, no hands, no feet, and I still can do it."[16] One woman, then a forty-two-year-old student and housewife whose history Money presented in a 1990 research paper, said one of the appeals of being an amputee was "coping heroically."[17] A man told Money that his fantasy was that of "compensating or overcompensating, achieving, going out and doing things that one would say is unexpectable."[18] One of my wannabe correspondents wrote that what attracted him to being an amputee was not heroic achievement so much as "finding new ways of doing old tasks, finding new challenges in working things out and perhaps a bit of being able to do things that are not always expected of amputees."

I AM ON the phone with Max Price, a graphic designer in Santa Fe, who has offered to talk to me about apotemnophilia. (He has asked me to change his name and the details of his life and history if I write about him, and I have.) Price is a charming man, articulate and well read, and despite my initial uneasiness about calling him, I am enjoying our conversation. I had corresponded by e-mail with a number of wannabes, but had not managed to talk to any of them until now. The conversation has taken on an easy intellectual tone, more like a discussion between colleagues than an interview. Price is telling me about his efforts to get doctors to adopt some guidelines for deciding when a person with apotemnophilia should have surgery. I am tossing out ideas, trying out some of my thoughts, and I won-

der aloud about a relationship between apotemnophilia and obsessive-compulsive disorder. I ask Price whether he feels that his desire
is more like an obsession, a fantasy, or a wish. He says, "Well, it was
definitely like an obsession. Until I cut my leg off, of course."

That brings me up short. I had been unaware that he had actually
gone ahead with an amputation. "Ah," I say. I pause. Should I ask? I
decide I should. "May I ask how you did it?" Price laughs. "It was
kind of messy," he says. "I did it with a log splitter." He then
explains, in a thoughtful, dispassionate manner, the details of his
"accident" ten years ago—the research he had done on anesthesia
and wound control, how he had driven himself to the emergency
room after partially amputating his limb, the efforts of the hospital
surgeons to reattach it. He lived with the reattached leg for six
months, he said, until medical complications finally helped him persuade another surgeon to amputate it.

I met Price through an Internet discussion listserv called
"amputee-by-choice," one of the larger lists. At first I had simply
prowled through the archives and listened to the ongoing conversation. I found many of the archived messages very creepy. Here were
people exchanging photographs of hands with missing fingers; spec-
ulating about black-market amputations in Russia; debating the merits of industrial accidents, gunshot wounds, self-inflicted gangrene,
chain-saw slips, dry ice, and cigar cutters as means of getting rid of
their limbs and digits. When I introduced myself to the active electronic group, however, the discussion abruptly stopped, like the conversation in a village pub when a stranger walks in. For several days
only a handful of new messages were posted. But I had invited
wannabes to get in touch with me individually, telling them that I was
a university professor working on apotemnophilia, and over the next
few days a dozen or so people responded. Some, like Price, were
insightful and articulate. Some had become mental-health professionals, in part as a way of trying to understand their desires. The few
who had managed an amputation seemed (somewhat to my surprise)
to have made peace with their desires. But others obviously needed
help: they were obsessive, driven, consumed. Many seemed to have
other psychiatric problems: clinical depression, obsessive-compulsive
disorder, eating disorders, transvestism of a type that sounded any-

thing but playful or transgressive. They did not trust psychiatrists. They did not want medication. They wanted to know if I could find them a surgeon. I felt like an ethnographer in a remote country, unfamiliar with the local customs, whom the natives believe can help them. I began to understand how Robert Smith must have felt. I also began to wonder at the strength of a desire that would take people to such lengths.

By all accounts, the Internet has been revolutionary for wannabes. I can see why. It took me months to track down even a handful of scientific articles on the desire for amputation. It took about ten seconds to find dozens of Web sites devoted to the topic. Every one of the wannabes and devotees I have talked with about the Internet says that it has changed everything for them. "My palms were actually sweating the first time I typed 'amputee' into a search engine," one wannabe wrote to me. But the results were gratifying. "It was an epiphany," she wrote. When Krafft-Ebing was writing *Psychopathia Sexualis*, people with unusual desires could live their entire lives without knowing that there was anyone else in the world like them. Today all it takes is a computer terminal. On the Internet you can find a community to which you can listen or reveal yourself, and instant validation for your condition, whatever it may be. This same wannabe told me that she has never spoken about her desire for amputation with a friend, a family member, or a mental-health professional, and that she never will. Yet she is a frequent anonymous participant on the wannabe discussion listserv.

"The Internet was, for me, a validation experience," writes a wannabe who is also a transsexual. She says she found herself thinking less about amputation after logging on, because her desire was no longer such a dark secret. "When one is afraid of discovery, I think one thinks rather more about the secret in order to guard against accidental revelation." She also points out that the Internet helped her get information on how to lose her legs. Another wannabe, a therapist, says that discovering the Internet was a mixed blessing. "There was a huge hole to be filled," she told me, and the Internet began to fill it. To discover that she was not alone was wonderful— but it also meant that a desire she had managed to push to the back of her mind now shoved its way to the front again. It occupied her conscious thoughts in a way that was uncomfortable. She says she knows wannabes who subscribe to as many as a dozen wannabe and devotee on-line mailing lists and spend hours every day wading through electronic messages.

In his book *Stigma*, Erving Goffman writes about the way that most stigmatized groups, even as they are set apart from mainstream society, will find a group of people who share their particular standpoint in the world.[19] So that at the same time that the stigmatized person is cut off from the world of so-called normal people, who see the stigmatized person as deviant or subnormal, this group of sympathetic others reassure him that he is essentially human and normal despite his own self-doubts. We applaud this if the stigma comes from being part of a racial minority, or from being deaf, from having AIDS, but we worry if the stigma is something like dangerous drug use or pedophilia. Wannabes appear to be finding this kind of sympathetic group on the Internet. They thought they were alone, they thought they were crazy, and this group reassures them that they are not. From a therapeutic point of view, this kind of community-building may have mixed results. It gives the wannabes solidarity, but it also nourishes and shapes a desire that might otherwise wither away or take another form.

Sociologists and media theorists have named these on-line groups "virtual communities."[20] But if these groups are communities, they are a very odd kind of community. They are really more like clubs, in that they are bound up around a particular interest or characteristic, or the participants come together for a particular purpose. In the 1950s, the anthropologist Victor Turner described a phenomenon called "cults of affliction."[21] Turner's fieldwork was in Zambia, among a group called the Ndembu. In the Ndembu cosmology, sickness and misfortune were caused by sorcerers, witches, or ancestor-spirits. If a person was sick it was because a spirit had "caught" him in some misdemeanor or another. The way to deal with the sickness was to perform what Turner called a "ritual of affliction." Different ancestor-spirits caused different afflictions: one caused leprosy, another caused menstrual problems, another caused twin births. Sometimes, if it was not obvious, a diviner was needed to tell you which spirit was causing your problems.

The interesting thing about these rituals, for Turner, was who took part in them. You needed a doctor, but the doctor had to gather together a group of people who had also been afflicted with the sickness. This group of people then performed a ritual on behalf of the sick person. The significant thing about these groups was that they transcended any other sort of grouping. They were not members of the same family, the same tribe, the same village, or the same clan. The only thing they had in common was that they had suffered from the same sickness, and had been treated by the same kind of group. This was what Turner called "cults of affliction."

Without trying to draw too tight a parallel here, some anthropologists have seen a similar phenomenon occurring in American culture today.[22] People with illnesses are coming together in support groups, self-help groups, and activist groups, all of which are organized solely around a particular illness or disability. They have different purposes, of course, different from one another and different from Turner's cults of affliction, but there is one important parallel, and that is the composition of the group. The members of these groups are not from the same family, don't work together, don't come from the same town or region, don't necessarily share a common ethnicity or religious background. What they do share is a common experience of illness.

Something similar may be occurring with wannabes. What they share is a desire—maybe a fetish, maybe an obsession, maybe a disorder—that has become a problem for them. It is a problem at least partly because it has to be kept secret. The Internet does a couple of things for them. First, because the desire is so rare, it is unlikely that most wannabes would ever spontaneously meet another wannabe. But the Internet brings the wannabes together, on-line if not in person. Second, on-line groups allow participants to take part in secret. Many wannabes participate in on-line groups anonymously. So they get both the comfort and satisfaction of being part of a group, and knowing they are not alone in the world, while also avoiding the potential shame of actually having to reveal themselves to anyone else face-to-face.

But how should their shared desire be characterized? Some argue that the desire to have a limb amputated is no different in principle from the desires motivating other enhancement technologies, like cosmetic surgery. In the same way that a person might want to have healthy tissue removed through breast-reduction surgery, so an amputee wannabe wants to have healthy tissue removed through amputation. Cosmetic surgery is certainly not prohibited by law, and the courts have even allowed healthy organs and other tissue to be removed for medical purposes deemed worthwhile, such as the transplantation of a kidney, bone marrow, or a liver lobe from a healthy donor into a needy recipient. (Courts have allowed such transplantations even when the donor is a child or a mentally impaired adult.) [23] But others believe that the desire to have a limb amputated qualifies, at least in some cases, as a psychiatric illness, for which surgery is a potentially effective treatment. On purely pragmatic grounds, this second strategy may be the best way for wannabes to get surgeons to cooperate with them—to have the desire for amputation recognized as a mental disorder, codified in the forthcoming *DSM-V*, reported on in respected medical journals, and legitimated with diagnostic instruments, reimbursement codes, and specialty clinics.

SOME CLINICIANS DO not like to admit it, but even wannabes who describe the desire for amputation as a wish for completeness will often admit that there is a sexual undertone to the desire. "For me having one leg improves my own sexual image," one of my correspondents wrote. "It feels 'right,' the way I should always have been and for some reason in line with what I think my body ought to have been like." When I asked one wannabe (who also happens to be a psychologist) if he experiences the wish to lose a limb as a matter of sex or a matter of identity, he disputed the very premise of the question. "You live sexuality," he told me. "I am a sexual being twenty-four hours a day." Even ordinary sexual desire is bound up with identity, as I was reminded by Michael First, a psychiatrist at Columbia University, who was an editor of the fourth edition of the American Psychiatric Association's *Diagnostic and Statistical Manual*. First is undertaking a study that will help determine whether apotemnophilia should be included in the fifth edition of the *DSM*. "Think of the fact that, in general, people tend to be more sexually attracted to members of their own racial group," he pointed out. What you are attracted to (or not attracted to) is part of who you are.

It is clear that for many wannabes, the sexual aspect of the desire is much less ambiguous than many wannabes and clinicians have publicly admitted. A man described seventeen years ago in the *American Journal of Psychotherapy* said that he first became aware of his attraction to amputees when he was eight years old. That was in the 1920s, when the fashion was for children to wear short pants. He remembered several boys who had wooden legs. "I became extremely aroused by it," he said. "Because such boys were not troubled by their mutilation and cheerfully, and with a certain ease, took part in all the street games, including football, I never felt any pity towards them." At first he nourished his desire by seeking out people with wooden legs, but as he grew older, the desire became self-sustaining. "It has been precisely in these last years that the desire has gotten stronger, so strong that I can no longer control it but am completely controlled by it." By the time he finally saw a psychotherapist, he was consumed by the desire. Isolated and lonely, he spent some of his time hobbling around his house on crutches, pretending to be an amputee, fantasizing about photographs of war victims. He was convinced that his happiness depended on getting an amputation. He desperately wanted his body to match his self-image: "Just as a transsexual is not happy with his own body but longs to have the body of another sex, in the same way I am not happy with my present body, but long for a peg-leg."[24]

The comparison of limb amputation to sex-reassignment surgery comes up repeatedly in discussions of apotemnophilia, among patients and among clinicians. "Transsexuals want healthy parts of their body removed in order to adjust to their idealized body image, and so I think that was the connection for me," psychiatrist Russell Reid stated in the BBC documentary "Complete Obsession." "I saw that people wanted to have their limbs off with equally as much degree of obsession and need and urgency."[25] The comparison is not hard to grasp. When I spoke with Michael First, he told me that his group was considering calling it "amputee identity disorder," a name with obvious parallels to the gender-identity disorder that is the diagnosis given to prospective transsexuals. The parallel extends to amputee pretenders, who, like cross-dressers, act out their fantasies by impersonating what they imagine themselves to be.

But gender-identity disorder is far more complicated than the "trapped in the wrong body" summary would suggest. For some patients seeking sex-reassignment surgery, the wish to live as a member of the opposite sex is itself a sexual desire. Ray Blanchard, a psychologist at the University of Toronto's Center for Addiction and Mental Health, has studied men being evaluated for sex-reassignment surgery. He has found an intriguing difference between two groups: men who are homosexual and men who are heterosexual, bisexual, or asexual. The "woman trapped in a man's body" tag fit the homosexual group relatively well. As a rule, these men had no sexual fantasies about being a woman; only a small percentage say they are sexually excited by cross-dressing, for example. Their main sexual attraction is to other men.[26]

Not so for the men in the other group: almost all are excited by fantasies of being a woman. Three-quarters of them are sexually excited by cross-dressing. Blanchard coined the term "autogynephilia"—"the propensity to be sexually aroused by the thought or image of oneself as a woman"—as a way of designating this group. Note the suffix -philia. Blanchard thought that a man might be sexually excited by the fantasy of being a woman in more or less the same way that people with paraphilias are sexually excited by fantasies of wigs, shoes, handkerchiefs, or amputees. But here sexual desire is all about sexual identity—the sexual fantasy is not about someone or something else, but about yourself. Anne Lawrence, a transsexual physician and a champion of Blanchard's work, calls this group "men trapped in men's bodies."[27]

If sexual desire, even paraphilic sexual desire, can be directed toward one's own identity, then perhaps it is a mistake to try to distinguish pure apotemnophilia from the kind that is contaminated with sexual desire. Reading Blanchard's work, I was reminded of a story that Peter Kramer tells in his introduction to *Listening to Prozac*. Kramer describes a middle-aged architect named Sam who came to him with a prolonged depression set off by business troubles and the deaths of his parents. Sam was charming, unconventional, and a sexual nonconformist. He was having marital trouble. One of the conflicts in his marriage was his insistence that his wife watch hard-core pornographic videos with him, although she had little taste for them. Kramer prescribed Prozac for Sam's depression, and it worked. But one of the unexpected side-effects was that Sam lost his desire for hard-core porn. Not the desire for sex: his libido was undiminished. Only the desire for pornography went away.[28]

Antidepressants like Prozac have long been used to treat compulsive desires, and some clinicians are also starting to use them for patients with paraphilias and sexual compulsions.[29] Can an antidepressant selectively knock out an aberrant or unwanted sexual desire, while leaving ordinary sexual desire intact? Even more interesting, though, is the way in which Sam came to view his desire. Before treatment he had thought of his taste for porn simply as part of who he was—an independent, sexually liberated guy. Once it was gone, however, it seemed as if it had been a biologically driven obsession. "The style he had nurtured and defended for years now seemed not a part of him but an illness," Kramer writes. "What he had touted as independence of spirit was a biological tic." Does this suggest that erotic desire is simply a matter of biology? Not necessarily. What it suggests is that an identity can be built around a desire. The person you have become may be a consequence of the things you desire. This may be as true for wannabes as it was for Sam, especially if their desires have been with them for as long as they can remember.

The link between identity, deformity, and erotic desire is explored in Katherine Dunn's *Geek Love*, a novel that occasionally pops up on devotee and wannabe book lists.[30] *Geek Love* tells the story of a carnival family conceived through the ingenuity of Al and Lil Binewski. Lil, the family matriarch, has ingested pesticides, radioactive materials, and a variety of drugs in order to produce children who are special: Iphigenia and Electra, piano-playing conjoined twins; Olympia, the bald albino hunchback dwarf who narrates the story; Chick, who has telekinetic powers; and Arturo the Aqua Boy, who was born with flippers instead of arms and legs. Arty, the undisputed star of the carnival, swims and frolics in an aquarium and then preaches dark, enigmatic sermons to his assembled admirers. "If I had arms and legs and hair like everybody else, do you think I'd be happy? NO! I would not!" he shouts to his audience. "Because then I'd worry did somebody love me! I'd have to look outside myself to find out what to think of myself!"

Arty's charisma eventually propels him into the leadership of an Arturan Cult, whose members tithe parts of their body in order to become more like him. His assistant, a rogue surgeon by the name of Dr. Phyllis, amputates the digits and limbs of enthusiastic Arturans. Off come toes and fingers, then hands and feet, and finally, as converts approach ecstatic completeness, all four limbs in their entirety. "Can you be happy with the movies and the ads and the clothes in the stores and the doctors and the eyes as you walk down the street all telling you there is something wrong with you?" Arty asks a blubbering fat woman in the audience, like a preacher making an altar call. "No. You can't. You cannot be happy. Because, you poor darling baby, you believe them." Soon his caravan is trailed by thousands of armless and legless disciples, living in tents, begging for food, waiting patiently for another turn in the operating room with Dr. Phyllis.

Geek Love is an odd choice for a devotee or wannabe reading list. It is brutal in its mockery of amputee wannabes. Yet it makes sense of a darker side of American life that often goes unexplored in the mainstream media. The media generally treat the desire for body modification either as the well-worn terrain of fashion slaves and social strivers, who buy cosmetic surgery in an endless quest for beauty and perpetual youth, or as something bizarre and unexplainable, like genital mutilation or masochistic fetishes. *Geek Love* makes the desire for amputation plausible by setting it against the bland, cheery aesthetic of mainstream American beauty. *Geek Love* may mock amputee wannabes, but it does not mock them for their poor taste. The aesthetic sensibility of *Geek Love* comes straight out of a carnival sideshow. Its heroes are not "norms," as ordinary Americans are called in the book, but the freaks of the Binewski Carnival Fabulon. "We are masterpieces," Olympia says when asked if she would like to be a norm. "Why would I want to change us into assembly-line items? The only way you people can tell each other apart is by your clothes."

The *Geek Love* aesthetic is not as marginal as the mainstream media might lead us to think. To browse even a handful of devotee Web sites and discussion groups is to be made aware of an immense amount of pop culture imagery surrounding amputation and disability. Much of it is innocent, of course (Captain Hook, Long John Silver, Barbie's wheelchair-bound friend Becky), and perhaps even more concerns the legitimate needs of involuntary amputees and other disabled people. But a surprising amount of it skirts close to the erotic interests of devotees and wannabes. Take the 1927 silent film *The Unknown*, for example, in which Lon Chaney plays a circus performer who amputates his arms to win the love of Joan Crawford. Or the 1968 film *Beguiled*, where Clint Eastwood plays a Union soldier who is wounded and nursed back to health in a girl's school in the South during the war. When one of the girls seduces him, the headmistress drugs him and amputates his leg. The South, in fact, seems to be an especially fertile place for amputee imagery. In "The Man with the Hardest Belly" by the South Carolina poet Paul Allen, a family travels to the riverside to hear a sermon by a quadruple amputee preacher. ("Nail me to the cross!" the preacher shouts. "Nails wouldn't work," murmurs a man in the congregation. "Toggle bolts might work.") A famous Flannery O'Connor story, "Good Country People," concerns a traveling Bible salesman who seduces a pretentious Georgia amputee in order to steal her prosthetic leg.

The world that comes closest to the darkly comic *Geek Love* aesthetic may be that of extreme body modification: piercing, scarification, tattooing, tongue-splitting, hook suspensions, and genital modifications.[31] For many years this kind of body modification was associated mainly with pornography and sadomasochism, but over the past decade or two it has blossomed into a thriving subculture. Many of the ritual adornments associated with extreme body modification are consciously borrowed from indigenous peoples—Maori facial tattoos, for instance, or the southeast Asian ampallang, a barbell stud inserted through the head of the penis. I have found little evidence of limb amputations within the extreme body modification movement, but some people have had digit amputations, penectomies, or castrations. Many modifications have an erotic element to them (nipple piercing, labial rings, penis studs) and also a strong social element, especially as Internet communities have gathered momentum. But as the godfather of the "modern primitives" movement, Fakir Musafar, points out, there is a spiritual element too. The mission statement for The Church of Body Modification, an interna-

tional organization whose members practice "ancient body modification rites," says that it "was formed for the body modification community to reconnect with the roots of our spirituality within our
culture."[32] Some "modern primitives," in imitation of (or tribute to)
the Plains Indian sun dance rituals, insert hooks in their chests or
backs and suspend themselves from trees as a means to achieve spiritual transcendence. Raelyn Gallina, a San Francisco piercer, says,
"I'd say 95 out of 100 people will end up saying it's (piercing) been
a spiritual act."[33]

The language of identity is as common with extreme body modification as it is elsewhere in the culture. When Anton LaVey, founder of
the Church of Satan in San Francisco, was asked in the late '80s why
people get piercing or tattoos, he could have been quoting Arty in
Geek Love. "[I]f a person feels alienated," said LaVey, "if they didn't
happen to be *born* looking freaky or strange, then activities like getting a tattoo are a way of stigmatizing one's self. . . . In other words,
people set up a certain stigma that says, 'Watch out for me—I'm dangerous!'—like the hourglass on the black widow's belly."[34] Extreme
body modifications are often intended to shock others; unlike cosmetic surgery, which people often undertake so that they can become
ordinary and blend in, people who undergo extreme body modification often do it to stand out.[35] Much of it has a strong element of
showmanship and public display. Suspensions and hook pullings are
videotaped; tattoos and studs are placed on the most visible parts of
the body; photographs are taken of genital modifications and posted
on the Web. This desire for display sets extreme body modification
apart from the amputations desired by many wannabes. Wannabes
usually harbor their desires in secret, and often have no wish to go
public.

Yet over the past ten years or so the aesthetic backdrop to all these
body modifications has changed dramatically. In the late 1980s,
LeVay could talk about "stigmatizing" himself with a tattoo or a
facial piercing and still be taken seriously. Today boutique surgical
clinics sell labial modifications to upscale California suburbanites,
and the smiling teenager behind the counter at the grocery store
probably has an eyebrow ring and a tongue stud. The book *Modern
Primitives*, once an underground guide to procedures like the "Prince

Albert," in which a ring is inserted through the urethra at the base of
the penis head, or the even more alarming "split Jimmy," is now
available at my local public library. "Oh, I haven't seen this book for
ages!" said the smiling librarian when I checked it out. She had
orange hair, a lip ring, and a tattoo on the back of her hand. For a
recent seminar on enhancement technologies, I invited an articulate
young student at a local Lutheran liberal arts college. His tongue was
split in two; the skin under his arm was filled with Teflon beads; and
tattoos and studs covered his face and tongue. As he showed us a
video of himself dangling from a tree by hooks in his back, he casu-
ally threaded a pencil through the hole in the septum of his nose.
Such are the rhythms of American life. In 1989, it was sadomasochism, underground porn, and the Church of Satan. In 2002, it
is Lutheran college students and Midwestern librarians.

EVEN IF WE assume that the obsessive desire for amputation is
evidence of a psychiatric disorder, it is unclear why such a desire
should be growing more common just now. Why do certain psychopathologies arise, seemingly out of nowhere, in certain societies
and during certain historical periods, and then disappear just as suddenly? Why did young men in late-nineteenth-century France begin
lapsing into fugue states, wandering the continent with no memory of
their past, coming to themselves months later in Moscow or Algiers
with no idea how they got there? What was it about America in the
1970s and 1980s that made it possible for thousands of Americans
and their therapists to come to believe that two, ten, even dozens of
personalities could be living in the same head? One does not have to
imagine a cunning cult leader to envision alarming numbers of desperate people asking to have their limbs removed. One has only to
imagine the right set of historical and cultural conditions.

So, at any rate, suggests the philosopher and historian of science
Ian Hacking, who has attempted to explain just how "transient mental illnesses" such as the fugue state and multiple-personality disorder arise.[36] A transient mental illness is by no means an imaginary
mental illness, though in what ways it is real (or "real," as the social
constructionists would have it) is a matter for philosophical debate.
A transient mental illness is a mental illness that is limited to a cer-

tain time and place. It finds an "ecological niche," as Hacking puts it. In the same way that the idea of an ecological niche helps to explain why the polar bear is adapted to the Arctic ecosystem, or the chigger to the South Carolina woods, Hacking's ecological niches help to explain the conditions that made it possible for multiple-personality disorder to flourish in late-twentieth-century America and the fugue state to flourish in nineteenth-century Bordeaux. If the niche disappears, the mental illness disappears along with it.

Hacking does not intend to rule out other kinds of causal mechanisms, such as traumatic events in childhood and neurobiological processes. His point is that a single causal mechanism isn't sufficient to explain psychiatric disorders, especially those contained within the boundaries of particular cultural contexts or historical periods. Even schizophrenia, which looks very much like a brain disease, has changed its form, outlines, and presentation from one culture or historical period to the next. The concept of a niche is a way to make sense of these changes. Hacking asks: What makes it possible, in a particular time and place, for this to be a way to be mad?

Hacking's books *Rewriting the Soul* and *Mad Travelers* are about "dissociative" disorders, or what used to be called hysteria. He has argued, I think very persuasively, that psychiatrists and other clinicians helped to create the epidemics of fugue in nineteenth-century Europe and multiple-personality disorder in late-twentieth-century America simply by the way they viewed the disorders—by the kinds of questions they asked patients, the treatments they used, the diagnostic categories available to them at the time, and the way these patients fit within those categories. He points out, for example, that the multiple-personality-disorder epidemic rode on the shoulders of a perceived epidemic of child abuse, which began to emerge in the 1960s and which was thought to be part of the cause of multiple-personality disorder. Multiple personalities were a result of childhood trauma; child abuse is a form of trauma. It seemed to make sense that if there were an epidemic of child abuse, we would see more and more multiples.

Sociologists have made us familiar with the idea of "medicalization," which refers to the way that a society manages deviant behavior by bringing it under the medical umbrella.[37] A stock example of medicalization is the way that homosexuality was classified by the

American Psychiatric Association as a psychiatric disorder until the 1970s. Many enhancement technologies become popular only when they are conceptualized as treatments for medicalized conditions, such as Ritalin and Adderall for Attention Deficit Disorder (medicalized distractibility) or Paxil and Nardil for social phobia (medicalized shyness). Many technologies (including some of those used to treat medicalized conditions) are also used as "normalizing" procedures. Normalizing procedures bring a deviant behavior, characteristic, or personality type back within a range considered normal, or at least aesthetically acceptable. Cosmetic facial surgery for children with Down's syndrome is a normalizing procedure, in that it is performed not for medical reasons but to make the child look more like an ordinary child. Both "normalization" and "medicalization" are related to the processes that Hacking describes, but Hacking is onto something slightly different. By "transient mental illnesses" he does not have in mind new descriptions of old conditions so much as conditions that look new in themselves.[38]

Crucial to the way that transient mental illnesses arise is what Hacking calls "looping effects," by which he means the way a classification affects the thing being classified. Unlike objects, people are conscious of the way they are classified, and they alter their behavior and self-conceptions in response to their classification. Look at the concept of "genius," Hacking says, and the way it affected the behavior of people in the Romantic period who thought of themselves as geniuses. Look also at the way in which their behavior in turn affected the concept of genius. This is a looping effect: the concept changes the object, and the object changes the concept. To take a more contemporary example, think about the way that the concept of a "gay man" has changed in recent decades, and the way this concept has looped back to change the way that gay men behave. Looping effects apply to mental disorders too. In the 1970s, Hacking argues, therapists started asking patients they thought might be multiples if they had been abused as children, and patients in therapy began remembering episodes of abuse (some of which may not have actually occurred). These memories reinforced the diagnosis of multiple-personality disorder, and once they were categorized as multiples, some patients began behaving as multiples are expected to behave.

Not intentionally, of course, but the category "multiple-personality disorder" gave them, as Hacking provocatively puts it, a new way to be mad.

I am simplifying a very complex and subtle argument, but the basic idea should be clear. By regarding a phenomenon as a psychiatric diagnosis—treating it, reifying it in psychiatric diagnostic manuals, developing instruments to measure it, inventing scales to rate its severity, establishing ways to reimburse the costs of its treatment, encouraging pharmaceutical companies to search for effective drugs, directing patients to support groups, writing about possible causes in journals—psychiatrists may be unwittingly colluding with broader cultural forces to contribute to the spread of a mental disorder.

Suppose doctors started amputating the limbs of wannabes. Would that contribute to the spread of the desire? Could we be faced with an epidemic of people wanting their limbs cut off? Most people would say, Clearly not. Most people do not want their limbs cut off. It is a horrible thought. The fact that others are getting their limbs cut off is no more likely to make these people want to lose their own limbs than state executions are to make people want to be executed. And if by some strange chance more people did ask to have their limbs amputated, that would be simply because more people with the desire were encouraged to "come out" rather than suffer in silence.

I'm not so sure. Clinicians and patients alike often suggest that apotemnophilia is like gender-identity disorder, and that amputation is like sex-reassignment surgery. Let us suppose they are right. Fifty years ago the suggestion that tens of thousands of people would someday want their genitals surgically altered so that they could change their sex would have been ludicrous. But it has happened. The question is, Why? One answer would have it that this is an ancient condition, that there have always been people who fall outside the traditional sex classifications, but that only during the past forty years or so have we developed the surgical and endocrinological tools to fix the problem.

But it is possible to imagine another story, that our cultural and historical conditions have not just revealed transsexuals but created them. That is, once "transsexual" and "gender-identity disorder" and "sex-reassignment surgery" became common linguistic currency, more people began conceptualizing and interpreting their experience in these terms. They began to make sense of their lives in a way that hadn't been available to them before, and to some degree they actually became the kinds of people described by these terms.

I don't want to take a stand on whether either of these accounts is right. It may be that neither is. It may be that there are elements of truth in both. But let us suppose that there is some truth to the idea that sex-reassignment surgery and diagnoses of gender-identity disorder have helped to create the growing number of cases we are seeing. Would this mean that there is no biological basis for gender-identity disorder? No. Would it mean that the term is a sham? No. Would it mean that these people are faking their dissatisfaction with their sex? Again, no. What it would mean is that certain social and structural conditions—diagnostic categories, medical clinics, reimbursement schedules, a common language to describe the experience, and, recently, a large body of academic work and transgender activism— have made this way of interpreting an experience not only possible but more likely.

Whether apotemnophilia (or, for that matter, gender-identity disorder) might be subject to the same kind of molding and shaping that Hacking describes is not clear. One therapist I spoke with, an amputee wannabe, believes that the desire for amputation, like multiple-personality disorder, is often related to childhood trauma. This is only one person's hypothesis, of course, and it may be wrong. But it is clear that sexual desire is malleable. It doesn't seem far-fetched to imagine that amputated limbs could come to be more widely seen as erotic, or that given the right set of social conditions, the desire for amputation could spread. For a thousand years Chinese mothers broke the bones in their daughters' feet and wrapped them in bandages, making the feet grow twisted and disfigured. To a modern Western eye, these feet look hideously deformed. But for centuries Chinese men found them erotic.

Hacking uses the term "semantic contagion" to describe the way in which publicly identifying and describing a condition creates the means by which that condition spreads. He says it is always possible for people to reinterpret their past in light of a new conceptual category. It is also possible for them to contemplate actions that they may not have contemplated before. When I was living in New Zealand, ten years ago, I had a conversation with Paul Mullen, who was then the chair of psychological medicine at the University of Otago, and who told me that he was a member of a government committee whose job it was to decide whether pornographic materials should be allowed into the country. I bristled at the idea of censorship, and asked him how he could justify being a part of something like that. He just laughed and said that if I could see what his committee was banning, I would change my mind. His position was that some sexual acts would never even occur to a person in an entire lifetime of thinking about sex if not for seeing them pictured in these books. He went on to describe to me various alarming acts that, it was true, had never occurred to me. Mullen was of the opinion that people were better off never having conceptualized such acts, and in retrospect, I think he may have been right.[39]

This is part of what Hacking is getting at, I think, when he talks about semantic contagion. The idea of having one's legs amputated might never even enter the minds of some people until it is suggested to them. Yet once it is suggested, and not just suggested but paired with imagery that a person's past may have primed him or her to appreciate, that act becomes possible. Give the wish for it a name and a treatment, link it to a set of related disorders, give it a medical explanation rooted in childhood memory, and you are on the way to setting up just the kind of conceptual category that makes it a treatable psychiatric disorder. An act has been redescribed to make it thinkable in a way it was not thinkable before. Elective amputation was once self-mutilation; now it is a treatment for a mental disorder. Toss this mixture into the vast fan of the Internet and it will be dispersed at speeds unimagined even a decade ago.

Michael First is aware of this worry. When I asked him how the *DSM* task force decides what to include in the manual, he told me there were three criteria. One, a diagnosis must have "clinical relevance"—enough people must be suffering from the condition to warrant its inclusion. Thus more data must be gathered on apotemnophilia before a decision is made to include it in the next edition. Two, a new diagnostic category must not be covered by existing categories. This may turn out to be the catch for apotemnophilia, because if the data suggest that it is a paraphilia, it will be subsumed into that category. "People have paraphilias for all kinds of things," First says, "but we do not have separate categories for all of them." Three, a new diagnostic category must be a legitimate "mental disorder." What counts as a disorder is hard to define and, in fact, varies from one age and society to the next. One way that *DSM-IV* marks off disorders from ordinary human variation is by saying that a condition is not a disorder unless it causes a person some sort of distress or disability.

However, the fuzziness around the borders of most mental disorders, along with the absence of certainty about their pathophysiological mechanisms, makes them notoriously likely to expand. A look at the history of psychiatry over the past forty years reveals startlingly rapid growth rates for a wide array of disorders—clinical depression, social phobia, obsessive-compulsive disorder, panic disorder, attention-deficit/hyperactivity disorder, and body dysmorphic disorder, to mention only a few. In trying to pinpoint the causes for this expansion one could, depending on ideological bent, point to the marketing efforts of the pharmaceutical industry (more mental disorder equals more profits), the greater diagnostic skills of today's psychiatrists, a growing population of mentally disordered Americans, or a cultural tendency to look to psychiatry for explanations of what used to be called weakness, sin, unhappiness, perversity, crime, or deviance. But the fact is that none of these disorders could have expanded as they have unless they looked a lot like ordinary human variation at their edges. Mild social phobia looks a lot like extreme shyness, and attention-deficit disorder can look a lot like garden-variety distractibility. The lines between mental dysfunction and ordinary life are not as sharp as some psychiatrists like to pretend.

Which makes me wonder how sharply the lines around apotemnophilia can be drawn. The borders between pretenders, wannabes, and devotees do not look very solid. Many wannabes are also devotees or pretenders. A study published in 1983, which surveyed 195 customers of an agency selling pictures and stories about amputees, found that more than half had pretended to be amputees and more than 70 percent had fantasized about being amputees.[40] Nor do the lines look very clear between "true" apotemnophiles (say, those for whom the desire is a fixed, long-term part of their identities) and those whose desire has other roots, such as an interest in extreme body modification. We also need to remember that even if a core group of people with true apotemnophilia could be identified, their diagnosis could come only from what they report to their psychiatrists. There is no objective test for apotemnophilia. People seeking amputation for other reasons—sexual gratification, for example, or a desire for extreme body modification—could easily learn what they need to say to doctors in order to get the surgery they want. Specialists working in gender-identity clinics were complaining of something similar with their patients as early as the mid-1970s. Intelligent, highly motivated patients were learning the symptoms of gender dysphoria and repeating them to clinicians in order to become candidates for sex-reassignment surgery.[41]

I WILL CONFESS that my opinions about amputation as a treatment have shifted since I began talking to wannabes. My initial thoughts were not unlike those of a magazine editor I approached about writing a piece on the topic, who replied, "Thanks. This is definitely the most revolting query I've seen for quite some time." Yet there is a simple, relentless logic to these people's requests for amputation. "I am suffering," they tell me. "I have nowhere else to turn." They realize that life as an amputee will not be easy. They understand the problems they will have with mobility, with work, with their social lives; they realize they will have to make countless adjustments just to get through the day. They are willing to pay their own way. Their bodies belong to them, they tell me. The choice should be theirs. What is worse: to live without a leg or to live with an obsession that controls your life? For at least some of them, the choice is clear—which is why they are talking about chain saws and shotguns and railroad tracks.

And to be honest, haven't surgeons made the human body fair game? You can pay a surgeon to suck fat from your thighs, lengthen your penis, augment your breasts, redesign your labia, even (if you are a performance artist) implant silicone horns in your forehead or split your tongue like a lizard's. Why not amputate a limb? At least Robert Smith's motivation was to relieve his patients' suffering.

It is exactly this history, however, that makes me worry about a surgical "cure" for apotemnophilia. Psychiatry and surgery have had an extraordinary and very often destructive collaboration over the past seventy-five years or so: clitoridectomy for excessive masturbation, cosmetic surgery as a treatment for an "inferiority complex," intersex surgery for infants born with ambiguous genitalia, and—most notorious—the frontal lobotomy. It is a collaboration with few unequivocal successes. Yet surgery continues to avoid the kind of ethical and regulatory oversight that has become routine for most areas of medicine. If the proposed cure for apotemnophilia were a new drug, it would have to go through a rigorous process of regulatory oversight. Investigators would be required to design controlled clinical trials, develop strict eligibility criteria, recruit subjects, get the trials approved by the Institutional Review Board, collect vast amounts of data showing that the drug was safe and effective, and then submit their findings to the U.S. Food and Drug Administration. But this kind of oversight is not required for new, unorthodox surgical procedures. (Nor, for that matter, is it required for new psychotherapies.) New surgical procedures are treated not like experimental procedures but like "innovative therapies," for which ethical oversight is much less uniform.

The fact is that nobody really understands apotemnophilia. Nobody understands the pathophysiology; nobody knows whether there is an alternative to surgery; and nobody has any reliable data on how well surgery might work. Many people seeking amputations are desperate and vulnerable to exploitation. "I am in a constant state of inner rage," one wannabe wrote to me. "I am willing to take that risk of death to achieve the needed amputation. My life inside is just too hard to continue as is." These people need help, but when the therapy in question is irreversible and disabling, it is not at all clear what that help should be. Many wannabes are convinced that amputation is the only possible solution to their problems, yet they have never seen a psychiatrist or a psychologist, have never tried medication, have never read a scientific paper about their problems. More than a few of them have never even spoken face to face with another human being about their desires. All they have is the Internet, and their own troubled lives, and the place where those two things intersect. "I used to pretend as a child that my body was 'normal' which, to me, meant short, rounded thighs," one wannabe wrote to me in an e-mail message. "As a psychology major, I have analyzed and reanalyzed, and re-reanalyzed just why I want this. I have no clear idea."

10

BRINGING UP BABY

And that's the news from Lake Wobegon,
where all the women are strong, all the men
are good-looking, and all the children are
above average.

—Garrison Keillor

In every period of Western history, writes Philippe Aries in his magisterial *Centuries of Childhood*, there seems to correspond a privileged age of human life.[1] In the seventeenth century it was youth, a period closer to what today we would call middle age. In the twentieth century, it was adolescence. But in the nineteenth century it was childhood, and it was during this period that childhood moved to the center of family life. As historian John Gillis tells us, it was during the Victorian period that children's birthdays, Christian confirmation, and Jewish bar mitzvah became major family occasions. Middle-class Victorian homes began to display children's photographs and family portraits. Children began to stay at home longer, and when they left, their toys were stored away and their rooms preserved like shrines. The calendar began to fill with newly invented family events.[2] Today, when someone asks a man or woman if they have a family, the question typically means not "Do you have a partner?" or "Are your parents still living?" but rather, "Do you have children?"

It has become common for Americans to complain that children

are being robbed of their childhood. No doubt there are grounds
for this complaint, but we shouldn't forget that what children are
being robbed of is a comparatively recent invention. In medieval
society, according to Aries, the concept of childhood did not exist.
As soon as a child was weaned he or she became the natural com-
panion of adults. Children were dressed in adult clothes and
played adult games. It was not uncommon for families to give
identical names to all their children, distinguishing between them
only by their birth order.[3] Medieval painters portrayed children
with adult proportions and adult muscles; look at a medieval
painting of Jesus gathering the children to him and you will see
Jesus surrounded by a group of bantam-sized grown-ups. A great
number of children in medieval times were not even brought up by
their own families. Some were given as presents to monasteries.
Many worked as servants in other people's homes. As late as the
eighteenth century, one-quarter of all children in Toulouse, France,
were turned over to the care of others. The picture of childhood as
a time of innocence and vitality, a carefree preface to the serious
business of life, dates only to the nineteenth century. As Jackson
Lears puts it, the Victorians transformed children from miniature
adults to superior pets.[4]

Despite all our worries about childhood, it is not a privileged time
of life for us, as it was for the Victorians. From the early twentieth
century to the present, we have been preoccupied with adolescence.
This preoccupation first became evident at the turn of the twentieth
century, when the opinions of young people on social issues began
to be taken seriously. Many people sensed that young people had
values that differed from those of their elders, and that these values
were capable of rejuvenating an aging, sclerotic society. Adolescents
were admired for their strength and spontaneity. During World War
I the gap between young and old became more widely apparent still,
as the younger servicemen at the front staunchly opposed their elders in the rear. After the war, writes Aries, adolescence expanded; it
encroached upon childhood in one direction, maturity in the other.
Adolescents grew both younger and older. Soon not even marriage
put a stop to adolescence, as it had in the nineteenth century. Instead,
writes Aries, "the married adolescent was to become one of the most

prominent types of our time, dictating its values, its appetites and its customs."[5]

Whether you believe with Aries that our own privileged time of life is adolescence, or, as I suspect, that it has shifted to a period slightly later, it is pretty evident that our "values, appetites and customs" now converge on a time of life sometime after childhood but before middle age. Certainly this is most evident on the far side of youth, in our relentless efforts to postpone the physical signs of aging. But it can be seen on the other side of youth as well. In the clothes they wear, the music they listen to, the way they spend their free time, the way they speak and joke and carry themselves, American children emulate the styles and tastes of adolescents. But adolescents are for children merely the closest stand-in for the age to which adolescents themselves aspire, which is young adulthood, a time between twenty and thirty that is seen by young and old as the prime of life, a period of maximal freedom and sexual desirability, the inhabitants of which rule like sovereign monarchs over matters of style, slang, humor, and pop culture. Unlike Victorian children, children today now dress like adults, eat like adults, talk like adults, and play adult games and sports—which are watched, refereed, and supervised by adults. The older, sentimental picture of the child as innocent, uncorrupted, and cloyingly sweet, so characteristic of the Victorian period, now ends at roughly the age of kindergarten.

When Americans say that children are being robbed of childhood, they usually mean that we have become like the medieval portraitists Aries described, turning children into miniature grown-ups. Critics of Ritalin, for example, often argue that the rowdiness Ritalin is used to correct is just part of being a healthy American kid. There is something to this criticism, I agree, but it is both too narrow and slightly off-center. The problem is not just that we are trying to turn children into young adults, but also that our concerns about children's welfare are so tied up with preoccupations of young adults: physical attractiveness, sexual desirability, the possibility of marriage or domestic partnership, finding a job or career. When we debate enhancement technologies for children—not just Ritalin, but also synthetic growth hormone, orthodontia, and cosmetic surgery—we cannot help but see the debate framed in terms of these adult issues. We may be obsessed with childhood, but we are obsessed because we think child-hood is such a crucial period for the young adult that the child will later become.

IF YOU WERE A casual reader of medical journals in the middle and late 1980s, you might have concluded that pediatricians were excessively preoccupied with the psychological effects of growing up short. The proximate cause of this debate was the development of synthetic human growth hormone, a laboratory-produced version of the natural pituitary hormone that is necessary for normal growth. Some children, for various reasons, do not produce enough human growth hormone themselves. Consequently they do not grow at a normal rate. These short children often turn out to be very short adults. This deficiency had been treated with growth hormone extracted from animals since the 1960s, but this type of natural growth hormone proved to be expensive and occasionally even dangerous. The development of synthetic growth hormone in the mid-1980s raised hopes for a safe, steadily available, ever less expensive remedy.

The ethical debate over growth hormone, like other debates about enhancement technologies, took what has now become a predictable shape: a lot of back-and-forth over the nature of illness, the proper business of medicine, and exactly what condition human growth hormone was being used to treat. First there were worries about who should get the hormone. Some pediatricians asked whether the hormone should be used to treat children who were short not because of any growth hormone deficiency, but simply because of the number they happened to draw in the genetic lottery. Most short children are short simply because they come from a family of short people. Should they get growth hormone too? If so, does this mean that shortness is a disease? And while we are at it, does anyone actually know how well growth hormone will work in genetically short children? (Not very, as it turns out; but this was not obvious until later.)

Then there were worries about giving growth hormone to children who are short because of a bona fide disease, but a disease that does not happen to be growth hormone deficiency. Take children with chronic kidney disease, for example. Some of these children do not grow normally, and it looked as if they might benefit from growth hormone. The same went for children with Turner syndrome, a genetic disorder that results in short stature. So the question became, Does any disease associated with short stature qualify you for growth hormone, or does it have to be growth hormone deficiency?

Predictably, pediatricians also began to worry about using medicine to treat social problems. "Isn't social prejudice against short boys the real problem here?" asked the critics. ("Yes," replied parents, "but while you are fixing that problem, I want *my* child to have growth hormone.") Perhaps we could reserve treatment only for children who are *very, very* short, said some pediatricians, children whose stature is a serious problem—say, children in the bottom 1 percentile for height. But there will always be a bottom 1 percentile, came the reply. Short and tall are relative concepts. The short will always be with us, unless we are all the same height. Men want to be tall, but for there to be tall men there must also be short men. As Gore Vidal once said, "It is not enough to succeed. Others must fail."

All in all, a pretty predictable debate. Yet for all its predictability, the debate is still worth considering more carefully, not for what was said as much as for what did not need saying. The debate may have been about whether shortness constituted a disease, but the real issue was how *bad* it is to be short. And how bad it is to be short, in turn, seemed to depend on two things: the damage shortness causes to the child's self-esteem, and the setbacks suffered by short people in the competition for partners and jobs. To judge by the growth hormone debate, the purpose of a boy's childhood is to prepare himself for the extended, bloody contest that lasts from adolescence through young adulthood, during which he will do battle with other young men for careers and sexual partners. Being short, it was argued, handicaps a man in the competition for schools, jobs, income, and "mates."[6] Parents seek growth hormone to give their children a "competitive edge" because more height means better "chances of success in the marital and job markets."[7] The title of a paper in a prominent pediatric journal put the case bluntly: "The Disability of Short Stature."[8]

For girls, of course, the problem was reversed: the disability was tall stature. Unlike boys, whose self-esteem is allegedly damaged if they are too short, the self-esteem of girls is allegedly damaged if they are too tall. This is why, beginning in the late 1950s, pediatric endocrinologists prescribed estrogens as growth-suppressants for tall girls. Estrogens speed up the maturation of bones during puberty and slow a girl's growth. Endocrinologists reasoned that estrogen pills taken by a girl would result in a shorter adult woman. A survey in 1978 suggested that as many as one-half of pediatric endocrinologists offered estrogens to girls whose adult height was predicted to be greater than 6 feet 1 inch.[9] Today estrogens as growth-suppressants have gone out of fashion, but they are not completely obsolete. A recent survey found that over one-fifth of pediatric endocrinologists had treated at least one girl for "tall stature" during the preceding five years.[10]

Somebody in a novel I once read (and have since forgotten) remarked that when he was a young man he was obsessed with sex; in middle age he was obsessed with food; and now in old age, he was obsessed with sleep. In thinking about the well-being of children, apparently, we do not look far beyond youth. Neither tall girls nor short boys, we believe, can "compete successfully for mates." The most striking thing about the growth hormone debate was not how often the metaphor of life as a competition was used, but the object of that competition: sexual partners. In the great homecoming dance of life, how does a short boy get a date with the head cheerleader?

If sex and marriage are the main preoccupations of American young adulthood, closely behind are their Protestant cousins, the preoccupations of work. By this I mean the cluster of questions that typically gather around a person's choice of vocation, and which grow increasingly urgent toward the beginning of young adulthood: What should I do for a living? How will I support myself? Should I have a career? This is the other competition in which short boys and tall girls are said to be handicapped. Partisans in the growth hormone debate were quick to point out that short men typically make less money than tall men, have a harder time in electoral politics, and compete less successfully in professional enterprises such as courtroom law and business. Advocates of estrogens for tall girls noted that in jobs such as "ballet dancer, military or airline pilot, or air hostess, there are official upper limits of stature."[11] In fact, work is still the battleground for debates over enhancing children. Ritalin advocates typically point out that children with attention-deficit/hyperactivity disorder often do worse than other children in school, and that doing poorly in school usually translates into fewer and poorer opportunities on the job market later.

I do not mean to suggest, of course, that vocational success and physical attractiveness are exclusively the concerns of youth. Sex and money cast a wide net in America, as elsewhere, and it is getting wider all the time. Nor should we minimize the social handicaps that short men may suffer (though it should be pointed out that at least one British study has found the self-esteem of short children to be no worse than that of children of average height).[12] The point is, like middle age for food and old age for sleep, youth is typically the time when marriage and career are thought to be most crucial. The fact that they feature so prominently in a debate about children (conducted, incidentally, by doctors who have probably reached middle age or later) simply indicates the importance of youth, and the issues of youth, in the way we Americans think about our lives.

PERHAPS ONE REASON it is hard for independent-minded, autonomy-driven Americans to think clearly about children is that children do not possess the values we steer by. Children are not yet autonomous or independent. Whatever interests adults have in (say) making their own decisions, being left alone, or exercising any number of the other rights adults are said to have, those interests are just not there yet for children. This confuses the ethical issues around pediatric enhancements. Grown-ups have the right to do all sorts of odd things to their bodies, to have toxins injected into their foreheads, and fat sucked from their thighs, as long as nobody else is damaged by it. No harm, no foul; and if it is self-inflicted and self-sustained, no foul even when there is harm. But children, at least when they are very young, are often neither capable of making good judgments about their interests nor of articulating what their long-term interests are. So not only must parents (and health care workers) make decisions for children, they must also try to guess what the interests of the children are, now and in the future. Children are in a process of development, physically and psychologically. The person being enhanced is not just the child himself, as he exists at that given moment in time, but the adult that the child will become.

But the problem is even more complicated than this gloss might suggest. The desires of Americans for enhancement technologies today are tightly bound up with questions of identity—questions about finding the self, changing the self, improving the self, or betraying the self. We have become accustomed to this kind of vocabulary, and dependent on it as well. With children, though, this relationship between technology and the self is even more complex than it is for adults, because the self—at least the adult self, as we Westerners conceptualize it—is still in the process of being formed. With adults, for example, it seems possible to add height to the body without really changing the person who inhabits it. I may be taller, but I'm still me. With a child, however, this is not such an easy statement to make. When being short or tall will go into the process of how that child eventually thinks of himself, when it will contribute to making the kind of self that eventually emerges—say, a person who is at ease with himself or one who has a chip on his shoulder—then the question is not so much whether the technology is changing the self as what kind of self it is helping to produce. The technology will influence, for good or bad, the kind of adult the child grows up to be.

Perhaps this is most evident with a new technology that has been hotly debated in recent years, that of cochlear implants for deaf children.[13] A cochlear implant is an electronic device that simulates hearing. It consists of a speech processor, a headset transmitter, and a surgically implanted receiver-stimulator. The speech processor transmits spoken speech to the receiver-stimulator, which directly stimulates the auditory nerve. This allows the deaf person to "hear." One of the things that makes cochlear implants controversial, rather than simply an unalloyed good, is that the approximation of hearing they produce is not perfect. A child has to learn to hear with the implants, and so also to speak. This requires years of training and hard work. The implants also seem to work much better with people who have lost their hearing after having learned how to speak. For children who are born deaf, or who have lost hearing before learning to speak—the "prelingually deaf"—the results are not as impressive.

Yet if this were all there was to the debate it would simply be a matter of weighing the downside of the implants against their benefits, which seem to be growing greater and more evident as the technology progresses. What makes the debate so heated is the background to the procedure: hundreds of years of controversy over the way that deaf children should be brought up and educated. On one side are oralists, who have traditionally insisted that deaf children must learn how to speak and read oral languages, to read lips, and that they must be prevented—forcibly if necessary—from using the sign languages that inevitably emerge when deaf people are thrown together. On the other side are the oralism resisters, who insist that not only do Deaf people have their own manual languages, they also have a culture that has emerged in Deaf schools. Resisters speak of Deaf culture (in capitals) as a social heritage and way of living that has been transmitted over generations, with its own unique values, traditions, rituals, institutions, and stories, as well as its own languages. Since most Deaf children are born to hearing parents, who know little about Deaf culture, and are treated by hearing surgeons, the Deaf community worries about whether these parents are even aware that refusing the implant is a realistic option. Many see the widespread use of cochlear implants as a threat to their culture and their collective identity.

This confluence of viewpoints makes the debate over cochlear implants especially fierce. For parents, it is about doing right by your children, giving them the best chance in life that you can muster. For doctors, it is about fixing an obvious physical disability. But for members of the Deaf community, it is about identity. It is about language, and history, and how to preserve a cultural identity that is in danger of being lost. It is about an identity that is not passed down from parent to child but is transmitted by sign language taught in Deaf schools. Seen this way, the choice for or against a cochlear implant looks less like a choice about a surgical procedure than a choice about what country or region to live in, what church to attend, what language to speak at home. The debate about cochlear implants is a debate about what sort of person a child will grow up to be.

In a way, this is the moral issue that all the debates over enhancement technologies for children boil down to. What sort of person do you want this particular child to be? The issue at stake with cochlear implants and Deaf culture is somewhat unique, in that the choice is a

246 ■ CARL ELLIOTT

matter of cultural identity. But other choices may affect a child's sexual identity, gender, ethnicity, or social status. Parents must make choices about their child's future interests, and they must make them in the absence of sound knowledge about the future that awaits their child—a future that sometimes changes in unexpected ways.

Consider, for example, the ancient Chinese practice of footbinding. Footbinding began in the Chinese royal courts in the eleventh century, then spread gradually to commoners. A Chinese girl's feet were sometimes bound as early as three years of age, sometimes as late as early adolescence, depending on the region, the family, and the particular period in question. Mothers, and sometimes grandmothers, would wrap a girl's feet with bandages to prevent the foot from growing. The child's four smaller toes were crushed and bent underneath the sole of the foot, and her instep was arched so that the toes met the heel. The bones in the foot and toes were often broken. The foot was wrapped so tightly in bandages that the flesh putrefied. The bandages were intended never to come off permanently, and were removed only when the foot had to be washed. The result was an adult foot the size of an infant's, pointed and slim, and to a Chinese man, exquisitely erotic. The ideal foot, the *ne plus ultra* of bound feet, was the tiny, fragrant, perfectly-proportioned foot that was no larger than three inches in length: the "3-inch golden lotus."

To a modern Western eye, a bound foot looks grotesquely deformed. It is bent, twisted, and barely functional. Some women could not walk on their bound feet, and had to be carried or supported by others. Yet to Chinese men and women they were lovely: not just their tiny size, but also the right shape and proportions— arched, pointed, their curves soft and balanced. Elaborately decorated shoes were designed to show the feet in their best light. Poetry, ecstatic essays, classics of Chinese literature celebrated the beauty of bound feet, their historical significance, their transcendence of mere fashion. Chinese writers rhapsodized about the lovely gliding walk of the woman with lotus feet, the pleasures of fondling a woman's feet before making love. Even the distinctive rotting smell of bound feet was sexually charged. Smelling and tasting the tiny lotus foot was often compared to smelling and tasting a fine delicacy, and became a part of sexual foreplay. Gu Hongming, a Chinese scholar of the early twentieth century, claimed that the only beautiful feet were those that could be inserted halfway up the nostrils.[14]

For lotus lovers, such fantasies were not excessive. The most memorable scenes in Feng Jicai's satiric 1986 novel *The Three-Inch Golden Lotus* are the private contests staged for men who gush over the aesthetic pleasures of bound feet. In Feng's fanciful prose these lotus contests come off as two parts magic realism, one part Miss America pageant: one contestant leaves powdered, lotus-shaped designs in her wake as she walks across the stage, another kicks a shuttlecock into the air with her tiny red-shoed feet as robins fly out miraculously from under her dress. The women contestants are viciously competitive, but the male spectators are foot-obsessed buffoons. They beg the women for their secrets, recite bad poetry about feet, try drunkenly to toss chopsticks into a three-inch shoe and then slurp wine from it. "This is just like poetry, painting, song, dreams, mist, and wine; if it leaves us enchanted, intoxicated, mindless, even dead, it is worth it," sighs one. "If a person can enjoy tiny feet at this level, he needs nothing else in life!"[15]

The size of a Chinese woman's foot was traditionally seen as part of her sexual allure, but it was also a marker of class identity. A small foot symbolized beauty and aristocracy. Like many class markers that can be voluntarily acquired, bound feet also became a means of social mobility for the lower classes. A pair of tiny feet offered a woman the chance to attract a husband from a higher class or to move into a wealthier or more educated family, often as a concubine or maid.[16] A woman who was homely in every other way could still be considered beautiful if she had small feet. But if she had large feet, her marriage prospects were poor. She would be considered both ugly and common, and would face ridicule for having "peasant feet."[17] "If you love your son, don't go easy on his studies," goes an old Chinese saying. "If you love your daughter, don't go easy on her footbinding."[18]

For one thousand years this would have been good advice. So how could a Chinese mother at the start of the twentieth century know that very soon it would become profoundly bad advice—the very opposite of what a good mother should do? For within only a few decades, the near-universal practice of footbinding vanished. Chinese intellectuals began arguing that bound feet were a marker of backwardness. Natural foot societies emerged, pointing out to women how much easier work and travel would be with unbound feet. Anti-footbinding ditties and propaganda songs became popular. Christian missionaries made unbound feet a requirement for entry into mission schools. As China began to change from a feudal, agricultural society to a more industrial economy, a practice that disabled half the nation's workforce became much harder to defend. The government imposed fines on women who bound their children's feet. By the early twentieth century, women with bound feet had lost their social status as well as their beauty.[19] Today only a handful of women with bound feet remain, virtually all of them very old. It was as if American society were to suddenly develop a preference for "natural" teeth, and women who had gotten orthodontic work as children were now seen as homely and proletarian.

This kind of arbitrariness is built into any enhancement that depends on socially contingent standards of beauty and status. The standards can change, and individuals can even work together to bring about change. But change is rarely inevitable, or even all that predictable. Efforts to bring about change can backfire, and they can fail. This leaves many parents in the unenviable position of either buying into a standard they despise or protesting it through their children. So even as North American parents realize that a correction is "merely" cosmetic (straight teeth, proper height, the right-looking genitalia); even as they realize that the technology reinforces inequalities they cannot endorse (the rich get access, the poor do not); even as they deplore the cultural values that produce the desire for the technology (sexism reinforced by advertising and the media); even as they realize all these things, still they get the technology for their children. They might be willing to make the sacrifices for themselves, but they are not willing to sacrifice the interests of children who cannot make decisions on their own.

In the late 1990s, the American Medical Association set up a task force to look at the question of whether attention-deficit/hyper-activity disorder (ADHD) was being overdiagnosed. The task force was a response to public alarm about methylphenidate, or Ritalin. Unlike the ethical debate over synthetic growth hormone for short children, which was largely limited to pediatricians, the debate over Ritalin had made headlines. Ritalin had appeared on the cover of weekly magazines, led the evening news, and was being fiercely debated on radio talk shows and television news programs. Ritalin had become a national problem. Pediatricians blamed teachers for medicating rowdy children; teachers blamed parents for a lack of discipline at home; everyone blamed our buzzing, driven, video-obsessed culture.

In some ways, the attention was a little hard to understand. Ritalin is by no means a new drug. It was synthesized nearly sixty years ago, and the FDA approved it in 1955. When the outcry over Ritalin began, there had been no dramatic unforeseen side effects, no suicides, no manufacturer's warnings, no government investigations. Ritalin is still widely regarded as safe, and it appears to work well for children with ADHD. Nor was ADHD a newly discovered disorder, though it has been called different names over the years. Medical library shelves are filled with scientific papers on ADHD and its treatment. Even the public outcry over Ritalin in the 1990s was a repeat performance from the first Ritalin scare in the 1970s. Most Americans who were in school in the '60s and '70s can probably remember at least one wired-up kid in class who needed Ritalin to keep him in his seat.

Why all the worry then? Because in the 1990s, the rates at which Ritalin was being used and produced went through the roof. From 1990 to 1995, the annual U.S. production of Ritalin increased by 500 percent. In 1970, it was estimated that 150,000 U.S. children were taking some sort of stimulant medications; by 1995, 2.6 million Americans were taking Ritalin alone. Even toddlers were being medicated: one study found that among children aged two to four, the use of psychoactive medication in the early '90s tripled.[20] No other industrialized country of Europe or Asia saw any sort of increase in Ritalin use during the same period. (Canada's rates of Ritalin use quadrupled during the early '90s, but still remained less than half that of the United States.) By the late '90s, the United States was producing and consuming 90 percent of the world's supply of Ritalin.[21] One recent study found that 10 percent of elementary schoolchildren in one North Carolina county had been diagnosed with ADHD, and 7 percent were being medicated.[22]

The debate over Ritalin has followed the pattern of many other types of enhancement technologies: a steep rise in use, accompanied by an anxious public outcry over the question of whether a medical technology is being used to treat social problems. On one side of the Ritalin debate are those who charge that Ritalin is being overprescribed. They argue that not all the children who are being given the drug have a true medical problem. Teachers are tempted to recommend Ritalin for children who misbehave in overcrowded classrooms. Overstressed families are tempted to see their children's misbehavior as the result of ADHD when the real problems lie elsewhere. Achievement-obsessed parents want Ritalin to give their children a competitive edge in school. Ritalin is a mask for deeper social ills, these critics argue, and the rising rates of use are an indicator that these ills are becoming critical.

On the other side of the debate are distraught parents—and increasingly, adult users of Ritalin—who see in ADHD a genuine problem that can be treated effectively with the drug. These parents and adult users have organized themselves into a potent political force, and they have been joined by physicians who see the growing use of Ritalin as the simple and predictable result of better medical practice. These physicians suggest that the diagnosis of ADHD has become more common because clinicians have become better equipped to recognize it. As rates of diagnosis rise, so also will rates of treatment. In fact, some physicians think they may rise higher still. Many current studies estimate the number of school-age children suffering from ADHD at anywhere from 3 percent to 5 percent of the childhood population, but some specialists actually believe this figure is low, and some studies have put it as high as 17 percent.[23] Joseph Biederman, the chief of the Harvard Medical School Psychopharmacology Clinic, estimates the number of American children with ADHD at something closer to 10 percent. Far from being overprescribed, he suggests, Ritalin is not being prescribed often enough.[24]

The American Medical Association task force on ADHD would probably agree. Despite the alarming statistics, the task force found no evidence that ADHD was being overdiagnosed. The reason ADHD was being so widely diagnosed, it concluded, was a combination of a number of different factors. Both doctors and the general public know a lot more about ADHD than they did several years ago, for example, and thus are more likely to recognize it. Doctors also know more about Ritalin itself, worry less about the risk of abuse, and are more willing to prescribe it for longer, uninterrupted periods. The task force also pointed out that the range of behavior counted as evidence of ADHD is broader than it used to be, encompassing inattention as well as hyperactivity. Finally, adults, who have been made more aware that stimulants can help them concentrate and work more attentively, are starting to use the drugs in far greater numbers.[25]

All of which is probably true. Yet by framing the question in terms of diagnosis and treatment, the task force sidestepped the real criticism of Ritalin. For critics, the term "overdiagnosis" suggests that there is a correct rate of diagnosis. But the real question is whether the diagnosis itself is a way of medicalizing inattention and rowdiness. To suggest that there is a correct rate of Ritalin prescription is like suggesting that there is a correct rate of coffee consumption or alcohol use. The issue is not really whether ADHD is being overdiagnosed, but whether it is a good thing for one in ten schoolchildren to take stimulant drugs.

For Ritalin is an excellent stimulant, of course, like caffeine, nicotine, and cocaine. Chemically, it is very similar to amphetamines. That these drugs will make you feel more alert and attentive is not recent news. Cocaine was extracted from the coca plant in the late nineteenth century, and was widely prescribed until the 1920s. Sigmund Freud, an avid user of cocaine, and at one point in his life something of an evangelist for the drug, wrote that after taking it he felt more self-controlled, more vigorous, and (a key feature for today's stimulant users) more capable of work. "Long-lasting, intensive mental work can be performed without fatigue," Freud observed. "It is as though the need for food and sleep, which otherwise makes itself felt peremptorily at certain times of the day, were completely banished."[26]

The discovery that stimulants could actually improve a child's behavior came in the 1930s. Like the discovery of many new psychiatric drugs, this one came entirely by accident. Charles Bradley, a physician who worked at the Emma Pendleton Bradley Home in

Providence, Rhode Island, gave Benzedrine, an amphetamine, to thirty children with neurological and behavioral disorders who had undergone spinal taps. He thought that Benzedrine might relieve the headaches that spinal taps often produced. Benzedrine didn't relieve any headaches, but it had another unexpected effect. It calmed many of the children down. It made them less active, and to Bradley's surprise, it also improved their academic performance. Bradley described the improvements as "spectacular."[27] Ciba-Geigy synthesized Ritalin in 1944 in an effort to reproduce the sort of effects that Bradley and Freud wrote so enthusiastically about, but without the potential for abuse.

Clinicians have known for years that some children are extraordinarily active and distractible from a very early age. Childhood "hyperactivity" was described in the clinical literature nearly 100 years ago.[28] Clinicians have also known since Bradley's time that many of these children will behave much better if they are given stimulants. But it was not until the 1950s that the treatment and the disorder began to be paired up in a formal way. The disorder took various shapes and names at first: minimal brain dysfunction, hyperkinesis, and hyperactive disorder, among others. In 1968, the American Psychiatric Association's *Diagnostic and Statistical Manual of Mental Disorders* (*DSM-II*) identified "minimal brain damage" as a syndrome characterized by distractibility, inattentiveness, overactivity, and restlessness in children. By the mid-1970s, "hyperactivity" or "hyperkinesis" was being identified as the most common psychiatric disorder of childhood, and stimulants were the treatment of choice.[29]

Why should stimulants, of all things, calm a child down? For a long time this question puzzled clinicians. The calming effect was especially puzzling in the case of hyperactive children, in whom the results were even more dramatic. Some physicians theorized that in hyperactive children, stimulants had a "paradoxical effect," relaxing instead of stimulating the child. This theory also led many clinicians to believe that a dramatic response to stimulants was a way of diagnosing hyperactivity. If a child is calmed down by a stimulant, the clinical reasoning went, he must be hyperactive.

Today this theory is widely thought to be wrong. There is no paradox: the direction of changes brought about by stimulants in hyperactive children is the same as that of normal children, and it is the same as in adults.[30] All of them will become more attentive, less impulsive, less distractible, more able to attend to repetitive tasks, once they take a stimulant. This is why children appear to be calmer: they are more focused and less easily distracted. Hyperactive children are hyperactive precisely because they cannot pay attention to a particular task without constantly getting sidetracked. They have trouble restraining themselves from acting on any impulse that pops into their minds. According to current thinking, inattention, hyperactivity, and impulsivity are the triad of symptoms that make up ADHD.[31]

Nobody who has seen a child with classic ADHD respond to Ritalin can doubt that stimulants help, at least in the short term. When I was in college, I spent a summer working at a residential home for children. A few of the children were orphaned, some came from broken homes, many others had psychiatric problems of differing kinds. A handful of the children in my cottage took Ritalin regularly. I remember one boy in particular, about six or seven years old that summer, who seemed to change into a different child when he did not take his medication. Medicated, he was a charming, athletic boy, friendly and mindful. In the classroom, he would work diligently, coloring or practicing his writing, with little apparent frustration. If he did not take his medication, however—and occasionally he would not, hiding the pill under his tongue—he was transformed into a terror. One of the symptoms of ADHD listed in the *DSM-IV* is that a child acts as if he is "driven by a motor." This phrase does not sound terribly scientific, but it describes this boy perfectly. Not only could he not sit still; he could not even stand still. He was also as quick and agile as a monkey. Wild-eyed, combative, vibrating like an overheated boiler; sometimes he was beyond the reach of words. Often there was nothing to do but chase him down and keep him still as best you could, before he hurt another child or went out the window.

This child clearly worked and behaved better on Ritalin. The problem is that just about any child would. The right dose of a stimulant will probably improve the concentration and focus of any child who takes it. Or any adult, for that matter. This has been empirically demonstrated in controlled conditions, but sleep-deprived college students and long-distance truckers have known it for years.[32] Stimulants give you a sense of alertness and clarity. You can work longer hours at boring tasks. You can immerse yourself in mental work in a way that is otherwise hard to sustain. "In no time, I was typing like a madman, spraying sentences like a broken hose," writes the novelist Walter Kirn, describing his first dose of Ritalin after being diagnosed with adult ADHD. After taking the drug he felt clean, radiant, and powerful. He sat down at his desk and wrote for six uninterrupted hours. "On Ritalin the task at hand was the only task in the world, and the world was very, very small—the size of a computer screen." No wonder teachers like Ritalin so much, Kirn writes. On Ritalin, Johnny can "sit still and silent at his desk while his brain bores through textbooks like a power drill."[33]

Not everyone reacts this way to stimulants, of course. Just as people react in different ways to coffee, they also react in different ways to Ritalin, Dexedrine, and Adderall. Adults are more likely to feel a sense of euphoria, while often children say simply that the drug makes them feel "different."[34] While there is little doubt that stimulants can help children diagnosed with ADHD immediately do better at some of the tasks they are asked to do in school, it is less clear what effects stimulants have on them (or on non-ADHD children) in the long term. The fact is that even after a century of research on ADHD, the disorder is still not terribly well understood. Few studies have followed children treated with Ritalin into adulthood.[35] The pathophysiology of the disorder is still a mystery. Like most mental and behavioral disorders, ADHD is diagnosed not by any laboratory work or radiological test, or even a physical examination, but by behavioral criteria. The guidelines for diagnosing ADHD ask things such as whether a child has trouble paying attention, fidgets often in his seat, or fails to listen when spoken to. Most children will meet at least a few of these criteria. Some will meet quite a number of them. Virtually all of them will work more efficiently if they are given stimulants.

This is a lesson learned by many adults in the late 1990s, the period when the diagnosis of adult ADHD began to flourish. Unlike childhood ADHD, which is typically diagnosed by doctors through the reports of parents and teachers, adult ADHD is usually diagnosed by patients themselves. Adult ADHD sufferers often come to believe that ADHD is the cause of their own failures, usually at work, and they bring the diagnosis of ADHD with them to the doctor. Sociologist Peter Conrad calls adult ADHD "the medicalization of underperformance."[36] With a diagnosis of ADHD, adults can reinterpret past failures as the consequence of illness. "I used to beat myself up," says a former Nasdaq vice-president who has been divorced twice, recently quit his job, and came to understand that he had ADHD only when his children were diagnosed with the disorder. With the diagnosis of ADHD, he says, "I know this is not a personality flaw, I am not screwed up."[37] This is a typical narrative for adult ADHD sufferers. It allows them to shift responsibility for their underperformance from themselves to the illness. "I had 38 years of thinking I was a bad person," says one adult ADHD sufferer. "Now I'm rewriting the tapes of who I thought I was to who I really am."[38]

Which is, of course, a person with a diagnosable mental disorder. It is true that such a classification may carry certain advantages. It gives you a socially legitimate reason to take stimulants, for example. ADHD advocacy groups have lobbied hard (and in the end, successfully) to have ADHD counted as a bona fide disability under federal law.[39] But is the diagnosis worth the cost? A friend of mine—I'll call him Grady—recently started taking Dexedrine to help him stay on task in a boring bureaucratic job that he hated but needed desperately to keep, in order to support his daughter and his pregnant wife. A former musician, Grady told me, "Taking Dexedrine felt pretty benign to me—a lot like taking beta-blockers before a musical performance or a job interview." The big difference was that Dexedrine, unlike a beta-blocker, is a controlled drug. Doctors must account for every Dexedrine prescription to the Drug Enforcement Agency. So anyone who wants the drug, in effect, needs a diagnosis of ADHD. To Grady, taking Dexedrine before work seemed very similar to taking a beta-blocker before a concert or a talk. But the two drugs were treated very differently. As he explains, "With beta-blockers, I just say, 'This takes the edge off public speaking.' But with Dexedrine, I am pushed into saying, 'I have a minor mental disorder, possibly genetically influenced, for which there is treatment but no cure. Dexedrine is a standard therapy.' This is a much more demoralizing narrative."

In the long run, a diagnosis may also make people feel more responsibility for their condition. According to Grady, he began to think, "These strange things I do are not just quirks, nor are they permanent features of my character. They are just symptoms of a disorder that can be treated with medication and lifestyle changes. So goddammit, I'd better get to work fixing them and adapting to the culture." Every time he made a mistake at work, he would ask himself, "Am I taking my meds regularly? What about the dose?" Once he became familiar with the signs and symptoms of ADHD, he found it harder and harder to tolerate things that seemed symptomatic of the condition: forgetting to pick up groceries on the way home, taking a long time to leave the house every morning, failing to clean up his office or apartment. Before the diagnosis, these just seemed like permanent features of his character, but afterward he found himself saying, "Damn, it took me forty-five minutes to get out of the house today. Plus I zoned out at the meeting today. Are these meds working? Should I try something else? Day planners? Exercise? Less caffeine? More caffeine?" He says it became easier to see his habits as personal failures, and harder to see them as a natural reaction to his circumstances (i.e., "I took forty-five minutes to get dressed because I was taking care of a baby at the same time; I zoned out at meetings because they were boring and unproductive").

In fact, I suspect the lines between illness and identity may be even fuzzier than Grady suggests. My wife, Ina, for example, grew up in Germany, the eldest of three sisters. All three of the Radetzky sisters share what I think of as a typical Germanic virtue of "care" or "mindfulness." By this I don't have in mind the stereotypical German obsession with tidiness and efficiency, though that is probably connected. I'm thinking more about a sort of attentiveness to the world around you, the kind of attentiveness that leads you to remember to turn off the lights when you leave a room, to avoid spilling drinks on your clothes, to remember directions, and more generally, to lead an organized and well-planned life. It is also connected to an appreciation for craft and workmanship, of the attentiveness that goes into a job well done, an appreciation for things that are handmade and well-constructed. These virtues characterize the sisters Radetzky. They do not, however, characterize my brothers and me, all of whom were raised in South Carolina and who have an air of abstraction and carelessness. None of us have a sense of direction. When something breaks, we fix it with duct tape. We are all prone to forgetfulness and sloppiness. We tend to live in our own heads more than in the actual physical world. We are more likely to get lost, to forget things, to lose a thought in midsentence, to stare blankly off in the distance for minutes at a time. To Ina (and perhaps also to her sisters) this is a Bad Thing. Maybe not unambiguously bad—they are a tolerant bunch, and patient, and tend to roll their eyes and laugh rather than criticize directly—but still, it isn't something to be encouraged. For Ina, in fact, it is something that our children are in danger of inheriting (or learning) and which needs to be stamped out early. They must learn to be careful, pay attention, watch what they are doing.

My brothers and I could probably do better on Ritalin or Dexedrine. I have been tempted to give it a try. Yet at least part of the reason I resist is that I am not convinced that the abstracted end of the mindfulness spectrum is really such a bad place to be. In fact, I kind of like it here. The "care" and "mindfulness" and "attentiveness" that some people (even me) see as a virtue can often be redescribed as "pettiness" or "anal-retentiveness." It can easily slide into a kind of fetishism, an obsession with things that (at least to my brothers and me) shouldn't really matter: a dent in the car, a spot on the carpet, dishes in the sink, a wasted hour on a back road. The microwave oven is not heating things up as quickly as it should. So what? Lighten up, I am tempted to say. Keep your eyes off the clock. Don't sweat the details.

My point here is not to argue for a laid-back, southern aesthetic of shabby abstractedness (though since it is my own aesthetic, I do have some stake in it). Nor do I want to suggest that any German I know would actually consider medication to become more attentive. My point is that the very changes that some people might think of as unqualified "enhancements" (i.e., becoming more attentive and mindful) are not quite as unqualified as they may initially think; and that, moreover, these enhancements may well be changes critical to a person's identity, a person's sense of who he or she is. This need not be individual identity. It can also be family identity (Elliott abstractedness) or even cultural identity (southern amiability). The trait in

258 ■ CARL ELLIOTT

question might even affect identity in ways that we do not appreciate, like, say, professional identity. I sometimes wonder whether it is
an accident that of the three abstracted Elliott brothers, two have
graduate degrees in philosophy and the other is a psychiatrist.

Conventional wisdom has it that Ritalin is prescribed so widely
because of the pace of American life. Contemporary American life is
so hectic, so frantic, so speed-obsessed, that we don't know how to
relax. We live in a world of jump-cuts and sound bites, it is argued;
of TV and video games and express mail and the Internet; we work
to the constant background hum of cell phones and modems and fax
machines. Ritalin is just another way to speed things up, to make life
more novel, to keep things from getting dull. Yet it is hard to know
how to take this critique. Given that most of the world's Ritalin is
produced and consumed in the United States, a country whose hur-
ried pace of life has been remarked upon by foreign visitors for centuries, it is hard to dismiss it entirely. Yet it is not clear that Ritalin
actually speeds life up in the way that critics suggest. In fact, it seems
to slow kids with ADHD down. This is why early researchers
thought stimulants had a paradoxical effect. What stimulants help
children with ADHD do better are the sorts of things that you ordinarily do while sitting still, like reading a book carefully from cover
to cover.

A more likely explanation may be simply that these days more and
more Americans are doing exactly what I am doing at this very
moment: sitting in front of a computer. I have not taken any Ritalin,
but I have been here for perhaps three hours so far this morning, and
I am now on my fourth cup of coffee. I am by no means unusual.
Whiskey may do the trick for novelists and poets, but for academics
the drug of choice is caffeine. Go into a coffee shop in my neighborhood of Minneapolis and you will see tables spread with books, writing materials, and laptop computers. The reason is simple. Coffee,
like Ritalin, clears the head and focuses the attention. It helps the
ideas come faster and more furiously.

Until you have had too much, of course. With too much coffee I
become impatient, distractible, unable to concentrate or even to sit
still in my chair. A book on the shelf catches my attention; I get up to
have a look. That book leads me to another book. Then another one.

This one needs to go back to the library. What was I thinking about again? Oh yes: the paper I was writing. Must write paper. I sit down again. I stare out the window and drum my fingers. My leg is hopping up and down furiously. I check my e-mail for the fourth time in fifteen minutes. Nothing. Damn. I stare intently at the screen again. What is that little icon over there on the left? I double-click it. It brings up a program I have never seen before. Useless. For no good reason I fiddle with it for a minute or two and then shut it down. Then I click over to Netscape to check the library Web site for a book I am waiting for. Nope, still not there. Well, maybe I should try Amazon.com. I click to Amazon.com. Maybe while I am on Amazon.com I should see how my book is selling. Still selling at number 278,456. Damn. Let's look at Barnesandnoble.com. No better. Ah well. Let me check my e-mail again. Still nothing. Now what was I working on again? Oh yes: the paper.

Is this, I wonder, what it is like to have ADHD? To be constantly distracted, impulsive, unable to concentrate on a single thing for more than a minute at a time? If so, it is not hard to see why a drug like Ritalin is so popular, especially for people called upon to do work that requires sustained attention. Like schoolwork, for example. Or work at a computer. Or any of a number of information-driven jobs that the American economy is supposedly creating. Today the service industry is the largest sector of the economy. Temp agencies are thriving; short-term contracts and a "flexible work force" have become the norm. This kind of environment places employees under a tremendous amount of pressure. Employees who cannot rely on job security often feel as if they are constantly required to prove their value to their employers.[40] Many of these same employees spend most of their time sitting in front of a computer screen performing repetitive tasks that require sustained attention and concentration. Stimulants help them do this sort of work better, for longer periods of time, without succumbing to boredom or mental exhaustion.

One of the reasons why people with ADHD have such a hard time with this sort of work is because they have trouble controlling their impulses. A thought comes into their minds; they immediately act on it. Impulsivity is one of the defining marks of the ADHD diagnosis.

Researchers have had children diagnosed with ADHD take computer tests where they are expected to distinguish between situations where they should hit a button and those where they must refrain. Children with ADHD make impulsive mistakes; they hit the button when they should wait. Give them even small doses of Ritalin, however, and they do much better on the test. They can prevent themselves from immediately hitting the button.[41]

Anyone who has tried to work at a computer while overcaffeinated will know that inattention and impulsivity are no small handicaps. With the Internet only a click away, and a new game or program only one more click, distraction is always beckoning at the gate. Critics of Ritalin sometimes argue that computers and video games are part of the ADHD problem, but in fact, the evidence shows that children with ADHD are worse at playing video games than unaffected children. Children with ADHD may be attracted by the stimulation video games provide, but this does not mean they are any good at them. More likely these flashing, beeping, buzzing games are merely a high-stimulus barrier against boredom.[42]

Perhaps, as Malcolm Gladwell suggests, Ritalin is simply a drug in tune with the needs of contemporary life. A century ago America was a far more rural society. Only 7 percent of children aged fourteen to seventeen were actually in school.[43] Stimulants may have been enjoyable, but they were rarely necessary. Yet in a society that rewards intellectual sharpness and concentration, where children are taught the values of achievement and self-control from a very early age, often against their natural impulses, stimulants have a much clearer social function. Certainly Ritalin is a safer stimulant than cigarettes and cocaine.

Yet one can still worry that this new world will have no room for some kinds of children. Perhaps some people are simply temperamentally unsuited to life at this fever pitch—drinking espresso in front of a computer screen, fax humming, speakerphone on, e-mail zipping in and out, lunch at the desk, people popping in and out of the office. Not everyone wants to live their life as if they were on the trading floor of the New York Stock Exchange, even if they could handle the pace. Maybe those who worry about Ritalin are really worrying that we have sped up the rhythm of American life to such a frenzied drum roll that those who march to the beat of a different drummer—or rather, who idle slowly rather than march—will simply be left behind.

O NE THING THAT virtually all debates over pediatric enhancement technologies have in common, no matter what the specifics of the technology are, is the child's self-esteem. Every commentator, regardless of the side he takes in the debates, points out that children are teased, mocked, bullied, picked on, discriminated against, and joked about by other children. In the growth hormone debate, for example, it was routinely written that short stature carries social stigma; and stigma, everyone agreed, is a terrible thing. It damages the child's sense of self-worth, leads to social isolation, and produces feelings of inferiority and shame. For some, it is shortness itself that will diminish the child's self-esteem; for others, it is the fact of taking growth hormone, which may lead the child to believe his shortness is an illness or a personal failing. But few commentators, pro growth hormone or contra, ignored the issue of self-esteem, or the way that stigmatization can damage it. Extremely short stature, wrote one commentator in *The New England Journal of Medicine*, is "psychologically disabling."[44]

The dominant vision of American childhood seems to be something like the following. The world is a cruel, vicious place, from which home and family are the only barriers. Very early childhood may still be a time of Victorian innocence, but that innocence ends the moment the child goes out the front door. Parents need to be especially vigilant about the terrors that await children in school, particularly junior high school and afterward. There, children will be ridiculed and humiliated. The ridicule children need to be protected from is not limited to being short. Children can be ridiculed for crooked teeth (for which orthodontia is the answer), big noses and ears that stick out (for which cosmetic surgery is the answer), misbehavior in class (for which Ritalin in the answer), and potentially embarrassing genitalia (for which normalizing surgery and hormonal treatment are the answers).

Given the American propensity to see life as a competition, it is striking that so many of these particular horrors seem to be located in school gyms and sports fields: the worries all seem to circle around being seen naked in the locker room, being bullied by sadistic coaches and gym teachers, or being picked last for the basketball team. Here is the downside of the American ethic of self-reliance and independence. If your vision of the world outside the family is one where you make your own way alone, stopping only occasionally to go knuckle-to-knuckle with rivals as you try to build a family of your own, then how do you make conceptual room for children, who are neither completely self-reliant nor independent? You will naturally be quite terrified for them. You will try to protect them as fiercely as you can, until they learn how to protect themselves. It is a cold, dangerous world out there, you tell them. Keep your privates protected and always lead with your left.

Maybe this is a realistic vision of American childhood, maybe not. Most people tend to see the experience of children through the lens of their own childhood, and this particular vision may be less of American childhood in general than of the childhood of people who write articles in medical journals. Still, it is probably fair to say that this sort of story rings a bell or two for Americans of a certain age. My wife can watch a string of Hollywood movies about American junior high and high schools, with all their gossipy plotting and scheming, their cliques and in-factions, the competitiveness, the relentless teasing of kids who are fat, or effeminate, or short, without seeing anything recognizable from her own schooling in Germany. Whereas Americans watch these movies and say, "Yes, that's exactly right. God, wasn't junior high awful?"

When American anthropologist Margaret Mead went to Bali in the 1930s, she was baffled that Balinese children could survive the relentless teasing that they underwent in childhood. Not only did Balinese children survive it; in fact, they seemed to thrive. Western visitors to Bali from the 1920s onward have noticed how happy and well-behaved Balinese children are. Mead says that during the two years she spent in Bali she never saw a child or adolescent fight. Hickman Powell, an American journalist who lived in Bali in the 1920s, says that he never even saw a Balinese child *cry,* with the exception of a single small child who was hurt. Of all the marvelous and exotic stories that he took back to America, he says, this was the single thing about Bali that his American friends refused to believe.

Yet from the time they are babies, Mead writes, Balinese children are teased. Everybody joins in, "flipping their fingers, their toes, their genitals, threatening them, playfully disregarding the sanctity of their heads." Mothers will borrow the babies of other women and hold them close in order to make their own children jealous. This kind of teasing is never brought to a climax; as the child grows tenser and more excited, the teaser inevitably turns away. Mead wonders: Why doesn't this relentless needling, threatening, and poking traumatize the child? In a tone of mild astonishment, she observes, "It is a child-hood training which, if followed here, would seem certain to bring out schizoid trends in the child's character."[45]

Yet it doesn't, of course; and this, for an American anyway, needs an explanation. Mead believes that the explanation lies in the way that art, in Bali, mirrors life—or perhaps better, the way that life and art in Bali merge. In the West, she writes, we have no ritualized way of dealing with childhood trauma. Children are traumatized in strange new ways, and later in their lives they are expected to deal with the consequences of that trauma by themselves. But for the Bali-nese, she writes, this traumatic conflict is communal, theatrical, and ritualized. The Balinese child constantly sees conflict enacted on stage, in the shadow plays, and in the elaborate, stylized Balinese dances. There, even as children are gently, relentlessly prevented from quarreling with their brothers and sisters, they see magnificent battles being fought on stage. Even as mothers tease children "in the eerie, disassociated manner of a witch," the children will see the witch defeated in the *wayang kulit*. "Over and over again, as babies in their mothers's arms, as toddlers being lifted out of the path of a pair of dancing warriors, as members of the solemn row of children who line the audience square, they see it happen—the play begins, mounts to intensity, and ends in ritual safety."[46]

But it would be misleading to compare this experience directly to that of an American child at the theater or the movies. The Balinese do not make the sharp divisions between art and life that we make in the West. For one thing, writes Mead, the Balinese do not separate ritual role and everyday role: "the artist, the dancer, the priest, is also the husbandman who tills his rice fields."[47] Nor do they rigidly sepa-rate professionals from amateurs, or rehearsals from performances.

In Bali, life and theater merge—in flamboyant religious ceremonies, ritualized public forms, and obsessive concern with the aesthetics of social behavior. "The whole of life," writes Mead, "is seen as a circular stage on which human beings, born small, as they grow taller, heavier and more skilled, play predetermined roles, unchanging in their main outlines, endlessly various and subject to improvisation in detail."[48] It is onto this stage that children are born, entering temporarily from the world of the dead, a human soul born into the same family every fourth generation. Once its turn on the stage is finished, that soul returns again to the other world.

Thus a Balinese life, writes Mead, is shaped not like a line but like a half-circle, in which newborns and the elderly are the beings closest to the other world, and middle age, being the farthest away, is the most secular. Balinese people do not grow in stature and importance as they age, as they might in a culture in which time is seen as sequential. "Newborns are treated as celestial creatures entering a more humdrum human existence and, at the moment of birth, are addressed with high-sounding honorific phrases reserved for gods, the souls of ancestors, princes, and people of a higher caste." No task is seen as impossible or inappropriate for a child. Children, she writes, are called "small human beings."[49]

For Mead, the reason why Balinese children are not, like American children, traumatized by this relentless teasing (and the reason why even Balinese parents, teased themselves as children, join in so enthusiastically) is that they learn early on to trust the arts. They learn that the teasing is a safe game. Life in Bali takes place on stage, and if that stage is anything like the one that the child watches from the earliest age onward, the conflicts enacted there will be ritually and safely resolved.

Perhaps Mead is right (although looking back on her explanation from a distance of seventy-five years, at a time when American children watch violent conflicts on television with ritualized regularity, it may sound less persuasive now than it did in the 1930s). Yet surely another reason for the difference between contemporary America and 1930s Bali lies in the relative importance (or lack of it) placed on the characteristics of the individual. The background to American teasing—indeed, teasing seems too mild a word; better to call it ridicule or humiliation—is one of extreme individualism: of the American's disposition "to get wrapped up in himself," as Tocqueville put it. We insist that parents make sure their child's self-esteem is not damaged, that the child realizes that she is valuable and loved; we worry when the child is mocked and teased by others, and what this will do to her self-conception. But the background to this insistence and worry is the mere fact that the individual child *herself* is the focus of all this attention: it is her personality, her appearance with which she needs to come to terms. She is taught that everyone is looking at her, evaluating her, making judgments about the way she looks and carries herself and behaves. These are judgments not about the way life is, the turns a plot might take, the characteristics associated with a certain dramatic role, but about the individual child herself—that singular bundle of looks and smarts and personality that constitute "me."

Personality and appearance are essential to the American self, not accidental: they are who we are, our very identity. To be teased or mocked about how we look and act will naturally cut us to the quick. If these cuts are made when the self is being formed, during childhood and adolescence, they will naturally be harder to heal. Yet contrast our self-conception with the Balinese notion that the self is merely the temporary inhabitant of an atemporal dramatic role, and in particular, the Balinese tendency to mute, as Clifford Geertz puts it, "anything that is uniquely characteristic of the individual physically, psychologically or biographically, in favor of his assigned role in the drama of Balinese life."[50] If, as Mead writes, "Personality characteristics are accidents, held gently constant through any given incarnation, that dissolve at death," then it would be no surprise if the kind of mockery that for Americans is so traumatizing is rather less so for the Balinese.[51] The less importance attached to individual appearance and personality, the less central to selfhood they are, and the less wounding this mockery will be. So incidental are these things, writes Mead, that a Balinese often cannot describe the character or looks of someone who has died only a few years ago.

If this is right, or even close, then the problem for American children is not just teasing, not even just ridicule or mockery, but the entire Western (and especially American) view of who persons are and how they are placed in the grand scheme of things. It is the fact that for us, ultimate meaning is essentially about who we are and what we make of ourselves in this life. As long as the individual is the locus of such value, as long as a person's looks and personality count for so much—and, importantly, something that he or she can do something about—then we will have to live with this kind of jealousy, resentment, and covetousness. The teasing could be gentler, of course, more playful and less wounding. But shadow puppets are not going to do the trick for American children, any more than will growth hormone, estrogens, or cosmetic surgery.[52]

ONE OF THE many pleasures of raising children is reading them books from your own childhood. Ina and I have a sort of informal competition going at home, each of us reading our kids our own favorites, hers in German, mine in English. The books are, to put it mildly, rather different from each other. Show an American of my generation the kind of stories many Germans are raised on and he will be taken aback by their brutality. We may like our television violent, but we prefer our fairy tales sweet. The fairy tales collected by the Grimm Brothers look especially shocking to Americans like me, who were brought up on the sanitized Disney-cartoon versions. In the German originals, the endings are not always happy; nor, for that matter, are the beginnings; and the middles are often filled with abandoned children, self-mutilation, and unhappy death. In the non-Disney Cinderella (or *Aschenputtel*, as the Grimm Brothers called it) there is no fairy godmother; Cinderella gets her dresses magically from her mother's grave; and Cinderella's stepsisters amputate their toes and heels in order to make their feet fit into the prince's glass slipper. Their scheme is given away by their blood-filled shoes. In these tales, the mice don't sing, the witches don't always lose, and the dead are not always resurrected. Trolls eat children. Princesses die. The bad guys win. *So ist das Leben.*

Kids love it, of course; and, I confess, so do I. What is a little harder to swallow, at least with some of these German stories, is a certain authoritarian tone. The two that my children love most, *Max und Moritz* and *Struwwelpeter*, were both written in the nineteenth century. *Max und Moritz* is a comic strip story about two young scamps who are always playing practical jokes on their neighbors—stealing chickens, sawing bridges, or putting gunpowder in a man's pipe. Pretty standard stuff for cartoon kids, and if it were left at that, there would be nothing for an American to notice. But this sort of horseplay was apparently frowned upon in Wilhelmine Germany. By the end of the book, both Max and Moritz have been ground up into corn meal and fed to the ducks. The moral of the story: don't play jokes on grown-ups, or else.

Struwwelpeter, which is even more didactic than *Max und Moritz*, was written by a psychiatrist from Hessen named Heinrich Hoffman (and was translated into English by Mark Twain). *Struwwelpeter* does not play so well among younger German parents these days, but it must have been enormously popular at one point; I have seen kindergartens, parks, streets, and health food shops all named after Struwwelpeter, not to mention the Struwwelpeter Museum in downtown Frankfurt. The book itself is a series of instructional rhymes that read like a cross between Dr. Seuss, Dr. Spock, and Dr. Strangelove. Struwwelpeter is a wild-haired, demented-looking creature with grotesquely long fingernails. His picture appears on the cover of the book, and his rhyme is about what will happen to you if you do not let your parents brush your hair and cut your nails. (You will look as demented as he does and people will call you names.) Other rhymes—take note, Ritalin opponents—tell children what will happen to you if you are absent-minded and distracted (you will plunge into the ocean) or if you fidget too much at the table (you will fall over backward and bring the table crashing down upon you). My son says his favorite is the one about the boy who refuses to stop sucking his thumb. In that one, a determined-looking man rushes out the door with an enormous pair of scissors and lops the boy's thumb off clean.

The vast majority of what passes for children's literature in America is probably no less moralistic than this, though the morals it puts forward are usually less autocratic. American children's books are relentlessly cheery and sentimental, populated by friendly ghosts, environmentally sensitive gnomes, and train engines that can accomplish anything as long as they keep up a positive attitude. Yet the best

American children's books—the ones I use as a counterpoint to *Struwwelpeter*—are, to use Alison Lurie's word, subversive.[53] These books show children a world where grown-ups don't always know best. Huck floating downriver on his raft, Milo disappearing through the phantom tollbooth, Dorothy skipping down the yellow brick road, the Cat in the Hat letting Thing One and Thing Two out of the box, Max riding triumphantly on the back of a Wild Thing, scepter raised high above his head, leading a wild rumpus: these are worlds where the kids are in charge; or if they are not, they ought to be, because the grown-up world is so dull.

The masters of this genre are not American, but British. The great British writers seem to remember what it was like to be a child. A. A. Milne's *Winnie the Pooh* books, Kenneth Grahame's *Wind in the Willows*, Lewis Carroll's *Alice's Adventures in Wonderland* and *Through the Looking Glass*, J. M. Barrie's *Peter Pan*, Frances Hodgson Burnett's *The Secret Garden*, Hugh Lofting's *Doctor Dolittle*, Philip Pullman's *His Dark Materials* trilogy, anything by Roald Dahl, especially the malicious *Charlie and the Chocolate Factory*: these are blueprints for childhood rebellion. Unlike *Struwwelpeter* or *Max und Moritz*, here you can defy grown-ups and get away with it. Their message is that the ordinary adult world may not be the best one, that you should not always believe what adults tell you, and that conventional adult values are not always preferable. Peter Pan refuses to grow up. Doctor Dolittle prefers animals to people. Pooh, a Bear of Very Little Brain, eats too much and can't read or write. And Alice, of course, is far more sensible than any of the nutcase grown-ups she runs into when she goes down the rabbit hole.

Most enhancement technologies for children are not subversive in the sense that the best children's books are. What look like pediatric enhancements usually turn out really to be adult enhancements. They mirror the adult world, reflecting and reinforcing conventional adult values. These technologies make children taller, make their teeth straighter, make them concentrate better and sit still. They make children better citizens. Enhancement technologies *by* kids, rather than simply *for* them, would give children gifts like those of Dr. Dolittle, who can talk to animals, or Roald Dahl's Matilda, who uses her telekinetic powers to defeat the malevolent Mrs. Trunchbull.

It is sometimes said that great children's literature, unlike run-of-the-mill children's books, can also be read as serious adult literature. So while kids read *Huckleberry Finn* for Huck and Jim's adventures on the river, adults can read it as a social critique of slavery. While kids read Lewis Carroll's *Alice* books as fantasy, adults can read them for their logical puzzles and philosophical jokes. Maybe there is something to this argument, but it is also true that most mediocre children's books pay excessive attention to the concerns of adults while ignoring the child's point of view. Most children's books are simply watered-down parables for adults, with bears or elves substituted for the humans, and they reflect adult concerns of the day. Even the great Dr. Seuss was not immune to adult moralizing. His later books were often heavy-handed polemics against nuclear war or environmental destruction.

Or take, for example, *Higgledy Piggledy Pop*, Maurice Sendak's slender illustrated book for children of about three or four years of age. *Higgledy Piggledy Pop* is the story of a rich but dissatisfied dog by the name of Jennie. Jennie leaves home because she has everything she wants, and she decides there must be more to life than having everything. She goes out into the wide world and has adventures. However, the adventures she has turn out not to be real adventures at all, but elaborate auditions for a stage play into which she has accidentally wandered. She does very well in the play, is invited to join the acting troupe, and becomes famous. And once she is famous, she becomes very happy. End of story.

What exactly are we to make of this? The animal characters are standard fare for children, but the story is clearly about adult worries. It is a story about an alienated dog and the peculiar dissatisfaction that comes with having everything you want. The subtitle of the book is, "There Must be More to Life." Even the adult message of the book is oddly American. Money isn't everything, it teaches; fame is. The real secret to happiness is celebrity. With the adulation of others, your alienation will vanish. Even setting this peculiar message aside, it is hard to imagine a four-year-old child with these existential concerns.

The great children's books are first and foremost for children, and when we read them as adults, we remember something of what it was like, once upon a time, to be a child. If logical jokes and Victorian parody were all there were to Alice's adventures in Wonderland, they would be a pretty sterile exercise. What keeps the Alice books vivid is neither the logic nor the parody, but their singular view of the world, which for all its hallucinogenic quality is always a child's point of view. The worlds Alice encounters through the looking glass and down the rabbit hole are even stranger to a contemporary child than they would have been for a child in Victorian England, with their white knights and red queens, rabbits with pocket-watches, and Cheshire cats, but their strangeness is still made intelligible by the bemused detachment with which Alice sees them. The conventional reading of the Alice stories, as Adam Gopnik points out, is as quest tales: Alice goes off on a quest, has adventures, and comes back with knowledge and maturity. But this can't be right. As Gopnik puts it, Alice is already the most mature person in Wonderland when she arrives. When she leaves she does not say "There's no place like home" but rather, "I can't stand this any longer!"[54]

If I were asked to pick a children's book to serve as a parable for childhood enhancement technologies, though, it would not be *Alice's Adventures in Wonderland*, nor any of the American children's stories I read as a child. It would be Carlo Collodi's *Pinocchio*. Not the saccharine Disney version, but the dark, funny Italian original. Here is an actual enhancement, Pinocchio's metamorphosis from wood to flesh: Pinocchio is a puppet, but he wants to be a real boy. He loves his father-creator Geppetto, keeps talking again and again of how much he loves him and wants to be with him and wants to make him proud. But Pinocchio is a foolish, weak-willed puppet. He is constantly being fooled and tricked and cheated, and it is always because he is too gullible or too willing to take the easy way. When Geppetto sells his own coat to get the money for Pinocchio to buy schoolbooks, Pinocchio loses it to con men. When he promises to go to school, he is lured away to a place of perpetual fun. Again and again he promises to do right, and again and again he fails.

But how, in the end, does he become a real boy? Through love and heroic self-sacrifice. Pinocchio rescues Geppetto from the belly of the shark. Returning home to find Geppetto gone, Pinocchio tracks him down, goes to sea in a boat, finds him alive, but just barely, and risks his own life in order to save him. The child saves the father. It is a wonderful story for a father to read to a child, and it conveys a powerful message: that the way to be truly human is to show truly human attributes. But these truly human attributes are not the attributes that moral philosophers have suggested are the markers of personhood, like reason or language or the capacity for abstract thought. Truly human attributes are the capacity for love, sacrifice, and the call of family. Once Pinocchio really feels these things, he becomes human.

The parable also has a darker side, however, a side about which I feel some ambivalence. When Pinocchio becomes a real boy, it is only through his own virtue. His humanity is not something that is given to him, not something he possesses by right, but something that he has to earn. Pinocchio does not want to be superior. He does not want to compete with other children and win. He just wants to be normal. Yet normality, the story teaches, is not something that everyone deserves. It is something that you must earn. It must come only through hard work.

Perhaps Collodi's story helps explain why we feel no qualms about someone who works his way through his unhappiness or alienation through therapy, while remaining judgmental about the person who does it with Prozac. As Wittgenstein says, we feel they have to go the bloody hard way. A hard, muscled body through workouts in the gym is great, but do the same thing with steroids and you are banned from competition. This, we are told, is cheating. And maybe it is. But we generally condemn steroid use even when no competition is involved. Perhaps we simply see competition everywhere, so that the steroid-user is condemned for cheating in life. The correct way, the noble way, is the bloody hard way.

If we see *Pinocchio* as a cautionary tale about enhancement technologies for children, it is because of the contradictory feelings that we have about children and how to treat them. We value autonomy and independence, but children are not autonomous or independent. We want to resist cultural pressures, but not at the expense of our children's well-being. We may not see life as a competition for ourselves, but we see it as a competition for them; and we want to give them a leg up. Pinocchio is a model of this kind of ambiguity. In so ways Pinocchio is treated more like an adult than like a child.

goes off on adventures by himself. He rebels against his father. He is held accountable for his actions and at one point is even tossed in jail. Yet he is not completely like an adult because he is not completely mature. He is held responsible, but not fully responsible. He is forgiven for his failings. His character is being formed. He is being taught how to behave.

In the end, maybe the real lesson of *Pinocchio*, and the reason it has something to teach us about enhancement technologies, is that it shows us our limits as parents, despite what we tell ourselves. Pinocchio is not merely raised by Geppetto; he is created. He is literally carved out of a stick of wood. The story begins with magic: the stick simply starts talking, behaving in ways over which the puppet-maker has no control. As the stick becomes a puppet, and later as the puppet becomes an older, more willful puppet, he behaves in ways that the maker can neither understand nor manage. Here is the wonder of being a parent: how your children come to be the way they are. Try as you might to mold them and teach them, there is something there that resists. They are human beings. They have a nature and a will of their own. The material, contrary to what we sometimes like to think, is not infinitely pliable.

11

SECOND ACTS

Sometime I wonder why she put me out of doors
Yeah sometime I wonder why she put me out of
doors
You know my letter's gone dead,
and my pencil it won't write no more.
—Muddy Waters

What would it be like to have a second chance at youth? John Frankenheimer's 1966 film *Seconds* opens with a man making his way through a crowded train station. Middle-aged and paunchy, he wears a gray business suit, and his damp, waxy complexion suggests a nervous sweat. We see the man through the fish-eye lens of the camera that follows him, lurching in an oddly stiff way: the visual effect is that of a businessman being followed by a zombie. As the man boards the train, he is suddenly slapped on the shoulder. He spins around, and a note is thrust into his hand. The train starts to move. The man sticks his head out the window, staring as it pulls away from the station. We can see no one. When the man finally opens the note nervously, all that is written on it is an address.

When the commuter train stops, the man gets into a station wagon driven by his wife. The two stare vacantly through the windshield, exchange a few words of meaningless small talk, and drive home in silence to the suburbs. The emotional effect is deadly. We immediately understand what we are seeing: Arthur Hamilton, Organization

Man, commuting to and from his job at the bank every day, dictating vacuous memos to his secretary, then boarding a commuter train to his sterile suburban home. We can easily imagine Arthur Hamilton sleepwalking to his grave.

Then we learn about the note. Hamilton gets a phone call in the dead of night from a college friend long presumed dead. The friend explains that the address on the note is that of a secret company that arranges second chances. The company will fake a client's death, provide a look-alike corpse, and give the client extensive cosmetic surgery and physical rehabilitation. Then it will help the client start all over: new career, new friends, and new identity. At first Hamilton is stunned, then wary. When he eventually works up the nerve to visit the company, he sits down to a conversation with the owner, a folksy gentleman in a white suit. "Is there really any meaning left for you?" the man asks Hamilton. "Anything at all?" Hamilton pauses, struggles. He thinks first of his daughter, then he admits he rarely sees her anymore. He mentions his wife, but confesses that there is no longer much left between them. He tells the man about a possible promotion at work, his voice trailing off. "There's nothing, is there?" asks the man, not unkindly. Hamilton shakes his head. The man smiles and nods sympathetically. He says, "There never was a struggle in the soul of a good man that wasn't hard."

Once Hamilton agrees to this Faustian bargain, the process of getting a new identity gets quickly underway. Hamilton is given extensive facial surgery. He undergoes a punishing regimen of physical training. He gets new hair and a younger, tauter body. A psychological counselor decides that Hamilton should not be a banker anymore, but a painter. Hamilton emerges a new man, as dashing and fit as a young Olympian. Even the actor who plays Hamilton has changed. No longer is Hamilton played by the middle-aged John Randolph. Now he is a young Rock Hudson.

The company sends Hamilton to an elegant new house in California, where a butler caters to his every need. He spends his days painting abstracts by the water. He even meets a beautiful young woman, a free spirit who has left her husband and children to live by the Pacific. She is the '60s California counterpart to Hamilton's northern, 1950s life, the kind of woman who drives a convertible, reads tea leaves, and runs spontaneously into the ocean waves, laughing, to ask mystical questions of the sea. The woman invites Hamilton to an orgy-like festival in the forest whose celebrants play madrigals on medieval horns and pour wine into each other's mouths from goatskin flasks. At first Hamilton is mortified and self-conscious. He looks on embarrassed from the fringes of the celebration as everyone else discards their clothes. But soon the celebrants drag him into a giant vat of grapes, where he is surrounded by frolicking nude strangers. Hamilton finally starts to laugh ecstatically and dance, his lovely young girlfriend in his arms, shouting "Yes, Yes!" as the scene fades away.

If *Seconds* were a conventional Hollywood movie, it might have ended there. We would be left to conclude that American lives do have second acts; that the demands of self-fulfillment trump the responsibilities of family; and that the ideal human life would combine the wisdom of age with the energy of youth. Instead, Hamilton's new identity soon becomes as oppressive as his old one. The new Hamilton has everything that today's anti-aging therapies promise, yet he looks in the mirror with the same hollow-eyed desperation. The reflection staring back at him looks just as empty as before.

One evening at a cocktail party Hamilton drinks too much and begins to drop alcohol-inspired hints that he is not who he seems to be. He almost gives away the secret of his identity. Some guests seem merely puzzled, but others are alarmed. A group of men descend upon Hamilton and drag him away to a bedroom, where they reveal that they too are all "Reborns": products of the very same company that has sent Hamilton to California. Everything about Hamilton's new life is exposed as a fake, even the things he had assumed were genuine. His new girlfriend is a company employee. The Reborns circle Hamilton like the Satan-worshipers in *Rosemary's Baby*, looking menacingly down as he lies drunk on the bed.

But the most chilling scene in *Seconds* does not come until Hamilton escapes California and goes back to New York. Like Ebenezer Scrooge with the Ghost of Christmas Future, Hamilton visits his wife to quiz her about her dead husband, the old Arthur Hamilton. He finds his old house remodeled and his wife unperturbed. Not only does she fail to recognize him, she does not even seem sad about his presumed death. "Arthur lived as if he were a stranger here," she says. "There was always a look around his eyes as if he were trying to say something. I don't know what. A protest against whatever he'd surrendered his life to." She paces the living room quietly, walks to the mirror. "He fought so hard for what he'd been taught to want. And when he got it, he just got more and more confused. The silences grew longer. We never talked about it. We lived our lives in a polite, celibate truce." The old Arthur Hamilton has disappeared and left not a trace of regret.

If the darkness of *Seconds* comes partly from the social climate of the era—the menacing sense that someone (the company, the government, the establishment) is secretly in charge of our lives, pulling the strings behind the scene—it also hints at the larger difficulties with medical interventions aimed at postponing aging. Can youth really solve the problems of age? We have become accustomed to the idea that the tragedy of aging is physical and mental decline: the soul of a young person trapped in a debilitated, traitorous body. Often it is not Death that we fear so much as the instruments of torture that he carries with him: the degeneration and disability, the creaking joints and aching bones, the loss of stamina and sexual attractiveness. But what if it were possible to disarm Death—not just to prolong life, but also to extend youth? What if we could all live twice as long as we do now in good health, then wither away quickly at the end? A growing body of biological research suggests that the idea is not as outrageous as it might once have seemed. Would longer and younger lives be better lives? Or as *Seconds* suggests, would they simply be much the same as they are now, only longer?

I FIRST SAW *Seconds* fifteen years ago on video in a cramped student flat in Glasgow, Scotland, at the suggestion of one of my flatmates, David Gems. At that time David was a postgraduate student in molecular genetics from London. At various times we shared the flat with a Palestinian ophthalmologist, an Egyptian cardiologist, a Marxist economist from Ulster, a Canadian postgraduate studying urban planning, and a moody Irishman who spent large blocks of time locked in his room praying aloud. *Seconds* was one of a number of films that David would recommend to me over the years, the most recent of which were a BBC documentary that featured a man with a sexual fetish for cleaning toilet bowls with his tongue, and Volker Schlondorff's *Why Does Herr R Run Amok?*, the story of an alienated German who guns down his family and commits suicide. *Seconds* was a prophetic choice, though, because David went on to specialize in the genetics of aging. Today he holds a Royal Society Fellowship at University College London, where he spends his days studying a tiny nematode worm called *c. elegans*. By selectively breeding mutant worms, he and his colleagues can make them live for a startlingly long time. For example, David and his colleague Linda Riddle have shown that by breeding male nematodes with one mutation in a gene called *daf-2*, they can increase the worms' maximum life span over sixfold, from 31 days to 199 days.[1] Even more remarkably, these elderly worms do not show the physical decline that you might expect of an aging nematode. The old worms are just as vigorous as the young ones. If these worms were humans, they would be living for 700 years.[2]

It is a long leap from nematodes to humans, of course, as David is quick to point out. Yet he also notes that many of the mechanisms that govern aging in nematodes have counterparts in humans. It is not implausible, he believes, even by the standards of conventional science, to think that what can be done for nematodes might also be done someday for other organisms. In a recent paper in *Science*, David and colleagues at University College London showed that a particular genetic mutation extends lifespan in both nematodes and fruit flies.[3] A common mechanism for worms and flies may not sound like much, but this was the first hard evidence that the aging process might be governed by the same mechanism in different species. This evidence has generated speculation that aging may well be governed by similar genetic mechanisms in *all* species, including *homo sapiens*.

For many years, biologists assumed that aging was a matter of simple physical decline. The decline of the body seemed as inevitable as the decline of a train engine or a washing machine: at some point, the parts wear out, and the machine stops working. Yet there have always been problems for this view when it comes to biological organisms. Why do some animal species live longer than others? Why does the fruit bat live for thirty years and the fruit fly for four weeks? Why do some species, like the hydra, appear not to age at all? According to evolutionary theories of aging, it is implausible to see aging as a process of simple physical decline. Aging is better seen as a consequence of genetic mutations that have accumulated in the population over time.[4]

As David explains, the insight that led to the evolutionary theory of aging initially came from problems explaining the continued existence of genetic diseases. In evolutionary terms, it makes sense that most genetic diseases would be very rare. Most are caused by mutant recessive genes. This means that if a person carries a recessive gene for a disease, he or she may still not actually have the disease itself. To have the disease, a person must have two copies of that recessive gene, not just one. For example, cystic fibrosis is caused by a recessive gene, and carriers of the cystic fibrosis gene do not have the disease themselves. Nor will they ordinarily have children with cystic fibrosis—not unless they conceive children with another carrier of the cystic fibrosis gene, in which case the chances of each of their future children having cystic fibrosis are one in four.

This is why the disease is relatively rare. In the first place, it is unlikely that two carriers of such a rare gene will meet and have children together. But secondly, even if they do meet and have children with the disease, those children are less likely than healthy children to survive to adulthood and have children of their own. Natural selection is working against them. Evolutionary theory predicts that the number of copies of the gene for cystic fibrosis in the general population should go down over time in comparison to the healthy gene, keeping cystic fibrosis rare.

But here is the puzzle. What about genetic diseases caused by dominant genes? With these genetic diseases, everyone who has the gene will have the disease. Their children will have one chance in two of carrying the gene, which (since the gene equals the disease) translates to one chance in two of having the disease. If the disease is lethal, then evolutionary theory would predict that it should be very rare. Natural selection should root it out. By the logic of evolutionary biology, for example, Huntington's disease should have disappeared from the population long ago. Not only is Huntington's disease caused by a dominant gene, it is also debilitating and eventually lethal. Those who suffer from it become mentally ill, suffer serious neurological problems, and often die a very painful death. Yet Huntington's disease, by the standards of genetic diseases, is still relatively common. It strikes one in 15,000 people of European descent. Why haven't evolutionary forces eliminated the Huntington's disease gene from the population?

This was the question asked in the 1940s by English biologist J. B. S. Haldane, whose early work laid the groundwork for evolutionary theories of aging. The answer, Haldane thought, is that Huntington's disease does not affect its victims until middle age. The average age of onset is about thirty-five. The tragedy of Huntington's disease is that by the time a person begins to suffer from its effects, that person probably will have already had children. This is how the gene remains in the population, even though it kills its carriers: its effects are delayed until after reproduction.

This simple idea explains the persistence of Huntington's disease, but it also explains a lot more. It explains how all sorts of genetic mutations remain relatively common, despite the fact that they are damaging or lethal. If the pressure of natural selection is very weak when it comes to genetic mutations whose effects become apparent only after the age of reproduction, then it makes sense that all sorts of these genetic mutations might have persisted in living populations, despite the fact that they confer no selective advantage. In fact, since many genes have not one but many different effects, it might well be possible for a gene to enhance an organism's reproductive fitness yet still shorten its life. The very same gene might increase the odds that an organism will produce offspring, yet lessen the odds that the organism will live a long life after it has reproduced.

The evolutionary theory of aging has grown up around this simple but revolutionary idea: that the force of natural selection weakens with increasing age after the onset of reproduction.[5] According to evolutionary theory, it is wrong to think of aging as an inevitable consequence of getting old. Biological systems do not simply wear out. Aging is a by-product of the process of evolution, and it is controlled by genetics, like eye color. The processes we think of as natural decline and loss may instead be a range of genetic mutations that strike late in life, accumulated and stored away over the course of our evolutionary history. Thus the evolutionary theory of aging has tremendous implications for clinical genetics. If aging is a product of genetic mutations, then those mutations might also be subject to therapeutic intervention.

So is aging a "genetic disease"? This is the kind of question that philosophers like to ask, and it is deliberately provocative.[6] Calling something a disease not only puts it within the domain of medical practice but also suggests that it ought to be cured, controlled, even done away with entirely. In some ways, of course, the cure and control of aging is what many doctors do every day, when they prescribe drugs for arthritis or diabetes or heart disease. As a rule, people get sicker more often as they get older. But doctors generally think of this as the treatment of age-related diseases, not the treatment of aging itself. To embark on the treatment of aging itself sounds like hubris at best, and at worst, pure folly, like Ponce de Leon on his quest through the Florida Keys. Yet once it is clear that the purpose of treating aging would be not just to extend life but also to make that life healthier, the line between the treatment of aging and the treatment of age-related diseases becomes fuzzy. What could be wrong with aiming for a longer but healthier life?

One difficulty in answering that question has always been the difficulty of imagining how a dramatically extended life span would affect our basic social conditions. Many people worry that an increased human life span would result in massive overpopulation, that it would increase existing gaps in health and wealth, and that it would doom political institutions set up to care for the elderly, such as Social Security and Medicare. Other social questions are more slippery. Which stages of life would be extended? Would adolescence stretch out even further? Would retirement? In what ways might life extension change the structure of the family? Many people find it difficult to marry and live with a person for twenty or thirty years; think how much harder it would be for them to sustain a marriage that was expected to last three times as long.[7] How would families change if they were spread out over four or five generations and a child could expect to have sixteen living great-great-grandparents? What duties would members of these extended families have to one another?

A longer life might also come at a biological cost. One important area of genetic research involves potential trade-offs between life span and reproduction. As early as the 1950s, Maynard Smith, a one-time student of Haldane's, found that female fruit flies lived much longer if he bred them with a mutation that inhibited the development of their ovaries. Other researchers have gone on to show that fruit flies can be bred to live longer, but they lose their early surge of reproductive energy.[8] This kind of trade-off does not seem to apply to all species (not to nematodes, for example), but some evidence suggests it may apply to humans. In the 1960s, for example, physician James Hamilton looked at the medical records of 300 mentally retarded men who had been institutionalized in Kansas at the turn of the century. At that period in history, it was not uncommon for institutional authorities to castrate such men to prevent behavioral problems. Hamilton compared the records of these castrated men to 700 men in the same institution who had not been castrated. Remarkably, he found not just that castration had extended these men's lives, but also that it had extended them by an average of fourteen years. To get an idea of just how long that fourteen-year extension is, compare it to the estimated *three* extra years of life that the average American could expect from a cure for cancer.[9]

For women, some of these issues are currently being played out in a heated debate over hormone replacement therapy, which physicians prescribe to postmenopausal women with the aim of preventing age-related illnesses such as osteoporosis, heart disease, and Alzheimer's Disease. Hormone replacement therapy is used by 38 percent of post-menopausal American women, who spent $2.75 billion on it in 2001. Premarin (an estrogen replacement therapy) was America's third most commonly prescribed drug in 2001, with 45 million prescriptions.[10] While it is controversial whether hormone replacement therapy actually prevents some of these age-related diseases (and if it can, whether its benefits are outweighed by its risks), even skeptical clinicians often argue that it prevents unwanted symptoms associated with menopause, such as hot flashes, which are sometimes said to occur in as many as 85 percent of American women.[11]

Yet one of the most striking aspects of menopause is the extent to which it varies across cultures. Hot flashes, for example, are not universally experienced. In fact, many of the symptoms of menopause experienced by American women are not seen as problems, much less medical problems, in other parts of the world. For her book *Encounters with Aging*, anthropologist Margaret Lock conducted 105 in-depth interviews with Japanese women ranging in age from forty-five to fifty-five years.[12] Of all the women Lock interviewed, only twelve reported any symptoms that even resembled hot flashes. Not a single woman complained of a serious sleep disturbance, or of waking up with drenched sheets from night sweats, as many North American women do.[13] Lock also conducted a much larger survey comparing over 1,300 Japanese women to ones from Canada (from Manitoba) and the United States (from Massachusetts.) Here, the differences were just as striking. While 75 percent of the North American women had experienced a hot flash at some point in their past, this was true of only 25 percent of the Japanese women. Asked what symptoms of menopause they had experienced over the past two weeks, the North Americans were nearly three to five times as likely as the Japanese to complain of night sweats or cold sweats, and two to three times as likely to complain of hot flashes.[14] Even Japanese doctors rarely reported patients who complained of hot flashes. In fact, when asked about a whole range of symptoms—shortness of breath, backache, headache, stomachache, dizziness, irritability, depression, insomnia, among others—the North American women were virtually guaranteed to have experienced the symptoms more often than the Japanese. The only symptoms Japanese women were significantly more likely to have experienced were diarrhea or constipation.

What accounts for these dramatically different experiences of menopause? For Lock, the most importance differences are cultural. Japanese women, for instance, neither fear nor dread menopause the way that North American women do. In fact, some of them even look forward to it. To get older in Japan is to advance in a social hierarchy, and this advancement is accompanied by more responsibility and greater maturity.[15] It is said that a person is not recognized as fully mature in Japan until the age of fifty.[16] Japanese women, writes Lock, see middle age as "relatively inviting, a transition from which individuals can both look back over the previous fifty years and look forward to the next thirty and, given financial security, usually report good fortune and happiness."[17]

Contrast this view of aging with our own, in which the middle years are seen not as a marker of maturity, but as the beginning of a slow, downward decline into old age. For women, menopause means the loss of fertility, which, in a society where normality for women is defined in terms of physical beauty and reproductive capacity, translates into abnormality. For all the American media propaganda about the "golden years," many North Americans desperately fear old age, which we treat as a stage of life somehow unconnected to all that has preceded it. Once we reach old age we are given special names ("seniors," "retirees," "the elderly"), special living spaces (retirement villages, nursing homes), special clubs, activities, organizations, and magazines, most of which center on no other aspect of our identities than the fact that we have reached the age of sixty-five. According to the philosopher Alasdair MacIntyre, we have such a distorted view of aging because we no longer see the end of a human life as part of a story that began much earlier.[18] Nor do we see ourselves as connected in any meaningful way to the past. So those who connect us to the past have lost their importance too. Old people are no longer repositories of wisdom, because wisdom is no longer about tradition or the shared history of a community. Once people pass a certain age, they are assumed to leave the rest of their identities behind and become, simply, "old." What else is there for the old but to fantasize about youth?

A consistent part of North America's infatuation with cosmetic anti-aging procedures is to embrace the procedures while passionately criticizing the cultural attitudes that make the procedures seem necessary. Faced with the prospect of middle age, many women try to stop the biological clock with treadmill workouts, constant dieting, and an occasional tune-up with a plastic surgeon, all the while criticizing the society that says female beauty means youth. It's not hard to understand the hostility provoked by the spread of cosmetic procedures such as Botox injections for aging skin; the more they are used, the more that people feel compelled to use them, and unlike most cosmetic surgery, the "need" for it is close to universal: unless we die early, all of us get old. Yet there is an air of futility about a lot of this criticism, as if a society could simply replace an aesthetic preference for smooth skin with one for wrinkles, given enough media advertising and better roles for sexy older women in Hollywood films. Perhaps we can do better, but the problem is not simply an aesthetic ideal in favor of youth; it is an absence of desirable cultural space for women apart from being objects of attraction. Southern writer Florence King has criticized American women for desperately trying to inspire passion in their old age. Older Southern women, in contrast, have always tried to inspire terror. King writes, "A country without a tradition of redoubtable battle-axes is a country that does not offer its young women any positive images for female old age."[19]

Contrast North American with Japanese women who, despite the fact that they live longer than anyone else in the world, do not wish for lives nearly as long as those that North American women wish for themselves. In Lock's survey, only 8 percent of Japanese women said that, given the choice, they would choose to live past the age of eighty. Fully 41 percent said they would settle for a life of less than seventy years. Canadian women, of course, wanted to live far longer. Twenty-nine percent wanted to live to eighty, and another 26 percent wanted to live past eighty-five.[20] In fact, when these menopausal women were asked what age they felt themselves to be, nearly a quarter said they felt younger than thirty. Japanese women said they felt quite close to their actual chronological ages.[21] While sweeping generalizations would be unwise here, the composite picture that emerges from this survey is striking: a middle-aged, fifty-five-year-old woman from Winnipeg who feels twenty-five on the inside, and wants to live until the age of eighty-five.

IN 2001, AFTER three years of retirement from basketball, Michael Jordan returned to the NBA. In many ways his return was remarkable. Even at the advanced age of thirty-eight, practically ancient for a professional basketball player, Jordan performed at a level well above that of most other players in the league. Yet as the season wore on it became clear that, despite occasional flashes of brilliance, Jordan was only a shadow of the player he used to be. He was simply not as quick or athletic as many of the muscled twenty-five-year-olds he was facing. Watching Jordan struggle through a grueling season, missing shots and making crucial turnovers, I could understand a little of his frustration. I am nearly two years older than Jordan, and unlike the vast majority of the people I grew up playing basketball with in high school, I still manage to play a regular pick-up game. It is not easy. Basketball is a young man's game. Most guys my age have given it up for golf or poker. To play pick-up basketball at age forty is not just to risk humiliation. It is also to risk being patronized by a teenager with a nose stud and a snake tattooed on his shoulder who was not even born when you started playing the game.

Professional athletes face a problem that some of us never have to think about. In many jobs people work their way up the career ladder, earning more money and more respect as they get older. But professional athletes often reach their peaks in their twenties, or even earlier. A thirty-year-old professional basketball player is a seasoned veteran, and a thirty-five-year-old is nearing the end of his career. Basketball players may get craftier as they get older, they may learn a few new tricks, but they are at the mercy of their physical skills. Many athletes simply flounder once they can no longer play competitively, squeezing out an unhappy existence at the margins of the sport. When a doctor retires at age seventy, the arc of his career has run roughly parallel to the arc of his life. But when an athlete retires at age thirty-five, he can see a long future stretching out in front of him with no career to fill it. It is no wonder Jordan felt compelled to come back.

Academic philosophers who have speculated on life extension have worried that a longer life would be a more boring life, like Sisyphus rolling the boulder up the mountain again and again.[22] Their worry is related to that of *Seconds*: that a second chance at youth in a society of alienation would simply produce longer, more alienated lives. But this worry may say more about the kinds of lives typically led by academic philosophers than it does about life extension. The typical academic career takes a strikingly predictable path when it is successful: college, graduate school, a job in a university department, maybe a few moves before gaining tenure, then years of teaching and writing about the same subjects until retirement. The most dramatic career change a successful academic can expect is to move into university administration. Academic career paths are designed for stability and specialization. Change is usually associated with failure:

unsuccessful job searches, rejected tenure applications, and the occasional sexual harassment charge. Academics do not face the same problems that professional athletes do because we do not have jobs that require us to learn how to do anything dramatically new in midlife. Our problem is not how to start over again with something new, like the professional athlete, but how to face a life where starting over again seems so remote a possibility.

David Gems suggests that the real tragedy of aging may be a kind of "ontological diminution." By "ontological" he means a flattening of the conditions that sustain our existence. As we move into old age, our senses dim, our minds get slower, our sexual desire diminishes, and our bodies lose their physical capacities. Our experience of the world gradually grows dimmer and narrower. As the end of life grows closer, even the future begins to look constricted. The range of possibilities open to us seems to close up, not only because we cannot do as much as before, but also because we do not *want* to. To be relieved of some desires can be a blessing, of course. But a future completely devoid of desire can seem like an especially depressing prospect. To be the kind of person who does not want to do anything whatsoever strikes many people as the worst kind of fate: a kind of volitional castration, lived out in a purgatory of dead routine.

For David, the promise of anti-aging therapies is not that of living a longer and healthier life, but living a richer and more interesting life. Anti-aging therapies could prevent the diminishing range of experience that aging seems to bring. What would life be like if old age offered youth's energy, enthusiasm, and flexibility? In our conversations, David wonders about a life dedicated not just to more of the same thing, but also to the opportunity to do more and experience more, like Dustin Hoffman in *Little Big Man*. What would it be like to have not one career, but three or five or ten? What would it be like to live not in one country, but in four or five? To learn more languages and more skills, to cultivate different kinds of relationships, to experience a fuller variety of things ordinarily prohibited by a life of conventional length and health?

Occasionally people live these kinds of lives within a conventional life span. Before going into genetics, for example, David played in a London punk band, dug graves in Nicaragua, and worked in a fish packaging plant in Iceland. When I finished medical school in South Carolina I gave up medicine, moved to Scotland to study philosophy, married a German, then spent the next decade working in New Zealand, South Africa, and Quebec. But David and I did most of these things before we turned thirty. Life since then has been much more conventional. The question is whether there is something about aging—biologically, socially, or culturally—that makes this kind of change so rare later in life. Many people simply do not see any fun or glamour in starting a new life at age forty-five. Others would like to start over in midlife, but are less willing to take risks as long as they have a family to support. Some people simply find that they cannot perform as well as younger people. It is well known that some mental abilities, such as language acquisition, peak in childhood. Many researchers have wondered whether other mental abilities decline with advancing age, especially those required for mathematics and physics. Einstein was only twenty-six when he devised his theory of special relativity, and Newton began his revolutionary work in physics and calculus before he turned thirty.[23] Is there something about aging that puts a damper on creative thought?

The classic book on the topic is Harvey Lehman's 1953 *Age and Achievement*, which attempted to map the relationship between age and "outstanding performance" in fields as diverse as bacteriology, astronomy, hymn-writing, and duck-pin bowling.[24] Lehman's research methods were varied and, at least by some accounts, somewhat questionable. His favored technique started with compiling a "best of" list for a particular field. For the sciences, he compiled lists of great discoveries from prominent histories of science; for literature, he relied on a book called *One Thousand Best Books*; for golf, he simply looked at the winners of the various U.S. and British golf championships. Once Lehman had his "best of" list, he matched up each great achievement with the age at which the person in question achieved it. The result is a series of charts mapping the great achievements with five-year spans of the achievers' lives.

For anyone over the age of forty, Lehman's charts make for profoundly depressing reading. Though there are exceptions, Lehman finds that the performance of most creative thinkers parallels the performance of athletes. Their best work is usually done before age forty, and often before thirty. After that, it is a fast downhill ride to the cemetery. And while it may not be terribly upsetting to learn that you have little chance to become a pistol-shooting champion or a first-rate hymn writer after age thirty-six, how many chemists will be happy to know that their peak years came between ages twenty-six and thirty, back when they were in graduate school? The "golden years" for creative work, according to Lehman, usually fall between thirty and forty. Billiards players, amateur bowlers, and writers of children's literature peak between the ages of thirty and thirty-four, while surgeons, geologists, and opera composers do their best work between thirty-five and thirty-nine. Only when Lehman turns his charts on factors such as earned income, industrial leadership, and membership in the British cabinet do the curves start to shift favorably toward the later stages of life. Philosophy professors, like surgeons and geologists, head downhill after age forty, but for us there is at least one small consolation: the ride down is much slower. The drop-off in quality of philosophical work is apparently not very steep until we reach our fifties and sixties. In fact, measured in terms of sheer quantity, the drop-off does not appear until a time very close to death. Many of us keep on writing philosophy well into our eighties, even if what we are writing is not much good.

Lehman's methodology has gotten its fair share of criticism. Lehman looked at only The Great Thinkers and Achievers, for example, not ordinary thinkers and achievers. Just because Austen, Burns, and Keats did their great work when they were young does not say anything about when ordinary writers are likely to do their best work. Great Thinkers and Achievers make up only a small proportion of the population of people involved in any given activity. It might well be that a disproportionate number of young people appear to do important work in a field simply because there are more young people working in that field. (Even Lehman notes that The Greats sometimes do great work when they are very old. Samuel Johnson published his *Lives of the English Poets* when he was seventy-two; Benjamin Franklin invented bifocal lenses at the age of seventy-eight; and Goethe finished *Faust* when he was eighty.) To get a better idea of what we really want to know about age and creativity, Lehman would need to follow a representative group of ordinary people in different careers over the course of their lives, and map the periods where these people did their best work. Yet even then, a cluster of good work in the early years would not necessarily mean that youth translates into natural creativity. It might be that scientists do their best work before age thirty-five because they have more energy and work harder when they are younger, or because this is the time when their tenure applications come due. Still, the idea that Lehman was trying to prove, however crudely, is one that is widely suspected, if not empirically confirmed: some human activities require skills at which young people excel, while others require long experience.[25] This is why anthropologist Clifford Geertz calls the Institute for Advanced Study at Princeton a nursery for mathematicians and a nursing home for historians.

Is A LOSS of creativity really what worries most people about mental aging? David Gems's phrase "ontological diminution" suggests a much broader and more nebulous problem, widely noticed but rarely studied: the inflexibility that age seems to bring. As we age, we seem to settle into grooves that get deeper and more rigid with time. The older we become, the more likely we are to listen to the same music, vacation at the same places, spend our evenings and weekends in the same ways, so that by the time we hit sixty, many of us are as dogmatic and inflexible as a first-grader who refuses to eat anything but hot dogs. This suggests not so much a loss of creativity as a loss of receptivity to new things, an unwillingness to change the channel. For older people, settled in their ways, this may simply look like good taste, but to many of us who have not quite gotten there yet, it carries the scent of existential dread. Anti-aging enthusiasts argue that a longer life would be a richer and fuller life, filled with new activities, new relationships, and new opportunities for self-fulfilment. But what if a longer life just means a longer retirement to fill with shuffleboard and mashed potatoes?

In recent decades psychologists have begun to measure a construct called "openness to experience." Openness to experience is one of the traits in the so-called five-factor model of personality, and is associated with characteristics such as flexibility, intellectual curiosity, artistic sensitivity, and unconventional attitudes.[26] Psychologist

Robert McCrae cites as a model of "experiential openness" Jean-Jacques Rousseau—the social philosopher, self-taught composer, father of Romanticism, and intellectual forebear of the French Revolution, who, late in life, flaunted his disregard for conventional attitudes by dressing in an Armenian cap and caftan.[27] (McCrae does not mention that Rousseau also abandoned his children, was frequently convinced that his friends were plotting to kill him, and had a fondness for exposing his backside to young female strangers.) Psychologists who have measured experiential openness across the life span have found that it does tend to diminish slightly with age, though not as much as one might expect.[28] According to this scale, people who are open at age thirty are apt to stay that way through old age.

Stanford neurobiologist Robert Sapolsky found something rather different in his (semi-serious) study of aging and receptivity to novel tastes.[29] As Sapolsky tells the story, his questions began with his administrative assistant, Paul. Paul was fresh out of college, and like many recent college graduates he listened to a lot of loud, popular music. Sapolsky found the music Paul played on his CD player irritating, but not because of the music itself. What was irritating was the way the music varied. One day Paul would be playing Sonic Youth; the next day, klezmer music; another day, Wagner overtures; the next day, Gregorian chants. John Coltrane, Shostakovich, Celtic folk music, Philip Glass, Puccini arias, and big-band hits: Paul was constantly trying out new styles of music, rejecting some styles and hanging on to others, methodically developing his musical tastes. To Sapolsky, Paul seemed extraordinarily open to novelty, and not just in his music. This open-mindedness extended to every part of Paul's life. He would watch a weekend's worth of Indian musicals, read contemporary Hungarian realist novels, dip into Chaucer or Melville, all for the sake of trying something new. For a time he would wear long hair and a beard, then one day report to work bald.

Sapolsky found Paul's open-mindedness both irritating and depressing. His irritation led him to reflect on his own musical tastes, and the way that they had seemed to ossify over the years. At the age of forty, he still listened to music constantly, but the music he generally listened to had not changed in a long time: it was always the same two Mahler symphonies, the same Bob Marley tape. This pattern seemed true of his other tastes as well. Lately, he seemed always to order familiar dishes at restaurants, for example. Why was this? Do people simply lose their receptivity to novel tastes as they get older? It's not an implausible thought. It certainly fits with our cultural stereotypes of older Americans. Not that there aren't exceptions, of course. But for every Alabama grandfather who decides to get a nipple ring at age sixty, there must be hundreds more whose cultural tastes have not changed much since they were thirty.

Or so we might guess. Sapolsky actually tested his hypothesis, in an informal, half-joking way. Sapolsky's theory was that most people have a window of opportunity to develop a cultural taste—in fashion, food, music—and that this window closes as a person gets older. As a way of estimating when people are likely to form their tastes in music, for example, Sapolsky and his research assistants called radio stations specializing in music of various periods. Some stations played only contemporary rock, others only fifties doo-wop, still others only seventies metal, and so on. Sapolsky asked each station manager for two pieces of information: the date when the style of music played by the station was first introduced, and the average age of the station's listeners. After talking to forty or so station managers, Sapolsky could see a pattern. Most people develop a taste for what will become their favorite style of music before they are twenty years old. In fact, according to Sapolsky's data, if a person is over thirty-five when a style of popular music is introduced, the odds are greater than 95 percent that this person will never choose to listen to it. So if you were in high school in the 1970s, you might well still be listening to Parliament, Aerosmith, or the Kinks. But if your children were the ones in high school, chances are you don't even know who these bands are. As Sapolsky puts it: by the time these bands were playing, that window of opportunity had closed.

Sapolsky got similar results when he looked at tastes in food and fashion. In order to investigate his "window of opportunity" hypothesis for food, Sapolsky called fifty sushi restaurants in the Midwest. He reasoned that sushi was probably different enough from what most Minnesotans and Nebraskans had been eating previously that it would take a fair bit of open-mindedness for them to try it. Again he asked for two pieces of information: the date when the sushi restaurant had opened, and the average age of the restaurant's non-Asian customers. And again, a pattern emerged. The typical non-Asian customer at a sushi restaurant had been less than twenty-eight years old when sushi arrived in town. If a person had been older than thirty-nine when sushi arrived, the odds were greater than 95 percent that he or she would never try it. The sushi window was closed.

For the fashion window Sapolsky chose body-piercing—navel rings, tongue studs, various bits of metal in the eyebrows, neck, or genitals. Body-piercing was a convenient fashion to measure because it had been introduced at a clearly identifiable period and was still relatively new. In addition, unlike tattoos or pierced ears for men, the cultural meanings of body-piercing had not yet changed dramatically since it was introduced. It seemed fair to guess that a person would need a fair degree of openness to novelty before he or she would choose to get a tongue stud. Again Sapolsky had his research assistants call body-piercing shops and ask the same two questions. When did your shop open, and how old is your average customer? After thirty-five shops had responded, it became clear that the window of opportunity here was very tight indeed. The typical body-pierced customer was eighteen years old or younger, and people who were older than twenty-three when the body-piercing shop had opened were unlikely ever to visit it. If you have not gotten your Prince Albert by age twenty-three, it is very improbable that you will get one later.

Sapolsky's informal research is unlikely to withstand scientific scrutiny, but there is something intuitively right (even depressingly right) about his conclusions. Most of us can see our lives taking more predictable patterns as we age, and we are generally happier with that predictability than we might have been at an earlier age. Even so, I am not sure that *all* tastes tend to harden with time. Fashion, for example, is a very public taste. It is driven by outer display. Part of the reason tastes in fashion are formed so early might be connected to the fact that, beginning in adolescence, young people are very self-conscious about impressing other young people. This self-consciousness does not go away as we get older, but it does (mercifully) seem to become less important. Maybe it is not simply that tastes in fashion ossify with age, but that fashion is driven by the cultural demands of the young. Part of the reason many older people would resist getting a tongue stud—or, for that matter, dreadlocks, skateboards, or those baggy pants that slip way down the hips—is that they want to resist being seen as vainly striving toward youth.

Private tastes seem different. In contrast to tastes in fashion, it does not seem so odd for a person to develop a brand new hobby at an advanced age—to start building model trains, learn to sail, or take up knitting. In fact, for some people it seems typical. (Alistair Cooke once said that the difference between America and Britain is that Americans live lives of frenetic activity and then retire into boredom, while the British live lives of boredom and retire into frenetic activity.) Nor does it seem nearly as odd for a person to develop new tastes in literature as they get older. If a new taste is truly private and less driven by outer display (such as tastes for food) then openness to novelty may be more likely. Of course, the distinction between public and private tastes is a fuzzy one, and somewhat artificial. Building model trains may look like a private taste, but it becomes public once you join a model train club. Yet it would be equally misguided to assume that the narrowing of tastes with age is a matter of biology rather than culture. At least part of the reason that tastes appear to narrow with age may be a result of the way that our lives change as we get older.

Perhaps it is not that aging people's lives narrow because their tastes narrow, but that their tastes narrow because their lives narrow. As I have moved from one country to another, I have probably been more receptive to local tastes than I would have been if I had stayed home. Balinese gamelan music seems much more appealing in Ubud; mealy meal and goat taste better if they are eaten somewhere in the Zambezi Valley. Something like this may also be true for the patterns of American life. Youth, as American culture has made it, is a time to experiment in music and fashion. It is less a time for experimenting with hobbies and literature. But this could be different, of course. There is no essential connection between youth and popular music; the connection is simply what our culture has made it to be (so much so, in fact, that American pop music is now almost entirely *about* the concerns of youth). In the same way, the fact that the younger end of middle age is the time when many Americans start to experiment with food probably says more about the shape of life in Middle

America than it does about the biology of taste. This is the time of life when many people find a partner, start to cook for themselves, and have the money to eat out in restaurants.

Looking at tastes as biological phenomena overlooks the contexts in which tastes are formed and in which they change, the way they fit into the shape of a life. Tastes are bound up with memory and nostalgia and the magic of repetition. Surely part of the reason why we hang on to certain tastes is the experience with which they are associated. I have all sorts of poor tastes to which I will happily confess (Moon Pies, beach music, *Evil Dead* 2) but which I'm unwilling to give up, simply because of the part they have played in my particular history. Maybe the reason we cling to certain tastes is not just that the window for new tastes has closed, but that we want to keep the old ones open. A taste for the old and familiar is the way we cling to the memories of a time of life that has passed.

To miss this is to miss the existential horror of *Seconds*. What made Arthur Hamilton's new life so terrifying—and as sterile, in its own way, as his old one—is its absolute erasure of the past. Hamilton had to give up everything about his old life. Hamilton regained youth, but it was not *his* youth: he became a completely different man. Whatever the evocations of music or food, or any kind of memory at all, he could not acknowledge them to others. By becoming a different man, Hamilton had to give up much of what gives aging its particular bittersweetness—all the accumulations of memory and character and taste that come from spending so many years on earth. No wonder Hamilton's new life seemed empty. It had literally been emptied out, drained of the very things that might make a longer life promise to be a fuller and richer one. What is the appeal of a life that stretches out endlessly into the future, but rolls up the past behind it?

Conclusion

THE TYRANNY OF HAPPINESS

> In America I have seen the freest and best edu-
> cated of men in circumstances the happiest to
> be found in the world, yet it seemed to me that
> a cloud habitually hung on their brow, and they
> seemed serious and almost sad even in their
> pleasures.
>
> —Alexis de Tocqueville

Thirty-five years ago, at the beginning of a twelve-year Senate inquiry into the drug industry, Senator Gaylord Nelson opened the session on psychotropic drugs by comparing them to the drugs in *Brave New World*. "When Aldous Huxley wrote his fantasy concept of the world of the future in the now classic *Brave New World*, he created an uncomfortable, emotionless culture of escapism dependent on tiny tablets of tranquility called soma."[1] Thirty-five years later, *Brave New World* is still invoked, time and again, as a warning against the dangers that await us if we embark on new enhancement technologies. News stories about psychotropic drugs, stem cells, reproductive technologies, or genetic engineering inevitably appear with headlines reading Brave New Medicine, Brave New Babies, Brave New Minds, or Brave New People. It is as if we have no other metaphors for these technologies, no competing visions of possible futures. Whatever the new technology of the moment happens to be, we hear the same cautionary tale: it will lead us to a total-itarian society where generic workers are slotted into castes and anesthetized into bliss. The people in these totalitarian societies are not so much unhappy as they are ignorant of what true happiness is, because they have been drugged and engineered to want nothing more than that which their station allows them.

We keep returning to this story, I suspect, partly because we like stories of individuals battling the forces of authority, and partly because it allows both teller and listener to collude in the shared sense that we, unlike our neighbors and coworkers and maybe even our family members, have figured out what is really bad about a technology that looks so good. This story says, "Our neighbors may have been sold a bill of goods, they may think that they have found happiness in a Prozac tablet and a Botox injection, but you and I know it's a crock. You and I are too smart to believe the cosmetic surgery Web sites, the drug companies peddling Sarafem and Paxil, and the psychiatrists who tell us we have adult ADHD." Yet as much as we like the *Brave New World* story, as many times as we read it and repeat it and write high school essays about it, somehow it never seems to apply to us. For men, the story of enhancement technologies is about the vanity of women; for women, it is about the sexual gaze of men; for Europeans and Canadians, it is about shallowness of American values; for Americans, it is about "other" Americans—the ones who are either too crooked or deluded to acknowledge what is really going on. If we blame anyone for the ill effects of enhancement technologies, it is either someone in power (the FDA, the media, Big Pharma, "the culture") or the poor suckers who have allowed themselves to be duped (Miss America contestants, neurotic New Yorkers, Michael Jackson). We imagine second-rate TV stars lining up for liposuction and anxious middle managers asking their family doctors for Paxil, and we just shake our heads and laugh. "Why can't they learn to accept themselves as they are?" we ask. Then we are asked to sing a solo in the church choir and can't sleep for a week, or our daughter starts getting teased at school for her buck teeth, and the joke doesn't seem so funny anymore.

We all like to moralize about enhancement technologies, except for the ones we use ourselves. Those technologies never seem quite so bad, because our view of them comes not from television or magazines but from personal experience, or the shared confidences of our troubled friends. There is often striking contrast between private conversation about enhancement technologies and the broader public discussion. In public, for example, everyone seems to be officially anti-Prozac. Feminists ask me why doctors prescribe Prozac more often for women than for men. Undergraduates worry that Prozac might give their classmates a competitive edge. Philosophy professors argue that Prozac would make people shallow and uncreative. Germans object that Prozac is not a natural substance. Americans say that Prozac is a crutch. Most people seem to feel that Prozac is creating some version of what historian David Rothman called, in a *New Republic* cover story, "shiny, happy people."

In private, though, people have started to seek me out and tell me their Prozac stories. They have tried Prozac and hated it; they have tried Prozac and it changed their life; they have tried Prozac and can't see what the big deal is. It has begun to seem as if everyone I know is on Prozac, has been on Prozac, or is considering taking Prozac, and all of them want to get my opinion. Most of all, they want me to try Prozac myself. "How can you write about it if you've never even tried it?" I can see their point. Still, it strikes me as a strange way to talk about a prescription drug. These people are oddly insistent. It was as if we were back in high school, and they were trying to get me to smoke a joint.

People who look at America from abroad often marvel at the enthusiasm with which Americans use enhancement technologies. I can see why. It is a jolt to discover the rates at which Americans use Ritalin or Prozac or Botox. But "enthusiasm" is probably the wrong word to describe the way Americans feel about enhancement technologies. If this is enthusiasm, it is the enthusiasm of a diver on the high platform, who has to talk himself into taking the plunge. Unlike Richard Nixon, I don't think Americans expect happiness in a handful of tablets. We take the tablets, but we brood about it. We try to hide the tablets from our friends. We worry that taking them is a sign of weakness. We try to convince our friends to take them too. We fret that if we don't take them, others will outshine us. We take the tablets, but they leave a bitter taste in our mouths.

Why? Perhaps because in those tablets is a mix of all the American wishes, lusts, and fears: the drive to self-improvement, the search for fulfillment, the desire to show that there are second acts in American lives; yet a mix diluted by nagging anxieties about social conformity, about getting too much too easily, about phoniness and self-deception and shallow pleasure. This is not a story from *Brave New World*. It is not even a story of enhancement. It is a story of flop sweat, sleepless nights, and the sting of casual insults. It is less a story about trying to get ahead than about the terror of being left behind, and the humiliation of crossing the finish line dead last, while the crowd points at you and laughs. You can still refuse to use enhancement technologies, of course—you might be the last woman in America who does not dye her gray hair, the last man who refuses to work out at the gym— but even that publicly announces something to other Americans about who you are and what you value. This is all part of the logic of consumer culture. You cannot simply opt out of the system and expect nobody to notice how much you weigh.

W HY HERE, WHY NOW? On one level, the answer seems obvious: because the technology has arrived. If you are anxious and lonely and a drug can fix it, why stay anxious and lonely? If you are unhappy with your body and surgery can fix it, why stay unhappy? The market moves to fill a demand for happiness as efficiently as it moves to fill a demand for spark plugs or home computers. It is on a deeper level that the question of enhancement technologies becomes more puzzling. What has made the ground for these technologies so fertile? The sheer variety of technologies on display is remarkable. Some people want their legs lengthened, while others want them amputated. Black folks rub themselves with cream to make their skin lighter, while white folks broil in tanning parlors to make their skin darker. Bashful men get ETS surgery to reduce blood flow above the neck, while elderly men take Viagra to increase blood flow below the belt. Each technology has its own rationale, its own cultural niche, a distinct population of users, and an appeal that often waxes or wanes with changes in fashion or the state of scientific knowledge. But do they have anything in common? Is there anything about the way we live now that helps explain their popularity?

The "self that struggles to realize itself," as philosopher Michael Walzer puts it, has become a familiar notion to most people living in the West today.[2] We tend to see ourselves as the managers of life projects that we map out, organize, make choices about, perhaps compare with other possible projects, and ultimately live out to completion. From late adolescence onward, we are expected to make important decisions about what to do for a living, where to live, whether to marry and have children, all with the sense that these decisions will contribute to the success or failure of our projects. Yet as Walzer points out, there is nothing natural or inevitable about this way of conceptualizing a life. Not everyone in the West today will think of their lives as planned projects, and most people at most times in history have probably thought of their lives differently. Marriages are arranged; educational choices are fixed; gods are tyrannical or absent. A life might be spontaneous, rather than planned; its shape might be given to us, rather than created. The shapes of lives can be determined not by the demands of personal values or self-fulfillment, but by those of God, family, social station, caste, or one's ancestors.

This notion of life as a project suggests both individual responsibility and moral uncertainty. If I am the planner and manager of my life, then I am at least partly responsible for its success or failure. Thus the lure of enhancement technologies: as tools to produce a better, more successful project. Yet if my life is a project, what exactly is the purpose of the project? How do I tell a successful project from a failure? Aristotle (for example) could write confidently about the good life for human beings because he was confident about what the purpose of being a human being was. Just as a knife has a purpose, so human beings have a purpose; just as the qualities that make for a good knife are those that help the knife slice, whittle, and chop, the qualities that make a human being better are those that help us better fulfill our purpose as human beings.

Our problem, of course, is that most of us don't have Aristotle's confidence about the purpose of human life. Good knives cut, that much we can see, but what does a good human being do, and how will we know when we are doing it? Is there even such a thing as a single, universal human purpose? Not if we believe what we are told by the culture that surrounds us. From philosophy courses and therapy sessions to magazines and movies, we are told that questions of purpose vary from one person to the next; that, in fact, a large part of our life project is to discover our own individual purpose and develop it to its fullest. This leaves us with unanswered questions not just about what kinds of lives are better or worse, but also about the criteria by which such judgments are made. Is it better to be a successful bail bondsman or a second-rate novelist? On what yardstick do we compare the lives of Reform Jews, high-church Episcopalians, and California Wiccans? Where exactly should the choices we make about our lives be anchored?

Many people today believe that the success or failure of a life has something to do with the idea of self-fulfillment. We may not know exactly what a successful life is, but we have a pretty good suspicion that it has something to do with being fulfilled—or at the very least, that an unfulfilled life runs the risk of failure. In the name of fulfillment people quit their jobs in human resources and real estate to become poets and potters, leave their dermatology practices to do medical mission work in Bangladesh, even divorce their husbands or wives (the marriage was adequate, but it was not fulfilling). Women leave their children in day care because they believe that they will be more fulfilled with a career; they leave their jobs because they believe that it will be more fulfilling to stay home with the kids. Fulfillment has a strong moral strand to it—many people feel that they *ought* to pursue a career, that they *ought* to leave a loveless marriage—but its parameters are vague and indeterminate. How exactly do I know if I am fulfilled? Fulfillment looks a little like being in love, a little like a successful spiritual quest; it is a state centered largely on individual psychic well-being. If I am alienated, depressed, or anxious, I can't be completely fulfilled.

If I am not fulfilled, I am missing out on what life can offer. Life is a short, sweet ride, and I am spending it all in the station. The problem is that there is no great, overarching metric for self-fulfillment, no master schedule that we can look up at and say, "Yes, I've missed the train." So we look desperately to experts for instructions—counselors, psychiatrists, advice columnists, self-help writers, life coaches, even professional ethicists. We read the ads on the wall for cosmetic dentistry, and we look nervously at the people standing next to us in line. Does she know something that I don't? Is she more fulfilled? How does my psychic well-being compare to hers?

The very nature of psychic well-being makes these comparisons both relentless and inconclusive. In his *Philosophical Investigations*, Ludwig Wittgenstein imagines a kind of philosophical game. "Suppose everyone had a box with something in it: we call it a 'beetle,' " writes Wittgenstein. "No one can look into anyone else's box, and everyone says he knows what a beetle is by looking only at *his* beetle."[3] It would be quite possible, Wittgenstein points out, for each person to have something different in his box. It would even be possible for the contents of the boxes to be constantly changing. In fact, it would even be possible for all the boxes to be empty—and still the players could successfully use the term "beetle" to talk about the contents of their boxes. There need not be any actual beetles in the boxes for the game to be played.

Wittgenstein's beetle box game makes an important point about the words we use to describe our inner lives—words such as "pain," "depression," "anxiety," "fulfillment," and so on. Like the word "beetle" in Wittgenstein's game, which does not refer to an insect but rather gets its meaning from the rules of the beetle-box game, words such as "depression" or "fulfillment" get their meanings not from the inner mental states they describe, but from the larger context in which they are used. We learn how to use these words not by looking inward and naming what we find there, but by taking part in the game. The players do not all need to be experiencing the same thing in order for the words to make sense. I say I am fulfilled, you say you are fulfilled, we both understand what the other means—yet this does not mean that our inner psychic states are the same. We can all talk about our "beetles," yet all have different things in our boxes.

To see why this matters, imagine a slightly different version of Wittgenstein's beetle-box game. In this version of the game each player still has access only to his or her box, the contents of which are called "beetle." But now some new players can win the game by persuading others that the "beetles" in their boxes are inferior. These players develop an entirely new vocabulary to describe and explain "beetles," the purpose of which is to distinguish between the quality of various "beetles." Because nobody can look into the box of another player, nobody has any way to compare his or her "beetle" to that of another player. But because of what they are being told by the new players, the players now have reason to suspect that their "beetles" could be inferior. So they begin to worry. How does my "beetle" measure up? Is my "beetle" healthy? Would I be happier with a different "beetle"?

The reason the new players in this game can successfully sow the seeds of doubt about "beetles," of course, is the fact that no player can look into another player's box. And this is precisely the reason it is possible to market successfully so many ways of improving psychic well-being, from psychoactive drugs and cosmetic surgery to self-help books and advice columns. If I never know for certain whether the quality of my experience matches up to yours, I am always susceptible to the suggestion that it could be improved. This is why I look so closely at the ads for Paxil and Viagra, read magazine articles about personal fitness and performance anxiety, and scan the shelves at Border's for books about depression, attention-deficit disorder, and the twelve-step method for achieving spiritual success. My inner life could be better; I could be more fulfilled; I could be psychologically healthier, if I could only find the right intervention.

In other times and places, success or failure in a life might have been determined by fixed and agreed-upon standards. You displeased the ancestors; you shamed your family; you did not accept Jesus Christ as your personal savior. You arrived late to the station, and the train left without you. But our situation today is different— not for everyone, of course, but for many of us. We have gotten on the train, but we don't know who is driving it, or where, some point off in the far distance, the tracks are leading. The other passengers are smiling, they look happy, yet underneath this facade of good cheer and philosophical certainty, a demon keeps whispering in our ears: "What if I have gotten it all wrong? What if I have boarded the wrong train?"

Tocqueville hinted at this worry over 150 years ago when he wrote about American "restlessness in the midst of abundance." Behind all the admirable energy of American life, Tocqueville saw a kind of grim relentlessness. We build houses to pass our old age, Tocqueville wrote, then sell them before the roof is on; we clear fields, then leave it to others to gather the harvest; we take up a profession, then leave it to take up another one or go into politics. Americans frantically pursue prosperity, and when we finally get it, we are tormented by the worry that we might have gotten it quicker. An American on vacation, Tocqueville marveled, "will travel five hundred miles in a few days as a distraction from his happiness."[4]

Tocqueville may well have been right about American restlessness, but it took another Frenchman, surrealist painter Phillipe Soupault, to put his finger on the form that it has taken today. According to Soupault, Americans see the pursuit of happiness not just as a right, as the Declaration of Independence states, but as a strange sort of duty. In the United States, he wrote, "one is always in danger of entrapment by what appears on the surface to be a happy civilization. There is a sort of obligation to be happy." Humans are born to be happy, and if they are not, something has gone wrong. As Soupault puts it, "Whoever is unhappy is suspect."[5] Substitute self-fulfillment for happiness and you get something of the ethic that motivates the desire for enhancement technologies. Once self-fulfillment is hitched to the success of a human life, it comes perilously close to an obligation—not an obligation to God, country, or family, but an obligation to the self. We are compelled to pursue fulfillment through enhancement technologies not in order to get ahead of others, but to make sure that we have lived our lives to the fullest. The train has left the station and we don't know where it is going. The least we can do is be sure it is making good time.

On the door of my office is a copy of a famous photograph taken in December 1970. It shows Elvis Presley shaking hands with Richard Nixon in the Oval Office. Elvis had written to Nixon requesting to be made a Federal Agent-at-Large in the Bureau of Narcotics and Dangerous Drugs. He told Nixon that he had studied communist brainwashing and the drug culture for over ten years. Nixon, worried as ever about happiness in a tablet, invited Elvis to the White House. He felt that people who use drugs were in the "vanguard of anti-American protest" and thought Elvis could help. And so here are Dick and Elvis doing a clasp-and-grin photo shot in the Oval Office, Elvis wearing sideburns, a gold necklace and enormous belt buckle, shirt unbuttoned halfway down his chest, shaking hands with a stiff, gray-suited Nixon. Nixon has a plastic smile on his face. Elvis stares blankly at the camera. That is why I love this photograph: Elvis, standing in the Oval Office, is obviously stoned.

I don't know which thought I like better: the idea that Elvis was so keen to wear an official FBI badge; the fact that Nixon believed that Elvis, now well into his sideburns-and-sequins phase, could improve his standing with the American counterculture; or the mere fact that Elvis would turn up at the White House baked. Do we really know who is in charge here? The story we tell ourselves, of course, is that the sovereign individual is in charge; that we would all be fine if the official authorities would just leave us alone. Society represents an authority to be challenged. What we tend to forget is that society doesn't just get in our way. Society helps make us who we are. America creates Americans, and it may well create profoundly alienated, unhappy Americans who are uncomfortable in their own skins. America creates Americans like Dick and Elvis, people whose desires are self-destructive, unhealthy, paranoid, or perverse. When Elvis died at the age of forty-two, lying face down on the bathroom floor with his silk pajamas around his knees, his toxicology report found Elavil, Aventyl, codeine, morphine, methaqualone, Valium, ethinamate, ethchlorvynol, amobarbital, Nembutal, Carbrital, and Sinutab, some in ten times their lethal doses.[6] This was not the result of any central authority slotting people into castes. It was the result of free choices made in a search for some peculiar kind of American happiness.

NOTES

INTRODUCTION

[1] Mickey C. Smith, *A Social History of the Minor Tranquilizers: The Quest for Small Comfort in an Age of Anxiety* (New York: Praeger, 1988), 182.

[2] Ibid., 186.

[3] See, for example, French Anderson, "Human Gene Therapy: Scientific and Ethical Considerations," *Journal of Medicine and Philosophy* 10 (1985): 275–91. For a thorough overview and analysis of the debate over genetic engineering, see John H. Evans, *Playing God? Human Genetic Engineering and the Rationalization of Public Bioethical Debate* (Chicago: University of Chicago Press, 2002).

[4] Erik Parens, ed., *Enhancing Human Traits* (Washington, D.C.: Georgetown University Press, 1996).

[5] Alexis de Tocqueville, *Democracy in America*, trans. George Lawrence, ed. J. P. Mayer (New York: Harper and Row, 1988), 430. This translation was first published in 1966, based on Tocqueville's 13th edition in 1850.

[6] Ibid., 510.

CHAPTER ONE: THE PERFECT VOICE

[1] Stephen Hawking, *Black Holes and Baby Universes* (New York: Bantam Books, 1993), 26.

[2] N. Katherine Hayles, *How We Became Posthuman: Virtual Bodies in Cyber-*

netics, Literature and Informatics (Chicago: University of Chicago Press, 1999), 84.

³ Parker Lee Nash, "My Fair Lady: Say Bye-Bye to Your Southern Accent," *Greensboro News and Record,* January 17, 1999; Woody Baird, "Learn to Take the South Out of Your Mouth, Y'all," *Palm Beach Post,* November 18, 1997; Art Harris, "Takin' the Drawl Outta Dixie," *Washington Post,* December 16, 1984.

⁴ Kathy Davis, *Reshaping the Female Body: The Dilemma of Cosmetic Surgery* (New York: Routledge, 1995), 70.

⁵ See Nash, "My Fair Lady."

⁶Alexis de Tocqueville, *Democracy in America,* trans. George Lawrence, ed. J. P. Mayer (New York: Harper and Row, 1988), 179.

⁷ Andrew Sullivan, "What We Look Up To Now," *New York Times Magazine,* November 15, 1998, Section 6, 59.

⁸ Ibid.

⁹ Tom Wolfe, "The Right Stuff" in *The Purple Decades* (London: Picador, 1993), 379.

¹⁰ Ibid., 379-80.

¹¹ John Honey, *Language is Power: The Story of Standard English and Its Enemies* (Boston: Faber and Faber, 1997), 31–32.

¹² I discuss beta-blockers at greater length in Chapter 4, "The Loneliness of the Late-Night Television Watcher."

¹³ Hayles, *How We Became Posthuman,* 210.

¹⁴ The quotations here come from a Yahoo e-group (electronic discussion group) called Transsexual Voice and Speech Therapy. The discussion group is intended to offer tips and techniques for male-to-female transsexuals who wish to have a more feminine voice. The discussion and the archives are open to anyone who wishes to subscribe. See http://groups.yahoo.com/group/voicets.

¹⁵ Hilde Lindemann Nelson, *Damaged Identities, Narrative Repair* (Ithaca, N.Y.: Cornell University Press, 2001), 125–26.

¹⁶ This story can be found on-line at: http://storymind.com/journeys/everything/voice.htm.

¹⁷ See the archives of the Transsexual Voice and Speech Therapy e-group.

¹⁸ M. Moerman, H. Vermeersch, J. Van Borsel, and P. Wallert, "Phonosurgery in Gender Dysphoria," *Acta Chirurgica Belgica* 100:2 (March–April, 2000), 58–61; M. Gross, "Pitch-Raising Surgery in Male-to-Female Transsexuals, *Journal of Voice* 13:2 (1999), 246–50; S. Kunachak, S. Prakunhunsit, and K. Suijalak, "Thyroid Cartilage and Vocal Fold Reduction: A New Phonosurgical Method for Male-to-Female Transsexuals," *Annals of Otology, Rhinology and Laryngology* 109:11 (November, 2000), 1082–6.

¹⁹ Good explanations of voice feminization can be found on-line at www.tsvoice.com and www.annelawrence.com.

²⁰ M. Brown, A. Perry, A. D. Cheesman, and T. Pring, "Pitch Change in Male-to-Female Transsexuals: Has Phonosurgery a Role to Play?" *International Journal of Language and Communication Disorders* 35:1 (2000), 129–36.

²¹ At the time this book went to press I was unable to find any reports of this pro-

cedure in the medical literature, but it was being discussed by male-to-female trans-sexuals. See, for example, a physician's description of the LAVA procedure on the Web site of Dr. Anne Lawrence at www.annelawrence.com/lava.html.

22 See the Transsexual Voice and Speech Therapy discussion group.

23 Ibid.

24 For a balanced account of some of these more speculative technologies, see Rodney Brooks, *Flesh and Machines: How Robots Will Change Us* (New York: Pantheon Books, 2002). See also Mark Dery, *Escape Velocity : Cyberculture at the End of the Century* (New York: Grove Press, 1996); Ed Regis, *The Great Mambo Chicken and the Transhuman Condition: Science Slightly Over the Edge* (Reading, Mass.: Addison-Wesley, 1990); Lauren Slater, "Dr. Daedelus: A Radical Plastic Surgeon Wants to Give you Wings," *Harper's* 303:1814 (July 2001), 57–67; Hans Moravec, *Mind Children: The Future of Robot and Human Intelligence* (Cambridge, Mass.: Harvard University Press, 1988).

25 Charles Horton Cooley, *Human Nature and the Social Order* (New York: Schocken Books, 1967; originally published in 1902), 254. See also George Herbert Mead, *Mind, Self and Society* (Chicago: University of Chicago Press, 1967; originally published in 1934), 136–37.

CHAPTER TWO: THE TRUE SELF

1 In a series of extraordinary books and essays, Charles Taylor has explored the historical and philosophical roots of the ideal of authenticity as well as its contemporary implications. My analysis here draws heavily on his work. His most concise summaries come in Charles Taylor, "The Politics of Recognition," in *Multiculturalism: Examining the Politics of Identity,* ed. Amy Gutman, (Princeton, N.J.: Princeton University Press, 1994), 25–73 and Charles Taylor, *The Ethics of Authenticity* (Cambridge, Mass.: Harvard University Press, 1991). For a more detailed and historically rich account, see Charles Taylor, *Sources of the Self* (Cambridge, Mass.: Harvard University Press, 1989). More recently, Alan Gewirth has examined related ideas in *Self-Fulfillment* (Princeton, N.J.: Princeton University Press, 1998).

2 Lionel Trilling, *Sincerity and Authenticity* (Cambridge, Mass.: Harvard University Press, 1971); Taylor, *Sources of the Self.*

3 Taylor, "The Politics of Recognition," 30.

4 Ibid., 28.

5 Jan Morris, *Conundrum* (New York: Harcourt Brace Jovanovich, 1974), 56.

6 Ibid., 41.

7 Ibid., 56.

8 Ibid., 106.

9 Ibid., 111.

10 Ibid., 141.

11 Ibid., 143.

12 The "trapped in the wrong body" narrative has been widely criticized, by trans-gendered writers and others. See, for example, Sandy Stone, "The Empire Strikes

Back: A Posttranssexual Manifesto," in *Sex/Machine: Readings in Culture, Gender and Technology*, ed. Patrick D. Hopkins (Bloomington: Indiana University Press, 1998), 322–41.

[13] Morris, *Conundrum*, 41, 104.

[14] Rollo May, *Man's Search for Himself* (New York: Dell, 1953), 14.

[15] Taylor, *The Ethics of Authenticity*, 16–17.

[16] Joan Jacobs Brumberg, *The Body Project: An Intimate History of American Girls* (New York: Random House, 1997), xxi.

[17] Ibid.

[18] Samuel Wilson Fussell, *Muscle: Confessions of an Unlikely BodyBuilder* (New York: Avon Books, 1991), 68. I learned about Fussell's memoir from Tod Chambers, who discussed it in a presentation called "Communities of Improvement" at a meeting of the Enhancement Technologies Group in Minneapolis (September 25, 1998). For an academic ethnography of bodybuilding subcultures, see Alan M. Klein, *Little Big Men: Bodybuilding Subculture and Gender Construction* (Albany: State University of New York Press, 1993).

[19] Fussell, *Muscle*, 69–70.

[20] Ibid., 127.

[21] Ibid., 122.

[22] Ibid., 123.

[23] Kathy Davis, *Reshaping the Female Body: The Dilemma of Cosmetic Surgery* (New York: Routledge), 77.

[24] Ibid., 78.

[25] Taylor, *The Ethics of Authenticity*, 47–48.

[26] Ibid., 46.

[27] W. E. B. Du Bois , *The Souls of Black Folk*, ed. David W. Blight and Robert Gooding-Williams (Boston: Bedford Books, 1997; originally published in 1903), 38.

[28] This appeared in print on April 20, 1959. The story and quotations come from Jay Stevens, *Storming Heaven* (New York: Harper and Row, 1987), 64–65. See also Mike Jay, ed., *Artificial Paradises* (London: Penguin, 1999), 258.

[29] Aldous Huxley, *The Doors of Perception and Heaven and Hell* (New York: Harper and Row, 1990; originally published in 1953), 18.

[30] Quoted in May, *Man's Search for Himself*, 23–24.

[31] David Riesman, Nathan Glazer, and Reuel Denney, *The Lonely Crowd: A Study of the Changing American Character* (New York: Doubleday, 1953; originally published in 1950), 31.

[32] Trilling, *Sincerity and Authenticity*.

[33] Arnold Ludwig, *How Do We Know Who We Are? A Biography of the Self* (Oxford: Oxford University Press, 1997), 247.

[34] Gail Sheehy, *New Passages: Mapping Your Life Across Time* (New York: Ballantine, 1996), 71.

[35] Robert Jay Lifton, *The Protean Self: Human Resilience in an Age of Fragmentation* (New York: Basic Books, 1995).

[36] Morris, *Conundrum*, 149.

38 Jerome Bruner, Acts of Meaning (Cambridge, Mass.: Harvard University Press, 1990), 99.

39 Lauren Slater, Prozac Diary (New York, Random House, 1999), 196.

40 This well-known philosophical point and the notion of "family resemblances," come from Ludwig Wittgenstein, Philosophical Investigations, ed. G. E. M. Anscombe (London: Macmillan, 1953); see especially §67.

41 This, as Wittgenstein would say, is a grammatical remark.

42 Kenneth Gergen, "The Healthy, Happy Human Being Wears Many Masks," in The Fontana Postmodernism Reader, ed. Walter Truitt Anderson, (London: Fontana, 1996), 138. My criticism of this remark notwithstanding, Gergen has done some fascinating psychological work on identity. See especially Kenneth Gergen, The Saturated Self: Dilemmas of Identity in Contemporary Life (New York: Basic Books, 2000).

43 Peter D. Kramer, Listening to Prozac (London: Fourth Estate, 1994), 219.

44 Sherwin Nuland, "The Pill of Pills," New York Review of Books 41:11 (June 9, 1994): 1–5; David Rothman, "Shiny Happy People," New Republic 210:7 (February 14, 1994): 34–38; David DeGrazia, "Prozac, Enhancement, and Self-Creation," The Hastings Center Report 30:2 (March 2000): 34–40.

45 See the case of "Philip" in Kramer, Listening to Prozac, 292.

46 Slater, Prozac Diary, 193.

47 Nikolas Rose, Governing the Soul: The Shaping of the Private Self (London: Routledge, 1990), 244 45.

CHAPTER THREE: THE FACE BEHIND THE MASK

1 John Marshall, Social Phobia: From Shyness to Stage Fright (New York: Basic Books, 1994), 5.

2 Ronald C. Kessler, Katherine A. McGonagle, et al., "Lifetime and 12-Month Prevalence of DSM-III-R Psychiatric Disorders in the United States: Results from the National Comorbidity Survey," Archives of General Psychiatry 51:1 (January 1994): 8–19; Lynne Lamberg, "Social Phobia: Not Just Another Name for Shyness," JAMA 280:8 (August 26, 1998): 685–86.

3 Harold I. Kaplan, Benjamin J. Sadock, and Jack A. Graeb, Kaplan and Sadock's Synopsis of Psychiatry, Seventh Edition (Baltimore, Md.: Williams and Wilkins, 1994), 971; David Healy, The Antidepressant Era (Cambridge, Mass.: Harvard University Press, 1997), 59–63; Peter D. Kramer, Listening to Prozac (London: Fourth Estate, 1994), 47–49.

4 Kaplan, Sadock, and Graeb, Synopsis of Psychiatry, 971.

5 M. R. Liebowitz, A. J. Fyer, J. M. Gorman, R. Campeas, A. Levin, "Phenelzine in Social Phobia," Journal of Clinical Psychopharmacology 6:2 (1986): 93–98; M. R. Liebowitz, J. M. Gorman, A. J. Fyer, R. Campeas, A. P. Levin, D. Sandberg, E. Hollander, L. Papp, and D. Goetz, "Pharmacotherapy of Social Phobia: An Interim Report of a Placebo-Controlled Comparison of Phenelzine and Atenolol," Journal of

Clinical Psychiatry 49:7 (1988): 252–57; M. R. Liebowitz, F. Schneier, R. Campeas, J. Gorman, A. Fyer, E. Hollander, J. Hatterer, and L. Papp, "Phenelzine and Atenolol in Social Phobia," *Psychopharmacology Bulletin* 26:1 (1990): 123–25.

[6] M. B. Stein, M. R. Liebowitz, R. B. Lydiard, C. D. Pitts, W. Bushnell, and I. Gergel, "Paroxetine Treatment of Generalized Social Phobia (Social Anxiety Disorder): A Randomized Controlled Trial, *JAMA* 280:8 (1998): 708–13; D. Baldwin, J. Bobes, D. J. Stein, I. Scharwachter, and M. Faure, "Paroxetine in Social Phobia/Social Anxiety Disorder: Randomised, Double-Blind, Placebo-Controlled Study, Paroxetine Study Group," *British Journal of Psychiatry* 175 (1999): 120–26.

[7] "Prescription Drugs and Mass Media Advertising 2000: A Research Report by The National Institute for Health Care Management Research and Educational Foundation," November 2001; available from NIHCM Foundation, 1225 19th St. NW, Suite 710, Washington DC 20036; on-line at www.nihcm.org.

[8] A. L. Montejo-Gonzalez, G. Llorca, J. A. Izquierdo, et al., "SSRI-induced Sexual Dysfunction: Fluoxetine, Paroxetine, Sertraline and Flovoxamine in a Prospective, Multi-Center, and Descriptive Study of 344 Patients," *Journal of Sex and Marital Therapy* 23 (1997): 176-94; M. H. Teicher, C. Glod, and J. O. Cole, "Emergence of Intense Suicidal Preoccupation During Fluoxetine Treatment," American Journal of Psychiatry 147 (1990): 207–10; P. Masand, S. Gupta, and M. Dewan, "Suicidal Ideation Related to Fluoxetine Treatment," *New England Journal of Medicine* 324 (1991): 420. See also H. Koizumi, "Fluoxetine and Suicidal Ideation," *Journal of the American Academy of Child and Adolescent Psychiatry* 30 (1991): 695; J. J. Mann and S. Kapur, "The Emergence of Suicidal Ideation and Behavior During Antidepressant Pharmacotherapy," *Archives of General Psychiatry* 49 (1991): 1027–33; R. A. King, M. A. Riddle, P. B. Chappell, et al., "Emergence of Self-Destructive Phenomena in Children and Adolescents During Fluoxetine Treatment," *Journal of the American Academy of Child and Adolescent Psychiatry* 30 (1991): 179–86; K. Dasgupta, "Additional Cases of Suicidal Ideation Associated with Fluoxetine," *American Journal of Psychiatry* 147 (1990): 1570; L. A. Papp and J. M. Gorman, "Suicidal Preoccupation During Fluoxetine Treatment," *American Journal of Psychiatry* 147 (1990): 1380; D. Healy, C. Langmaak, and M. Savage, "Suicide in the Course of the Treatment of Depression," *Journal of Psychopharmacology* 13 (1999): 94–99; D. Healy, "Antidepressant Induced Suicidality," *Primary Care Psychiatry* 6 (2000): 23–28.

[9] K. G. Orr, D. J. Castle, "Social Phobia: Shyness as a Disorder," *Medical Journal of Australia*, 16:2 (January 1998): 55–56; J. A. den Boer, "Social Phobia: Epidemiology, Recognition and Treatment," *BMJ* 315:7111 (1997): 796–800.

[10] Murray B. Stein, "How Shy is Too Shy?" *Lancet* 347:9009 (April 27, 1996): 1131–32.

[11] Den Boer, "Social Phobia," 796.

[12] Warren Susman, *Culture as History: The Transformation of American Society in the Twentieth Century* (New York: Pantheon Books, 1984), 271–85.

[13] Ibid., 277.

[14] Christopher Lasch, *The Culture of Narcissism: American Life in an Age of Diminishing Expectations* (New York: W. W. Norton, 1979), 57–58.

15 Ibid., 58. See also John Cawelti, *Apostles of the Self-Made Man* (Chicago: University of Chicago Press, 1965) on whose work Lasch draws.

16 Susman, *Culture as History*, 277.

17 Ibid.

18 Ibid.

19 Lasch, *Culture of Narcissism*, 93. See also Richard Sennett, *The Fall of Public Man* (New York: Knopf, 1977). Thorstein Veblen, writing in the late nineteenth century, makes similar observations in *The Theory of the Leisure Class*. See Thorstein Veblen, *The Theory of the Leisure Class* (New York: Viking, 1967; originally published in 1899), 86–87.

20 Susan Sontag, "Notes on Camp," in *Against Interpretation* (New York: Vintage, 1994; originally published in 1966), 280.

21 Lionel Trilling, *Sincerity and Authenticity* (Cambridge, Mass.: Harvard University Press, 1971), 10.

22 Clifford Geertz, *Local Knowledge: Further Essays in Interpretive Anthropology* (New York: Basic Books, 1983), 59. On personhood, see also the classic essay by Marcel Mauss, "A Category of the Human Mind: The Notion of Person; The Notion of Self," in *The Category of the Person: Anthropology, Philosophy, History*, ed. Michael Carrithers, Steven Collins, and Steven Lukes (New York: Cambridge University Press, 1985), 1–25.

23 Geertz, *Local Knowledge*, 61.

24 Kingsley Amis, *Lucky Jim* (London: Victor Gollancz Ltd., 1968; originally published in 1953), 15.

25 Ibid., 9.

26 Ibid., 230.

27 See, for example, Ray Monk, *Ludwig Wittgenstein: The Duty of Genius* (New York: Vintage, 1991).

28 Hisato Matsunaga, Nobuo Kiriike, Tokuzo Matsui, Yoko Iwasaki, Toshihiko Nagata, and Dan J. Stein, "Taijin Kyofusho: A Form of Social Anxiety Disorder That Responds to Serotonin Reuptake Inhibitors?" *International Journal of Neuropsychopharmacology* 4:3 (September 2001): 231–37.

29 Laurence Kirmayer, "The Place of Culture in Psychiatric Nosology: Taijin Kyofusho and DSM-III-R," *Journal of Nervous and Mental Disease* 179:1 (1991): 19–28.

30 Ryoei Takano, "Anthropophobia and Japanese Performance," *Psychiatry* 40:3 (August 1977): 259–69.

31 Kirmayer, "The Place of Culture in Psychiatric Nosology," 19–28.

32 Ruth Benedict, *The Chrysanthemum and the Sword: Patterns of Japanese Culture* (London: Secker and Warburg, 1947), 224.

33 Kirmayer, "The Place of Culture in Psychiatric Nosology," 22.

34 Lawrence Kirmayer, "The Sound of One Hand Clapping: Listening to Prozac in Japan," in *Prozac as a Way of Life*, eds. Carl Elliott and Tod Chambers (Chapel Hill: University of North Carolina Press, in press).

35 O. Tajima, "Mental Health Care in Japan: Recognition and Treatment of

Depression and Anxiety Disorders," *Journal of Clinical Psychiatry*, 62, Supplement 13 (2001): 39–44.

[36] David Healy, ed., *The Psychopharmacologists III: Interviews by Dr. David Healy* (New York: Oxford University Press, 2000), 286–87.

[37] Rudolf Hoehn-Saric, John R. Lipsey, and Daniel R. McLeod, "Apathy and Indifference in Patients on Fluvoxamine and Fluoxetine," *Journal of Clinical Psychopharmacology* 10:5 (October 1990): 344–48. At the time, she saw this simply as "letting steam off," but once her Luvox dosage was decreased, she found her behavior inappropriate and "out of character."

[38] E. Jane Garland and Elizabeth A. Berg, "Amotivational Syndrome Linked with SSRI Use in Youth for the First Time," *Journal of Child and Adolescent Psychopharmacology* 11 (2001): 181–86.

[39] W. Greil, A. Horvath, N. Sassim, N. Erazo, and R. Grohmann, "Disinhibition of Libido: An Adverse Effect of SSRI?" *Journal of Affective Disorders* 62 (2001): 227.

[40] Hoehn-Saric, Lipsey, and McLeod, "Apathy and Indifference in Patients on Fluvoxamine and Fluoxetine," 344.

[41] Ibid., 345.

[42] Ian Penman, "Prozac Zombie," *HQ*, July/August 1996, 104.

[43] Hoehn-Saric, Lipsey, and McLeod, "Apathy and Indifference in Patients on Fluvoxamine and Fluoxetine," 344.

[44] Lauren Slater, *Prozac Diary* (New York: Random House, 1999), 29.

[45] David Plath, *Long Engagements* (Stanford: Stanford University Press, 1980), 218.

CHAPTER FOUR: THE LONELINESS OF THE LATE-NIGHT TELEVISION WATCHER

[1] Bernardo J. Carducci, *Shyness: A Bold New Approach* (New York: Harper-Collins, 1999), 34.

[2] Charles Cooley, *Human Nature and the Social Order* (New York: Schocken Books, 1967; originally published in 1902), 247.

[3] Murray B. Stein, John R. Walker, and David R. Forde, "Public-Speaking Fears in a Community Sample: Prevalence, Impact on Functioning, and Diagnostic Classification," *Archives of General Psychiatry* 53:2 (February 1996): 169–74.

[4] Erving Goffman, "Embarrassment and Social Organization," *American Journal of Sociology* 62:3 (November 1956): 264.

[5] I. M. James, D. N. W. Griffith, R. M. Pearson, and P. Newbury, "Effect of Oxprenolol on Stage-Fright in Musicians," *The Lancet* 2 (November 5, 1977): 952–55.

[6] This may help explain why, at the annual meeting of the American College of Cardiology in 1983, 15 percent of speakers used beta-blockers or other drugs for anxiety before delivering their scientific presentations. See D. Gossard, C. Dennis, R. F. DeBusk, "Use of Beta-Blocking Agents to Reduce the Stress of Presentation at an International Cardiology Meeting: Results of a Survey," *American Journal of Cardiology* 54 (1984): 240–41.

[7] Joseph Himle, James Ableson, Hedieh Haghightou, Elizabeth Hill, Randolph Nesse, and Curtis George, "Effect of Alcohol on Social Phobia Anxiety," *American Journal of Psychiatry* 156:8 (August 1999): 1237–43.

[8] Lionel Trilling, *Sincerity and Authenticity* (Cambridge, Mass.: Harvard University Press), 85.

[9] Ibid.

[10] Robert Putnam, *Bowling Alone* (New York: Simon and Schuster, 2000), 217.

[11] Ibid., 223.

[12] John P. Robinson and Geoffrey Godbey, *Time for Life: The Surprising Ways Americans Use Their Time* (University Park: Pennsylvania State University Press, 1997), xvii.

[13] For a broad sample of some of this research, see the following: Randy M. Page, Jon Hammermeister, Andria Scanlan, and Ola Allen, "Psychosocial and Health-Related Characteristics of Adolescent Television Viewers," *Child Study Journal* 26:4 (1996): 319–31; Seth Finn and Mary Gorr, "Social Isolation and Social Support as Correlates of Television Viewing Motivations," *Communication Research* 15:2 (April 1988): 135–58; Mary Lynne Ditmar, "Relations Among Depression, Gender, and Television Viewing of College Students," *Journal of Social Behavior and Personality* 9:2 (June 1994): 317–28; Richard Perloff and Julia Krevans, "Tracking the Psychosocial Predictors of Older Individuals' Television Uses," *Journal of Psychology* 121:4 (July 1987): 365–72; Elizabeth Perse and Alan Rubin, "Chronic Loneliness and Television Use," *Journal of Broadcasting and Electronic Media* 34:1 (Winter 1990): 37–53; Richard Potts and Dawn Sanchez, "Television Viewing and Depression: No News Is Good News," *Journal of Broadcasting and Electronic Media* 38:1 (Winter 1994): 79–90.

[14] Putnam, *Bowling Alone*, 231.

[15] This observation has become a commonplace in media studies and cultural studies. Two of the better books on the influence of television are Cecilia Tichi, *Electronic Hearth: Creating an American Television Culture* (New York: Oxford University Press, 1991) and Neil Postman, *Amusing Ourselves to Death: Public Discourse in an Age of Show Business* (New York: Viking, 1985).

[16] See David Foster Wallace's brilliant essay, "E Unibus Pluram: Television and U.S. Fiction," in David Foster Wallace, *A Supposedly Fun Thing I'll Never Do Again* (Boston: Back Bay Books, 1997), 21–82. Wallace says everything I am trying to say here (and he says it with a lot more style).

[17] See David Lodge, "Dickens Our Contemporary," *Atlantic Monthly* 289:5 (May 2002): 92–101; Daniel Boorstin, *The Image: A Guide to Pseudoevents in America* (New York: Harper and Row, 1961); Chris Rojek, *Celebrity* (London: Reaktion Books, 2001). Rojek dates the birth of celebrity even earlier, to the late eighteenth century.

[18] David Giles, *Illusions of Immortality: A Psychology of Fame and Celebrity* (New York: St. Martin's Press, 2000); and Lodge, "Dickens Our Contemporary."

[19] Boorstin, *The Image*, 57.

[20] Ibid., 65.

[21] Warren Susman, *Culture as History: The Transformation of American Society in the Twentieth Century* (New York: Pantheon Books, 1984), 284–85. See also Stanley Cavell, *The World Viewed: Reflections on the Ontology of Film* (Cambridge, Mass.: Harvard University Press, 1979), 29–37.

[22] George W. S. Trow, *Within the Context of No Context* (New York: Atlantic Monthly Press, 1997; originally 1980), 48.

[23] I have discussed this at greater length in "Prozac and the Existential Novel: Two Therapies," in *The Last Physician: Walker Percy and the Moral Life of Medicine*, eds. Carl Elliott and John Lantos (Durham, N.C.: Duke University Press, 1999), 59–69.

[24] Quoted in Tichi, *Electronic Hearth*, 137.

[25] Patricia Priest, " 'Gilt by Association': Talk Show Participants' Televisually Enhanced Status and Self-Esteem," in *Constructing the Self in a Mediated World*, eds. Debra Grodin and Thomas R. Lindlof (Thousand Oaks, Calif.: Sage Publications, 1996), 68–83. See especially p. 80.

[26] See Charles Taylor, "The Politics of Recognition," in *Multiculturalism: Examining the Politics of Identity*, ed. Amy Gutman (Princeton, N.J.: Princeton University Press, 1994), 25–73.

[27] Leo Braudy, *The Frenzy of Renown: Fame and Its History* (New York: Vintage Books, 1997).

[28] Putnam, *Bowling Alone*, 217.

[29] See Wallace, "E Unibus Pluram."

[30] Atul Gawande wrote an excellent piece on Drury and chronic blushing for *The New Yorker*. A version of Gawande's article appears in his book *Complications: A Surgeon's Notes on an Imperfect Science* (New York: Metropolitan Books, 2002), 146–61. Drury has also appeared on the television show *Good Morning America*, and she was kind enough to let me have a videotape of that appearance. Another longer interview with Drury was broadcast on the radio program "Sound Medicine" in March 2002, and can be heard via the Internet at: http://soundmedicine.iu.edu/archive/2002/030202.html#segment_2. I have drawn on this interview and Gawande's essay for some of the information included here about Drury, ETS, and chronic blushing.

[31] Mark Leary, Thomas Britt, William Cutlip, and Janice Templeton, "Social Blushing," *Psychological Bulletin* 112:3 (1992): 452.

[32] Don Shearn, Erik Bergman, Katherine Hill, Andy Abel, and Lael Hines, "Blushing as a Function of Audience Size," *Psychophysiology* 29:4 (1992): 432–36.

[33] Leary et al., "Social Blushing," 449.

[34] See Ibid., 446–60. Though Leary and his colleagues described a pilot study on the creeping blush (see p. 457), that study was not published, and as far as I can tell, no one else has studied the phenomenon.

[35] P. D. Drummond, "The Effect of Adrenergic Blockade on Blushing and Facial Blushing," *Psychophysiology* 34:2, (March 1997): 163–68.

[36] C. Drott, G. Claes, L. Rex-Olsson, P. Dalman, and G. Gothberg, "Successful Treatment of Facial Blushing by Endoscopic Transthoracic Sympathicotomy," *British Journal of Dermatology* 138:4 (April 1998): 639–43; Timo Telaranta, "Treatment of

Social Phobia by Endoscopic Thoracic Sympathicotomy," *European Journal of Surgery,* Supplement 580 (1998): 27–32.

[37] See Drott et al., "Successful Treatment of Facial Blushing"; also P. D. Drummond, "A Caution About Surgical Treatment for Facial Blushing," *British Journal of Dermatology* 142 (2000): 195–96.

[38] A patient quoted in Canada's *National Post* says, "I feel it looks like I'm lying, and then I'll blush worse and because I avert my eyes to help make it stop—that makes me look even more shifty." See Samantha Grice, "It's a Crying Shame," *National Post,* May 31, 2001.

[39] This can be seen in the testimonials section of the Red Mask Foundation Web site at: www.redmask.org.

[40] On-line at: www.dreamwater.com/hyperhid/surgery.html.

[41] C. Castelfranchi and I. Poggi, "Blushing as a Discourse: Was Darwin Wrong?" *Shyness and Embarrassment: Perspectives from Social Psychology,* ed. W. R. Crozier (Cambridge: Cambridge University Press, 1990), 230–54.

[42] G. R. Semin and A. S. R. Manstead, "The Social Implications of Embarrassment Displays and Restitution Behavior," *European Journal of Social Psychology* 12 (1982): 367–77.

[43] On-line at: www.dreamwater.com/hyperhid/surgery.html.

[44] Alexander Gerlach, Frank Wilhelm, Karen Gruber, and Walton Roth, "Blushing and Physiological Arousal in Social Phobia," *Journal of Abnormal Psychology,* 110:2 (2001): 247–58.

[45] Sandra Mulkens, Peter J. De Jong, and Susan Boegels, "High Blushing Propensity: Fearful Preoccupation or Facial Coloration?" *Personality and Individual Differences* 22:6 (1997): 817–24; Sandra Mulkens, Peter J. De Jong, Annemiek Dobbelar, and Susan Boegels, "Fear of Blushing: Fearful Preoccupation Irrespective of Facial Coloration," *Behaviour Research and Therapy* 37 (1999): 1119–28.

CHAPTER FIVE: THE IDENTITY BAZAAR

[1] "Drug Firms Use Coupons in Marketing Blitz," *Houston Chronicle,* June 4, 2001.

[2] These figures come from a study by the nonprofit National Institute of Health Care Management, "Prescription Drugs and Mass Media Drug Advertising 2000." See also "Prescription Drug Expenditures in 2000: The Upward Trend Continues." Both reports are available on-line at www.nihcm.org or from the NIHCM Foundation, 1225 19th St. NW, Suite 710, Washington DC 20036.

[3] Thorstein Veblen, *The Theory of the Leisure Class* (New York: Viking, 1967; originally published in 1899), 148–49.

[4] Ibid., 171.

[5] Ibid., 74.

[6] Ibid., 114.

[7] Malcolm Cowley, *Exile's Return: A Literary Odyssey of the 1920s* (New York: Penguin, 1994; originally published in 1934), 61–62.

[8] Ibid., 59.

[9] Ibid., 65.

[10] Ibid., 49.

[11] Ibid., 65.

[12] Kathy Peiss, *Hope in a Jar: The Making of America's Beauty Culture* (New York: Henry Holt, 1998), 12.

[13] Ibid., 17.

[14] Ibid., 40.

[15] Hendrik Hertzberg, "The Parent Trap: How Did They Ever Raise Kids Without Magazines?" *The New Yorker* 75:20 (July 26, 1999): 91–92.

[16] Sander Gilman, *Making the Body Beautiful: A Cultural History of Cosmetic Surgery* (Princeton, N.J.: Princeton University Press, 1999).

[17] Peiss, *Hope in a Jar*, 145.

[18] Ibid., 162.

[19] Cowley, *Exile's Return*, 60.

[20] Peiss, *Hope in a Jar*, 146–48.

[21] Ibid., 142.

[22] Christopher Lasch, *The Culture of Narcissism* (New York: W. W. Norton, 1979), 92. See also Stuart Ewen, *Captains of Consciousness: Advertising and the Roots of Consumer Culture* (New York: McGraw Hill, 1976), 54–55.

[23] Malcolm Gladwell, "True Colors: Hair Dye and the Hidden History of Postwar America," *The New Yorker* 75:4 (March 22, 1999): 70–82.

[24] Ibid.," 77.

[25] John Seabrook, "Nobrow Culture," *The New Yorker* 75:27 (September 20, 1999): 109.

[26] V. Vale and Andrea Juno, *Modern Primitives: An Investigation of Contemporary Adornment and Ritual* (San Francisco: Re/Search Publications, 1989), 39.

[27] Susan Bordo, "Braveheart, Babe and the Contemporary Body," in *Enhancing Human Traits: Ethical and Social Implications*, ed. Erik Parens (Washington, D.C.: Georgetown University Press, 1998), 193.

[28] Laurie Zoloth, *Health Care and the Ethics of Encounter* (Chapel Hill: University of North Carolina Press, 1999), 96.

[29] Thomas Frank, *The Conquest of Cool: Business Culture, Counterculture, and the Rise of Hip Consumerism* (Chicago: University of Chicago Press, 1997), 155. Frank is the author and editor of a number of brilliant anticonsumerist polemics, including *One Market Under God: Extreme Capitalism, Market Populism, and the End of Economic Democracy* (New York: Anchor Books, 2001) and, with Matt Weiland, eds., *Commodify Your Dissent: Salvos from the Baffler* (New York: W. W. Norton, 1997).

[30] Frank, *Conquest of Cool*, 144.

[31] Ibid., 136.

[32] Grant McCracken, *Big Hair: A Journey into the Transformation of Self* (Woodstock, New York: Overlook Press, 1996), 2.

[33] Gina Bellafante, "Tan Is the New Black," *New York Times Magazine*, August 12, 2001, 13–14.

[34] Andrew Sullivan, "What We Look Up To Now," *New York Times Magazine*, November 15, 1998, Section 6, p. 59.

[35] National Institutes for Health Care Management, "Prescription Drugs and Mass Media Drug Advertising 2000."

[36] On-line at: www.drugdispensary.com/xenical.html.

[37] Sheryl Stolberg, "High-Tech Stealth Being Used to Sway Doctor Prescriptions," *New York Times*, November 16, 2000, A1.

[38] National Institutes for Health Care Management, "Prescription Drugs and Mass Media Drug Advertising 2000."

[39] Elizabeth Haiken, *Venus Envy: A History of Cosmetic Surgery* (Baltimore, Maryland: Johns Hopkins University Press, 1997). See also Gilman, *Making the Body Beautiful*, 264.

[40] Haiken, *Venus Envy*, 102.

[41] Ibid., 122.

[42] Peiss, *Hope in a Jar*, 155.

[43] Ibid., 155.

[44] Ibid., 155.

[45] John Pick, "Ten Years of Plastic Surgery in a Penal Institution: Preliminary Report, *Journal of the International College of Surgeons* 11:3 (May/June 1948): 315–18. See also Gilman, *Making the Body Beautiful*, 29; Haiken, *Venus Envy*, 109.

[46] David Healy, *The Antidepressant Era* (Cambridge, Mass.: Harvard University Press, 1997), 75–76.

[47] M. J. Grinfeld, "Protecting Prozac," *California Lawyer* 18:12 (December 1998): 36–40.

[48] Harold I. Kaplan, Benjamin Sadock, Jack Grab, *Kaplan and Sadock's Synopsis of Psychiatry*, 7th Edition (New York: Williams and Wilkins, 1994), 599. See also National Institute of Mental Health (NIMH) data on-line at: www.nimh.nih. gov/publicat/numbers.cfm#12.

[49] Edward Shorter, *A History of Psychiatry: From the Era of the Asylum to the Age of Prozac* (New York: Wiley, 1997), 320.

[50] W. E. Narrow, D. S. Rae, D. A. Regier, "NIMH Epidemiology Note: Prevalence of Anxiety Disorders. One-year prevalence best estimates calculated from ECA and NCS data. Population estimates based on U.S. Census estimated residential population age 18 to 54 on July 1, 1998." Unpublished. Information available at and provided by NIMH Public Inquiries, 6001 Executive Boulevard, Rm. 8184, MSC 9663, Bethesda, MD 20892-9663 U.S.A., or on-line at:www.nimh.nih.gov/publicat/numbers.cfm#12.

[51] "Focus on Social Anxiety Disorder," *Journal of Clinical Psychiatry* 59, Supplement 17 (1998).

[52] Joseph Glenmullen, *Prozac Backlash* (New York: Touchstone Books, 2001), 228–29.

[53] Healy, *The Antidepressant Era*, 180.

[54] Lawrence H. Diller, *Running on Ritalin* (New York: Bantam Books, 1998), 41.

[55] David Riesman, Nathan Glazer, and Reuel Denney, *The Lonely Crowd: A Study*

of the Changing American Character (New York: Doubleday, 1953; originally published in 1950), 142.

[56] T. J. Jackson Lears, *No Place of Grace: Antimodernism and the Transformation of American Culture* 1880-1920 (Chicago: University of Chicago Press, 1994), 4.

[57] Daniel Bell, *The Cultural Contradictions of Capitalism* (New York: Basic Books, 1978). For the link between self-liberation and consumerism, see also Philip Cushman, *Constructing the Self, Constructing America: A Cultural History of Psychotherapy* (Reading, Mass.: Addison-Wesley, 1995), 210–78.

CHAPTER SIX: THREE WAYS TO FEEL HOMESICK

[1] Edward Shorter, *A History of Psychiatry: From the Era of the Asylum to the Age of Prozac* (New York: John Wiley and Sons, 1997), 315–16; Mickey Smith, *Small Comfort: A History of Minor Tranquilizers* (New York: Praeger, 1985), 69–74.

[2] Shorter, *A History of Psychiatry*, 154–57. See also David Healy, *The Creation of Psychopharmacology* (Cambridge, Mass.: Harvard University Press, 2002), 67–68, 98–99.

[3] Walker Percy, *The Second Coming* (New York: Washington Square Press, 1980), 313.

[4] Susan Sontag, "The Anthropologist as Hero," in *Against Interpretation* (New York: Vintage, 1994, originally published in 1966), 69.

[5] Richard Ford, *Independence Day* (New York: Vintage, 1996), 9.

[6] Ibid., 94.

[7] Ibid., 156.

[8] Ibid., 37.

[9] Ibid., 44.

[10] Ibid., 57.

[11] Robert N. Bellah, Richard Madsen, William M. Sullivan, Ann Swidler, and Steven M. Tipton, *Habits of the Heart: Individualism and Commitment in American Life* (Berkeley: University of California Press, 1985), 334. See also Andrew Delbanco's moving book, *The Real American Dream: A Meditation on Hope* (Cambridge, Mass.: Harvard University Press, 1998).

[12] John Lukacs, "The Bourgeois Interior," *The American Scholar* 39:4 (Autumn 1970): 620–21.

[13] Ibid., 623; Witold Rybczynski, *Home: A Short History of an Idea* (New York: Penguin, 1987), 35–36.

[14] Lionel Trilling, *Sincerity and Authenticity* (Cambridge, Mass.: Harvard University Press, 1971), 24–25.

[15] Witold Rybczynski, "Beyond the Old Woman in the Shoe," *New York Times Magazine*, March 7, 1999, 70–73.

[16] Ibid., 70

[17] Walker Percy, *Lost in Cosmos: The Last Self-Help Book* (New York: Washington Square Press, 1983), 24.

[18] Alexis de Tocqueville, *Democracy in America*, trans. George Lawrence, ed. J. P. Mayer (New York: Harper and Row, 1988), 513.

[19] Bellah, *Habits of the Heart*, 89.

[20] Ibid., 47.

[21] Ford, *Independence Day*, 76.

[22] Joel Garreau, *Edge Cities: Life on the New Frontier* (New York: Anchor Books, 1991), 278.

[23] Ibid., 280.

[24] Richard Yates, *Revolutionary Road* (London: Methuen, 1961; 1986), 3.

[25] Ibid., 97.

[26] Ibid., 112.

[27] Ibid., 20.

[28] Ibid., 115.

[29] Louis Menand, "Holden at Fifty: 'The Catcher in the Rye' and What it Spawned," *The New Yorker* 77:29 (October 1, 2001): 82-88.

[30] Albert Borgmann, *Technology and the Character of Everyday Life* (Chicago: University of Chicago Press, 1984), 41.

[31] Charles Taylor, *Sources of the Self* (Cambridge, Mass.: Harvard University Press, 1989), 15.

[32] Ibid., 13.

[33] Ibid., 217. See also the powerful essay by Stanley Hauerwas, "Killing Compassion," in *Dispatches from the Front: Theological Engagements with the Secular* (Durham, N.C.: Duke University Press, 1994), 164–76.

[34] Max Weber, *The Protestant Ethic and the Spirit of Capitalism*, trans. Talcott Parsons (London: Routledge; 1992, originally published in 1930), 54.

[35] B. McNamara, J. L. Ray, J. Arthurs, and S. Boniface, "Transcranial Magnetic Stimulation for Depression and Other Psychiatric Disorders," *Psychological Medicine* 31:7 (October 2001): 1141–46; B. P. Bejjani, P. Damier, I. Arnulf, L. Thivard, A. M. Bonnet, D. Dormont, P. Cornu, B. Pidoux, Y. Samson, and Y. Agid, "Transient Acute Depression Induced by High-Frequency Deep-Brain Stimulation," *New England Journal of Medicine* 340:19 (May 13, 1999): 1476–80; R. Kumar, P. Krack, and P. Pollak, "Transient Acute Depression Induced by High-Frequency Deep-Brain Stimulation," letter, *New England Journal of Medicine* 341:13 (September 23, 1999): 1003–4.

[36] Walker Percy, "The Man on the Train," in *The Message in the Bottle* (New York: Farrar, Straus and Giroux, 1998; originally published in 1975), 85.

[37] Walker Percy, "The Delta Factor," in *The Message in the Bottle* (New York: Farrar, Straus and Giroux, 1998; originally published in 1975), 6.

[38] Walker Percy, *Love in the Ruins* (New York: Ivy Books, 1990; originally published in 1971), 325.

[39] James C. Edwards, "Passion, Activity and 'The Care of the Self,' " *The Hastings Center Report* 30:2 (March-April 2000): 31–35. Edwards has explored similar themes in a remarkable series of books as notable for their stylistic elegance as for

their philosophical acuity: *The Plain Sense of Things: The Fate of Religion in an Age of Normal Nihilism* (University Park: Pennsylvania State University Press, 1997), *The Authority of Language: Heidegger, Wittgenstein and the Threat of Philosophical Nihilism* (Tampa: University of South Florida Press, 1990), and *Ethics Without Philosophy: Wittgenstein and the Moral Life* (Tampa: University of South Florida Press, 1983).

[40] Edwards, "Passion, Activity and 'The Care of the Self,' " 33.

[41] The idea of Sisyphus on Prozac I owe to a conversation with Robin Downie. See also his article, R. S. Downie, "The Value and Quality of Life," *Journal of the Royal College of Physicians of London* 33:4 (July–August 1999): 378–81.

CHAPTER SEVEN: PILGRIMS AND STRANGERS

[1] Walker Percy, *The Last Gentleman* (London: Panther Books, 1985; originally published in 1965) 110–12. I use the old-fashioned terms "Negro" and "colored" because they are the terms that Percy uses in the novel.

[2] John Howard Griffin, *Black Like Me* (New York: Signet, 1996; originally published in 1961).

[3] Grace Halsell, *Soul Sister* (New York: World, 1969).

[4] Joshua Solomon, "Skin Deep: Reliving *Black Like Me*: My Own Journey into the Heart of Race-Conscious America," *Washington Post*, October 30, 1994, C1.

[5] Laura Browder, *Slippery Characters: Ethnic Impersonators and American Identities* (Chapel Hill, North Carolina: University of North Carolina Press, 2000).

[6] Tony Horwitz, *Confederates in the Attic* (New York: Random House, 1999), 7–8.

[7] Griffin, *Black Like Me*, 7.

[8] Ibid., 15.

[9] Ibid., 161.

[10] Ibid., 109. My italics.

[11] Ibid., 31.

[12] Ibid., 41.

[13] Ibid., 113.

[14] Ibid., 69.

[15] Ibid., 163. My italics.

[16] Eddy L. Harris, *Native Stranger: A Black American's Journey into the Heart of Africa* (New York: Vintage, 1993), 69.

[17] Gayle Wald, "A Most Disagreeable Mirror: Reflections on White Identity in Black Like Me," in *Passing and the Fictions of Identity*, ed. Elaine Ginsberg (Durham, N.C.: Duke University Press, 1996), 151–77.

[18] There are a number of good books about *The Wizard of Oz*, both the film and Baum's original book, and I have drawn on several of them here. See especially Salman Rushdie, *The Wizard of Oz: BFI Classics* (London: British Film Institute, 1992) and the extended discussion in William Leach, *Land of Desire: Merchants, Power, and the Rise of a New American Culture* (New York: Vintage, 1994).

[19] L. Frank Baum, *The Wonderful Wizard of Oz* (New York: Dover, 1960), 128.

[20] Percy, *The Last Gentleman*, 15.

[21] Ian Hacking, *Mad Travelers: Reflections on the Reality of Transient Mental Illnesses* (Charlottesville: University Press of Virginia, 1998).

[22] Robert N. Rudnicki, *Percyscapes: The Fugue State in Twentieth Century Southern Fiction* (Baton Rouge: Louisiana State University Press, 1999).

[23] Hacking, *Mad Travelers*, 7.

[24] Ibid., 26.

[25] Ibid., 62.

[26] Ibid., 61.

[27] Percy, *The Last Gentleman*, 17.

[28] Ibid., 14.

[29] Kathy Peiss, *Hope in a Jar: The Making of America's Beauty Culture* (New York: Henry Holt, 1998), 144.

[30] Deirdre McCloskey, "From Donald to Deirdre," *Reason* 31:7 (December 1999): 42.

[31] Quoted in Richard M. Levine, "Crossing the Line: Are Transsexuals at the Forefront of a Revolution—or Just Reinforcing Old Stereotypes about Men and Women?" *Mother Jones* 19:3 (May–June 1994), 43–48.

[32] Quoted in Jay Stevens, *Storming Heaven* (New York: Harper and Row, 1987), 49.

[33] Robert Bretall, ed., *A Kierkegaard Anthology* (Princeton, N.J.: Princeton University Press), 23–24.

[34] Walker Percy, *Lost in the Cosmos: The Last Self-Help Book* (New York: Washington Square Press, 1983), 151.

[35] Bretall, *A Kierkegaard Anthology*, 25.

CHAPTER EIGHT: RESIDENT ALIENS

[1] George Schuyler, *Black No More: Being an Account of the Strange and Wonderful Workings of Science in the Land of the Free, A.D. 1933–40* (Boston: Northeastern University Press, 1989; originally published in 1931), 27.

[2] A note of caution: these figures come from press releases by professional cosmetic surgery associations, with no explanation of their survey methods. See Scott Gottlieb, "Plastic Surgery Rockets as Baby Boomers Search for Youth and Beauty," *British Medical Journal* 322:7286 (March 10, 2001): 574; "Cosmetic Procedures Rise 66% to 4.6 Million in 1999, Says America Society for Aesthetic Plastic Surgery," *PR Newswire*, March 9, 2000; "American Society of Plastic Surgeons Reports Most Popular Cosmetic Surgery Procedures Just Became More Popular," *PR Newswire*, July 20, 2000; "Ninety-Seven Percent of Breast Augmentation Patients Happy with Results, According to Survey by the American Academy of Cosmetic Surgery," *PR Newswire*, June 26, 2000.

[3] Elizabeth Haiken, *Venus Envy: A History of Cosmetic Surgery* (Baltimore, Md.: Johns Hopkins University Press, 1997), 184. See also Sander Gilman, *Making the*

Body Beautiful: A Cultural History of Cosmetic Surgery (Princeton, N.J.: Princeton University Press, 1999) and Sander Gilman, *Creating Beauty to Cure the Soul: Race and Psychology in the Shaping of Aesthetic Surgery* (Durham, N.C.: Duke University Press, 1998).

[4] Haiken, *Venus Envy*, 175–227.

[5] Gilman, *Making the Body Beautiful*, 193.

[6] Haiken, *Venus Envy*, 186.

[7] Ibid., 182, 96.

[8] Ibid., 84.

[9] Ibid., 200–209; Gilman, *Making the Body Beautiful*, 98–111; Eugenia Kaw, "Medicalization of Racial Features: Asian American Women and Cosmetic Surgery," *Medical Anthropology Quarterly* 7 (1993): 74–89.

[10] Kathy Peiss, *Hope in a Jar: The Making of America's Beauty Culture* (New York: Henry Holt, 1998), 209. See also N. Jamiyla Chisholm, "Fade to White: Skin Bleaching and the Rejection of Blackness," *Village Voice*, January 22–28, 2001.

[11] Schuyler, *Black No More*, 13.

[12] Malcolm X, with the assistance of Alex Haley, *The Autobiography of Malcolm X* (New York: Ballantine Books, 1964), 61.

[13] Schuyler, *Black No More*, 59.

[14] Peiss, *Hope in a Jar*, 204.

[15] Ibid., 205.

[16] Ibid., 213.

[17] Schuyler, *Black No More*, 19. See also Ronald Hall, "The Bleaching Syndrome: African Americans' Response to Cultural Domination Vis-à-vis Skin Color," *Journal of Black Studies* 26:2 (1995): 172–84.

[18] Peiss, *Hope in a Jar*, 205.

[19] Margaret Olivia Little, "Cosmetic Surgery, Suspect Norms and the Ethics of Complicity," *Enhancing Human Traits: Ethical and Social Implications*, ed. Erik Parens (Washington, D.C.: Georgetown University Press), 166.

[20] Little, "Cosmetic Surgery, Suspect Norms and the Ethics of Complicity," 166. Her italics.

[21] For a sample of this debate, see Melvin Grumbach, "Growth Hormone Therapy and the Short End of the Stick," *New England Journal of Medicine* 319:4 (July 1988): 238–41; Douglas Diekema, "Is Taller Really Better? Growth Hormone Therapy in Short Children," *Perspectives in Biology and Medicine* 34:1 (Autumn 1990): 109–23.

[22] Erving Goffman, *Stigma: Notes on the Management of Spoiled Identity* (New York: Simon and Schuster, 1963), 128.

[23] I owe this point to Paul Brodwin.

[24] Kwame Anthony Appiah, "We Are All Multiculturalists Now," *New York Review of Books* 44:15 (October 9, 1997): 30–35. See also Ian Buruma, "The Joys and Perils of Victimhood," *New York Review of Books* 46:6 (April 8, 1999): 8; and Elizabeth Lasch-Quinn, *Race Experts* (New York: W. W. Norton, 2001).

[25] Nelson examines the notion of counterstories further in her fine book: Hilde Lindemann Nelson, *Damaged Identities, Narrative Repair* (Ithaca, N.Y.: Cornell University Press, 2001).

[26] Ruth Benedict, *The Chrysanthemum and the Sword: Patterns of Japanese Culture* (London: Secker and Warburg, 1947), 207.

[27] Henry Louis Gates Jr., *Colored People: A Memoir* (New York: Knopf, 1994), 187.

[28] Haiken, *Venus Envy*, 224.

[29] Kathryn Pauly Morgan, "Women and the Knife: Cosmetic Surgery and the Colonization of Women's Bodies," in *Sex/Machine: Readings in Culture, Gender and Technology*, ed. Patrick D. Hopkins (Bloomington: Indiana University Press, 1998), 278–79.

[30] Francis Fitzgerald, *Cities on a Hill* (New York: Picador, 1986), 54, 116.

[31] Goffman, *Stigma*, 123.

[32] Marya Mannes, "The Roots of Anxiety in the Modern Woman," *Journal of Neuropsychiatry* 5 (1964): 412.

[33] Philip Rieff, *Triumph of the Therapeutic: Use of Faith After Freud* (New York: Harper and Row, 1966), 32.

CHAPTER NINE: AMPUTEES BY CHOICE

[1] P. Taylor, "'My Left Foot Was Not Part of Me,' " *The Guardian*, February 6, 2000, 14; Tracey Lawson, "Therapist Praises Doctor's Bravery," *The Scotsman*, February 1, 2000; Clare Dyer "Surgeon Amputated Healthy Legs," *British Medical Journal* 320 (February 5, 2000): 332.

[2] J. H. Burnett, "Southside Man Uses Homemade Guillotine to Sever Arm," *Milwaukee Journal Sentinel*, October 7, 1999; Stephen McGinty and Sue Leonard, "Secret World of Would-Be Amputees," *Sunday Times*, February 6, 2000; Michelle Williams, "Murder Trial Opens for Fetish M.D.," *Associated Press*, September 29, 1999.

[3] Cherry Norton, "Disturbed Patients Have Healthy Limbs Amputated," *The Independent*, February 1, 2000.

[4] BBC2 Horizon, "Complete Obsession," Transcript of television documentary, screened in United Kingdom Feb 17, 2000; downloaded November 27, 2000 at: www.bbc.co.uk/science/horizon/obsession.shtm. More recently, the Australian radio program "Soundprint" broadcast a documentary on amputee wannabes, available on-line at: http://soundprint.org/radio/display_show/ID/232/name/Wannabes.

[5] J. Money, R. Jobaris, and G. Furth, "Apotemnophilia: Two Cases of Self-Demand Amputation as a Paraphilia," *Journal of Sex Research* 13:2 (May 1977): 114–25.

[6] P. L. Wakefield, A. Frank, R. W. Meyers, "The Hobbyist: A Euphemism for Self-mutilation and Fetishism," *Bulletin of the Menninger Clinic* 41 (1977): 539–52.

[7] W. Everaerd, "A Case of Apotemnophilia: a Handicap as a Sexual Preference," *American Journal of Psychotherapy* 37:2 (April 1983): 285–93; J. Money, "Paraphilia in Females: Fixation on Amputation and Lameness: Two Personal Accounts,"

Journal of Psychology and Human Sexuality 3:2 (1990): 165–72; R. L. Bruno, "Devotees, Pretenders and Wannabes: Two Cases of Factitious Disability Disorder," *Sexuality and Disability* 15:4 (Winter 1997): 243–60; Wakefield, Frank, and Meyers, "The Hobbyist." On acrotomophilia, see Grant Riddle, *Amputees and Devotees* (New York: Irvington Publishers, 1989).

[8] Keren Fisher, Robert Smith, "More Work Is Needed to Explain Why Patients Ask for Amputation of Healthy Limbs," letter, *British Medical Journal* 320 (April 22, 2000): 1147. Smith and Gregg Furth also recently published a book titled *Amputee Identity Disorder: Information, Questions, Answers, and Recommendations About Self-Demand Amputation* (Portland, Ore.: 1stBooks Library, 2000).

[9] Taylor, " 'My Left Foot Was Not Part of Me.' "

[10] Helen Rumbelow and Gillian Harris, "Craving That Drives People to Disability," *The Times* (London), February 1, 2000.

[11] See www.geocities.com/FashionAvenue/6914/ABOUT_ME_PAGE_1.html.

[12] L. E. Nattress, "Amelotasis: A Descriptive Study." Unpublished doctoral dissertation, Walden University, 1996.

[13] Katherine A. Phillips, *The Broken Mirror: Understanding and Treating Body Dysmorphic Disorder* (New York: Oxford University Press, 1996). Phillips is a psychiatrist at Brown University who has also published extensively on body dysmorphic disorder in the medical literature. The patients she describes generally do not much resemble amputee wannabes, but she does briefly mention a man who asked a surgeon to remove his nose (p. 289).

[14] J-J Sue, *Anecdotes Historiques, Littéraires et Critiques, sur la Médecine, la Chirurgie, & la Pharmacie* (Paris: Chez la Bocher, 1785). I am indebted to Dr. Price, who wrote to me about this text and generously sent me his translation, along with other materials on amputation.

[15] Richard von Krafft-Ebing, *Psychopathia Sexualis* (New York: Putnam, 1906; originally published in 1898), 234–38.

[16] B. Taylor, "Amputee Fetishism: An Exclusive Journal Interview with Dr. John Money of Johns Hopkins," *Maryland State Medical Journal* (March 1976): 35–38.

[17] John Money, "Paraphilia in Females: Fixation on Amputation and Lameness, Two Personal Accounts," *Journal of Psychology and Human Sexuality* 3:2 (1990): 165–72.

[18] Money, Jobaris, and Furth, "Apotemnophilia."

[19] Erving Goffman, *Stigma: Notes on the Management of a Spoiled Identity* (New York: Simon and Schuster, 1986; originally published in 1963).

[20] Howard Rheingold, *The Virtual Community: Homesteading on the Electronic Frontier* (New York: HarperCollins, 1993).

[21] Victor Turner, *The Drums of Affliction: A Study of Religious Processes among the Ndembu of Zambia* (Oxford: Clarendon Press, 1968).

[22] See Paul Rabinow, "Artificiality and Enlightenment: From Sociobiology to Biosociality," *Essays on the Anthropology of Reason* (Princeton, N.J.: Princeton University Press, 1996), 81–111. Thanks to Paul Baldwin for directing me to Turner and to Rabinow.

[23] Josephine Johnston has written about the legal aspects of healthy limb amputa-

tion for her master's dissertation at the University of Otago. She and I have also written about the issue in a forthcoming article in *Clinical Medicine*. For a comprehensive review of moral and legal aspects of organ and tissue donation by children, see Robert Crouch, "The Child as Tissue and Organ Donor" (Master's Dissertation, McGill University, Department of Philosophy, 1996); also R. Crouch and C. Elliott, "Moral Agency and the Family: The Case of Living Related Organ Transplantation," *Cambridge Quarterly of Healthcare Ethics* 8:3 (1999), 257–87. See also Sally Sheldon and Stephen Wilkinson, "Female Genital Mutilation and Cosmetic Surgery: Regulating Non-Therapeutic Body Modification," *Bioethics* 12:4 (1998): 263–85.

[24] Everaerd, "A Case of Apotemnophilia," 286–87.

[25] BBC2 Horizon, "Complete Obsession."

[26] R. Blanchard, "The Concept of Autogynephilia and the Typology of Male Gender Dysphoria," *Journal of Nervous and Mental Disease* 177:10 (October 1989): 616–23; R. Blanchard, "Clinical Observations and Systematic Studies of Autogynephilia," *Journal of Sex and Marital Therapy* 17:4 (Winter 1991): 235–51; R. Blanchard, "Nonmonotonic Relation of Autogynephilia and Heterosexual Attraction," *Journal of Abnormal Psychology* 101:2 (May 1992): 271–76.

[27] See Anne Lawrence's Web site at: http://www.annelawrence.com. Blanchard has also found that a subset of autogynephiles is sexually aroused by the thought of themselves not as complete women, but as having a mixture of male and female sex characteristics. He calls this group "partial autogynephiles." See R. Blanchard, "The She-Male Phenomenon and the Concept of Partial Autogynephilia," *Journal of Sex and Marital Therapy* 19:1 (Spring 1993): 69–76.

[28] Peter D. Kramer, *Listening to Prozac* (London: Fourth Estate, 1993), ix–xi.

[29] M. P. Kafka and J. Hennen, "Psychostimulant Augmentation during Treatment with Selective Serotonin Reuptake Inhibitors in Men with Paraphilias and Paraphilia-Related Disorders: A Case Series," *Journal of Clinical Psychiatry* 61:9 (September, 2000): 664–70; A. Abouesh and A. Clayton, "Compulsive Voyeurism and Exhibitionism: A Clinical Response to Paroxetine," *Archives of Sexual Behavior* 28:1 (February, 1999): 23–30; V. B. Galli, N. J. Raute, B. J. McConville, S. L. McElroy, "An Adolescent Male with Multiple Paraphilias Successfully Treated with Fluoxetine," *Journal of Child and Adolescent Psychopharmacology* 8:3 (1998): 195–97; R. Balon, "Pharmacological Treatment of Paraphilias with a Focus on Antidepressants," *Journal of Sex and Marital Therapy* 24:4 (October–December, 1998): 241-54; M. P. Kafka, "Sertraline Pharmacotherapy for Paraphilias and Paraphilia-Related Disorders: An Open Trial," *Annals of Clinical Psychiatry* 6:3 (September 1994): 189–95.

[30] Katherine Dunn, *Geek Love* (New York: Knopf, 1989).

[31] Marianne Torgovnik includes a good chapter on extreme body modification in her book *Primitive Passions: Men, Women and the Quest for Ecstasy* (Chicago: University of Chicago Press, 1996), 189–208. See also Eric Gans, "The Body Sacrificial," in *The Body Aesthetic: From Fine Art to Body Modification*, ed. Tobin Siebers (Ann Arbor: University of Michigan Press, 2000), 159–78. On-line, see the "Body Modification Ezine" at www.bme.freeq.com and the "Almost Complete Body Piercing Links List" at www.piercinglinks.com.

[32] Available on-line at www.churchofbodmod.com or by request from 3439 N.E. Sandy Blvd. Suite 601, Portland, OR 97232.

[33] V. Vale and Andrea Juno, *Modern Primitives: An Investigation of Contemporary Adornment and Ritual* (San Francisco: Re/Search Publications, 1989), 101.

[34] Ibid., 94.

[35] For sociological data on women getting cosmetic surgery to blend in, see Kathy Davis, *Reshaping the Female Body* (New York: Routledge, 1995). See also the European Commission Report on Bioethics by Ineke Bolt and Henri Wijsbek, *Beauty and the Doctor: Moral Issues in Health Care with Regard to Appearance* (Rotterdam: Erasmus University, Department of Medical Ethics, 2002).

[36] See especially Ian Hacking, *Mad Travelers: Reflections on the Reality of Transient Mental Illness* (Charlottesville: University Press of Virginia, 1998) and Ian Hacking, *Rewriting the Soul: Multiple Personality and the Sciences of Memory* (Princeton, N.J.: Princeton University Press, 1995).

[37] Ivan Illich, *Limits to Medicine* (London: Marion Boyars, 2002); Peter Conrad and Joseph W. Schneider, *Deviance and Medicalization: From Badness to Sickness* (Philadelphia, Pa.: Temple University Press, 1992); Allan V. Horwitz, *Creating Mental Illness* (Chicago: University of Chicago Press, 2002).

[38] What looks like an entirely new condition may on closer examination turn out to be a new variation on previously existing conditions. Hacking suggests, for instance, that some of the young men characterized as having fugue states would, in the terms of today, be characterized as having epilepsy or traumatic head injuries.

[39] Mullen is also the coauthor of an interesting paper on the emergence of the idea of "stalking" in recent years. See P. E. Mullen, M. Pathe, and R. Purcell, "Stalking: New Constructions of Human Behaviour," *Australian and New Zealand Journal of Psychiatry* 35:1 (2001): 9–16.

[40] Dwight Dixon, "An Erotic Attraction to Amputees," *Sexuality and Disability* 6:1 (Spring 1983): 3–19.

[41] Donald R. Laub and Patrick Gandy, eds., *Proceedings of the Second Interdisciplinary Symposium on Gender Dysphoria Syndrome* (Stanford, Calif.: Division of Reconstructive and Rehabilitation Surgery, Stanford Medical Center, 1973). See also Sandy Stone, *The Empire Strikes Back: A Posttranssexual Manifesto*, in *Sex/Machine: Readings in Culture, Gender and Technology*, ed. Patrick D. Hopkins (Bloomington: Indiana University Press, 1998), 330.

CHAPTER TEN: BRINGING UP BABY

[1] Philippe Aries, *Centuries of Childhood*, trans. Robert Baldick (London: Pimlico, 1996; originally published in 1960).

[2] John Gillis, *A World of Their Own Making: Myth, Ritual and the Quest for Family Values* (New York: Basic Books, 1996).

[3] Neil Postman, *The Disappearance of Childhood* (New York: Vintage, 1994), 43.

[4] Jackson Lears, *No Place of Grace: Antimodernism and the Transformation of American Culture, 1880–1920* (Chicago: University of Chicago Press, 1981), 144.

[5] Aries, *Centuries of Childhood*, 28.

[6] D. B. Allen and N. C Fost, "Growth Hormone for Short Stature: Panacea or Pandora's Box?" *Journal of Pediatric Surgery* 117:1 (July 1990): 16–21.

[7] D. S. Diekema, "Is Taller Really Better? Growth Hormone Therapy in Short Children," *Perspectives in Biology and Medicine* 34:1 (Autumn 1990): 109–23.

[8] C. M. Law, "The Disability of Short Stature," *Archives of Disease in Childhood* 62:8 (August 1987): 855–59.

[9] F. A. Conte and M. M. Grumbach, "Estrogen Use in Children and Adolescents: A Survey," *Pediatrics* 62 (1978): 1091.

[10] Neal D. Barnard, Anthony R. Scialli, and Suzanne Bobela, "The Current Use of Estrogens for Growth-Suppressant Therapy in Adolescent Girls," *Journal of Pediatric and Adolescent Gynecology* 15:1 (February 2002): 23–26.

[11] Andrea Prader and Milo Zachman, "Treatment of Excessively Tall Girls and Boys with Sex Hormones," *Pediatrics* 62 (1978): 1209.

[12] Bruce Downie, Jean Mulligan, Robert Stratford, Peter Bettes, and Linda Voss, "Are Short Children at a Disadvantage? The Wessex Growth Study," *British Medical Journal* 314:7074 (January 11, 1997): 97–100.

[13] There is a large and rapidly changing literature on cochlear implants and Deaf culture. See, for example, Robert Crouch, "Letting the Deaf Be Deaf: Reconsidering the Use of Cochlear Implants in Prelingually Deaf Children," *Hastings Center Report* 27:4 (1997): 14–21. On the potential benefits of cochlear implants, see Gerald O'Donoghue, "Hearing without Ears: Do Cochlear Implants Work in Children?: Yes, So Long as They Are Given to the Right Children Early Enough," *British Medical Journal* 318:7176 (January 9, 1999): 72–73. The classic work on Deaf culture and identity is Harlan Lane, *The Mask of Benevolence: Disabling the Deaf Community* (New York: Alfred A. Knopf, 1992). See also Oliver Sacks, *Seeing Voices: A Journey into the World of the Deaf* (New York: HarperCollins, 1990) and Nora Ellen Groce, *Everyone Here Spoke Sign Language: Hereditary Deafness on Martha's Vineyard* (Cambridge, Mass.: Harvard University Press, 1985).

[14] Wang Ping, *Aching for Beauty: Footbinding in China* (Minneapolis: University of Minnesota Press, 2000), 83.

[15] Feng Jicai, *The Three-Inch Golden Lotus* (Honolulu, Hawaii: University of Hawaii Press, 1986), 117.

[16] Ping, *Aching for Beauty*, 59.

[17] See, for example, Howard Levy, *Chinese Footbinding: The History of a Curious Erotic Custom* (New York: Bell Publishing, 1967).

[18] Ping, *Aching for Beauty*, 32.

[19] Ibid., 29–53.

[20] J. M. Zito, D. J. Sofer, S. dos Reis, et al., "Trends in the Prescrbing of Psychotropic Medication to Preschoolers," *JAMA* 283(8) (February 2000): 1025–30. Reported in Eliot Marshall, "Planned Ritalin Trial for Tots Heads into Uncharted Waters," *Science* 290, November 17, 2000, 1280–82.

[21] Lawrence H. Diller, *Running on Ritalin* (New York: Bantam), 35–36. Diller cites Barbara Crossette, "Agency Sees Risk in Drug to Temper Child Behavior," *New York Times*, February 29, 1996, A7; United Nations International Narcotics Control Board, *Report of the UN International Narcotics Control Board* 1994 (New York: United Nations Publications, 1995).

[22] Andrew S. Rowland, David M. Umbach, Lil Stallone, A. Jack Naftel, E. Michael Bohlig, and Dale P. Sandler, "Prevalence of Medication Treatment for Attention-Deficit Hyperactivity Disorder among Elementary School Students in Johnston County, North Carolina," *American Journal of Public Health* 92:2 (February 2002): 231–34.

[23] For recent reviews of drug treatment of ADHD, see Thomas D. Challman and James Lipsky, "Methylphendiate: Its Pharmacology and Uses," *Mayo Clinic Proceedings* 75:7 (July 2000): 711–21; Josephine Elia, Paul Ambrosini, and Judith Rapoport, "Drug Therapy: Treatment of Attention-Deficit-Hyperactivity Disorder," *New England Journal of Medicine* 340:10 (March 11, 1999): 780–88.

[24] Joseph Biederman, "Are Stimulants Overprescribed for Children with Behavioral Problems?" *Pediatric News* (August 1996), 26.

[25] Larry S. Goldman, Myron Genel, Rebecca J. Benzman, and Priscilla J. Slanetz, for the Council on Scientific Affairs, American Medical Association, "Diagnosis and Treatment of Attention-Deficit/Hyperactivity Disorder in Children and Adolescents," *Journal of the American Medical Association* 279:14 (April 8, 1998): 1100–7.

[26] Sigmund Freud "On Cocaine," 1884; the quotations are from *Artificial Paradises*, ed. Mike Jay (London: Penguin, 1999), 44–45.

[27] Charles Bradley, "The Behavior of Children Receiving Benzedrine, *American Journal of Psychiatry* 94 (1937): 577–88.

[28] Goldman et al., "Diagnosis and Treatment of Attention-Deficit/Hyperactivity Disorder in Children and Adolescents."

[29] Peter Conrad and Deborah Potter, "From Hyperactive Children to ADHD Adults: Observations on the Expansion of Medical Categories," *Social Problems* 47:4 (2000): 559–82.

[30] M. G. Aman, M. Vamos, and J. S. Werry, "Effects of Methyphenidate in Normal Adults with Reference to Drug Action in Hyperactivity," *Australian and New Zealand Journal of Psychiatry* 1 (1984): 86–88.

[31] Elia, Ambrosini, and Rapoport, "Drug Therapy: Treatment of Attention-Deficit-Hyperactivity Disorder."

[32] Aman, Vamos, and Werry, "Effects of Methyphenidate in Normal Adults with Reference to Drug Action in Hyperactivity"; Judith L. Rapoport, Monte S. Buchsbaum, et al., "Dextroamphetamine: Cognitive and Behavioral Effects in Normal Prepubertal Boys," *Science* 199 (1978): 560–63; Judith L. Rapoport, Monte S.

Buchsbaum, et al., "Dextroamphetamine: Its Cognitive and Behavioral Effects in Normal and Hyperactive Boys and Normal Men," *Archives of General Psychiatry* 37 (1980): 933–43; R. Elliott, B. J. Sahakian, K. Matthews, et al., "Effects of Methylphenidate on Spatial Working Memory and Planning in Healthy Young Adults, *Psychopharmacology* 131:2 (May 1997): 196–206.

[33] Walter Kirn, "Inside Ritalin," *GQ*, December 2000, 297–301.

[34] Rapoport, Buchsbaum, et al., "Dextroamphetamine."

[35] L. Hechtman, G. Weiss, and T. Perlman, "Young Adult Outcome of Hyperactive Children Who Received Long-Term Stimulant Treatment," *Journal of the Academy of Child and Adolescent Psychiatry* 23 (1984): 261–65; L. Hechtman, "Adolescent Outcome of Hyperactive Children Treated with Stimulants in Childhood: A Review," *Psychopharmacology Bulletin* 21 (1985): 178–94; J. E. Richters, L. E. Arnold, P. S. Jensen, et al., "NIMH Collaborative Multi-Site Multimodal Treatment Study of Children with ADHD, I: Background and Rationale," *Journal of the American Academy of Child and Adolescent Psychiatry* 34 (1995): 987–1000. A Canadian meta-analysis of 62 studies of Ritalin for ADHD found that most clinical trials lasted three weeks or less, and none lasted for more than seven months. Now that many adults are being given a diagnosis of ADHD, there is a real possibility that many people will take stimulants their entire lives, with little data on the long-term effects of the drugs. See Howard M. Schachter, Ba Pham, Jim King, Stephanie Langford, and David Moher, "How Efficacious Is Short-Acting Methylphenidate for the Treatment of Attention-Deficit Disorder in Children and Adolescents? A Meta-Analysis," *Canadian Medical Association Journal* 165:11 (November 27, 2001): 1475–88.

[36] Conrad and Potter, "From Hyperactive Children to ADHD Adults."

[37] Kathleen Phalen, "World of Distraction: Adult Attention-Deficit/hyperactivity Disorder," *American Medical News*, March 18, 2002.

[38] Claudia Wallis, "Life in Overdrive," *Time*, July 18, 1994: 43.

[39] Diller, *Running on Ritalin*, 146.

[40] See, for example, Richard Sennett, *The Corrosion of Character: The Personal Consequences of Work in the New Capitalism* (New York: W. W. Norton, 1998).

[41] B. L. Trommer, J. A. Hoeppner, and S. G. Zecker, "The Go-No Go Tests in Attention Deficit Disorder Is Sensitive to Methylphenidate," *Journal of Child Neurology* 6:Supplement (1991): S128–31.

[42] Malcolm Gladwell, "Is the Hectic Pace of Contemporary Life Really to Blame for A.D.D.?" *The New Yorker* 74:46 (February 15, 1999): 80–85.

[43] Postman, *The Disappearance of Childhood*, xii.

[44] Melvin Grumbach, "Growth Hormone Therapy and the Short End of the Stick," *New England Journal of Medicine* 319:4 (July 1988): 238–41.

[45] Margaret Mead, "Children and Ritual in Bali," in *Childhood in Contemporary Cultures*, eds. Margaret Mead and Martha Wolfenstein (Chicago: University of Chicago Press, 1955), 44.

[46] Ibid., 44, 45.

[47] Ibid., 40.

[48] Ibid., 47–48.

[49] Ibid., 40.

[50] Clifford Geertz, *Local Knowledge: Further Essays in Interpretive Anthropology* (New York: Basic Books, 1983), 62.

[51] Mead, "Children and Ritual in Bali," 41.

[52] I do not want to idealize the Balinese. I have omitted details about caste and identity, for example, for the sake of simplicity and the larger conceptual point.

[53] Alison Lurie, *Don't Tell the Grown-ups: The Subversive Power of Children's Literature* (New York: Back Bay Books, 1990).

[54] Adam Gopnik, "Wonderland," in *The Best American Essays 1996*, ed. Geoffrey Ward (Boston: Houghton Mifflin, 1996), 193–208.

CHAPTER ELEVEN: SECOND ACTS

[1] David Gems and Linda Riddle, "Genetic, Behavioral and Environmental Determinants of Male Longevity in *Caenorhabditis elegans*," *Genetics* 154 (2000): 1597–1610.

[2] David Gems, "Is More Life Always Better? Problems Arising from the New Biology of Aging," (forthcoming, *The Hastings Center Report*).

[3] David J. Clancy, David Gems, Lawrence G. Hirschman, Sean Oldham, Hugo Stocker, Ernst Hafen, Sally J. Leevers, and Linda Partridge, "Extension of Lifespan by Loss of CHICO, a *Drosophila* Insulin Receptor Substrate Protein," *Science* 292 (2001): 104–6. See also David Gems and Linda Partridge, "Insulin/IGF Signalling and Ageing: Seeing the Bigger Picture," *Current Opinion in Genetics and Development* 11 (2001): 287–91.

[4] Much of this section has come out of conversations with David, who was also kind enough to share his lecture notes and several unpublished papers with me. There is also an enormous popular literature on the science of aging, much of which concentrates on aspects other than the evolutionary explanations. One of the best is Steven Austad, *Why We Age* (New York: John Wiley and Sons, 1997). See also Tom Kirkwood, *Time of Our Lives: The Science of Human Aging* (New York: Oxford University Press, 1999); William R. Clark, *A Means to an End: The Biological Basis of Aging and Death* (New York: Oxford University Press, 1999); and S. Jay Olshansky and Bruce A. Chaney, *The Quest for Immortality: Science at the Frontiers of Aging* (New York: W. W. Norton, 2001).

[5] Gems, "Is More Life Always Better?"

[6] See, for example, Timothy P. Murphy, "A Cure for Aging?" *Journal of Medicine & Philosophy* 11:3 (1986): 237–55; Arthur Caplan, "Is Aging a Disease?" in *If I Were a Rich Man Could I Buy a Pancreas?* (Bloomington: Indiana University Press, 1992): 195–209.

[7] I owe this example to Chris Hackler, who discussed anti-aging therapies at a meeting of the Enhancement Technologies and Human Identity Project in Montreal (June 19, 1998).

[8] Austad, Why We Age, 108; Malcolm Gladwell, "The New Age of Man," The New Yorker 72:29 (September 30, 1996), 67.

[9] Austad, Why We Age, 104.

[10] N. L. Keating, P. D. Cleary, A. S. Rossi, A. M. Zalavsky, and J. Z. Ayanian, "Use of Hormone Replacement Therapy by Postmenopausal Women in the United States," Annals of Internal Medicine 130 (1999): 543–53; Denise Grady, "Weighing Risks and Benefits of Hormone Therapy," New York Times, April 30, 2002. For a comprehensive review of hormone replacement therapy, see J. E. Manson and Kathryn Martin, "Postmenopausal Hormone Replacement Therapy," New England Journal of Medicine 345:1 (2001): 34–40.

[11] Morris Notelovitz, "Estrogen Replacement Therapy: Indications, Contraindications and Agent Selection," American Journal of Obstetrics and Gynecology 161 (1989): 8–17. See also Manson and Martin, "Postmenopausal Hormone Replacement Therapy."

[12] Margaret Lock, Encounters with Aging: Mythologies of Menopause in Japan and North America (Berkeley: University of California Press, 1993).

[13] Ibid., 13.

[14] Ibid., 35.

[15] Ibid., 205.

[16] Margaret Lock, "Menopause in Cultural Context," Experimental Gerontology 29;3/4 (1994): 317.

[17] Lock, Encounters with Aging, 240.

[18] Alasdair MacIntyre, After Virtue (Notre Dame, Indiana: University of Notre Dame Press, 1984).

[19] Florence King, Southern Ladies and Gentlemen (New York: St. Martin's Press, 1993; originally published in 1975), 215.

[20] Lock, Encounters with Aging, 216, 396.

[21] Ibid., 378

[22] Bernard Williams, "The Makropulos Case: Reflections on the Tedium of Immortality," in Problems of the Self (Cambridge, U.K. University Press, 1973), 82–100; Leon Kass, "The Case for Mortality: Why Should We Age and Die?" American Scholar 52 (Spring 1983): 173–200.

[23] Stephen Cole, "Age and Scientific Performance," American Journal of Sociology 84:4 (January 1979): 958. See also Dean K. Simonton, "Career Landmarks in Science: Individual Differences and Interdisciplinary Contrasts," Developmental Psychology 27:1 (January 1991): 119–30; Dean K. Simonton, "Age and Literary Creativity," Journal of Cross-Cultural Psychology 6:3 (September 1975): 259–77.

[24] Harvey Lehman, Age and Achievement (Princeton, N.J.: Princeton University Press, 1953).

[25] According to the University of Chicago psychologist Mihaly Csikszentmihalyi, psychologists distinguish between two kinds of mental abilities: fluid intelligence and crystallized intelligence. Fluid intelligence is the ability to respond quickly to problems

and compute accurately, and is measured by tests asking people to draw inferences from logical relationships, recognize patterns, and memorize lists of numbers or letters. It is supposed to peak early in life and decline thereafter. Crystallized intelligence involves making sensible judgments, recognizing similarities across categories, and using logical reasoning and induction. Csikszentmihalyi says it is more dependent on learning than fluid intelligence, and improves or stays stable until age sixty or so. See Mihaly Csikszentmihalyi, *Creativity: Flow and the Psychology of Discovery and Invention* (New York: HarperCollins, 1996): 213.

[26] The other traits measured on the five-factor model are neuroticism, extroversion, agreeableness, and conscientiousness.

[27] Robert M. McCrae, "Social Consequences of Experiential Openness," *Psychological Bulletin* 120:3 (1996): 323–37.

[28] Paul T. Costa et al., "Cross-Sectional Studies of Personality in a National Sample: II. Stability in Neuroticism, Extraversion and Openness," *Psychology and Aging* 1:2 (June 1986): 144–49; Peter Warr, Anthony Miles, and Conall Platts, "Age and Personality in the British Population between 16 and 64 Years," *Journal of Occupational and Organizational Psychology* 74:2 (June 2001): 165–99.

[29] Robert M. Sapolsky, "Open Season: Why Do We Lose Our Taste for the New?" *The New Yorker* 74:6 (March 30, 1998), 57–72.

CONCLUSION: THE TYRANNY OF HAPPINESS

[1] Mickey Smith, *A Social History of the Minor Tranquilizers: The Quest for Small Comfort in an Age of Anxiety* (New York: Praeger, 1989), 178.

[2] Michael Walzer, *Thick and Thin: Moral Argument at Home and Abroad* (South Bend, Ind.: Notre Dame University Press, 1994), 23–24.

[3] Ludwig Wittgenstein, *Philosophical Investigations*, trans. G. E. M. Anscombe (New York: Macmillan, 1958), 293.

[4] Alexis de Tocqueville, *Democracy in America*, trans. George Lawrence, ed. J. P. Mayer (New York: Harper and Row, 1988), 536.

[5] Philippe Soupault, "Introduction to Mademoiselle Coeur Brise (Miss Lonelyhearts)" in *Nathanael West: A Collection of Critical Essays*, ed. Jay Martin (Englewood Cliffs, N.J.: Prentice-Hall, 1971), 112–13.

[6] Julie Baumgold, "Midnight in the Garden of Good and Elvis," in *The Best American Essays 1996*, ed. Geoffrey Ward (Boston: Houghton Mifflin, 1996): 51.

Acknowledgments

For the past five years I have had the good fortune to be part of a project called "Enhancement Technologies and Human Identity," which was funded by the Social Sciences and Humanities Research Council of Canada. The Enhancement Technologies Group has been like a traveling salon, meeting two or three times a year in Montreal, London, Berkeley, Minneapolis, or Charleston for several consecutive days of cloistered, nonstop discussion with invited guests about enhancement technologies. This book feels like an extension of discussions and arguments that began in that group. I am very grateful to the many guests who shared their work with us, but I am especially grateful to the core members of the group: Françoise Baylis, Tod Chambers, Alice Dreger, David Gems, Kathy Glass, Margaret Lock, and Laurence Kirmayer.

The book that I have written is not exactly the one that I intended to write, and a lot of what has wound up in the book I came across by pure chance. As the book progressed, I found myself spending less time in the library and more time talking to people who were actually involved with the technologies in question—some as clinicians, some as patients, some as consumers or clients. Many were friends or colleagues. Others approached me after hearing a lecture or reading an article I had written. Sometimes an e-mail correspondence with a person I knew would lead to another correspondence with someone I had never met before. Occasionally I sought out people on the Internet—authors of scholarly papers, people with home pages, participants in on-line discussion groups. At some point the question presented itself: when does this conversation and correspondence become formal "research," and how should it be handled from an ethical perspective? It seemed more than a little odd to ask an Institutional Review Board to render an ethical judgment on conversations I was having with my friends and colleagues, but Institutional Review Boards do monitor the empirical surveys, questionnaires, and ethnographies carried out to gather data for medical and psychological research. When should an e-mail conversation with a stranger for a book be considered empirical research, and when should it be considered journalism? Eventually I decided to treat it as journalism, not so much because I consider myself a journalist but out of fear that an Institutional Review Board would require me to approach everyone to whom I had ever spoken and ask them to sign an informed consent document detailing the risk/benefit ratio of our conversations. In the absence of Institutional Review Board oversight, I have done my best to treat these conversations and correspondences in a manner that is both loyal to the truth and respectful of the people who were kind enough to talk to me.

In the cases where I approached a person about a topic in the book, I explained that I was writing a book (or in some cases, an article) on enhancement technologies. I offered anonymity to anyone who wanted it. The people I have quoted have given me their permission to use their comments. I have tried to make sure that all the statements I have included from on-line sources are accurate. The remarks I have quoted from on-line discussion groups come only from groups that are open to anyone who wants to join, and thus available to anyone who logs on. I have included the URLs in my endnotes. In addition, I e-mailed each of the people who made the on-line remarks and asked permission to quote them. (No one refused, but in two cases I was unable to track down the original source of the remark.)

If not for the people who agreed to talk to me about their own personal experiences with these technologies, this would have been a very different book. I am deeply indebted to the people who spoke to me or corresponded with me off the record, as well as those who agreed to be quoted in the book, including Christine Drury, Lisa Stewart, Snowy Angelique Maslov, and Anne Lawrence. I am especially grateful to Kate Jirik, a remarkable person who has helped me think more clearly about many things beyond voice synthesizers.

I have had a lot of editorial help with this book, both formal and informal. Leigh Turner, Kathryn Montgomery, and John Lantos all read and commented on drafts of the entire manuscript—a thankless task for which they deserve much more than my thanks here. Rachel Toor advised me, read an early draft of the manuscript, and gave me some brutally candid remarks, which, once I recovered from the urge to slit my wrists, made the tone of the final version less shrill and moralistic. Cullen Murphy helped me polish a shortened version of "Amputees By Choice" and did me the great favor of publishing it in *The Atlantic Monthly* as "A New Way to Be Mad?" Jennifer Geddes and Joe Davis did the same for a version of "Pilgrims and Strangers," which appeared in *The Hedgehog Review* under the title "Dark Passage." I had no idea what to expect of a literary agent before Andrew Blauner got in touch with me, but he has proven to be a capable advisor and a thoughtful reader. Starling Lawrence, my editor at Norton, and his editorial assistant, Morgen Van Vorst, have made my entrance into the world of trade publishing a pleasure.

Many of the ideas in the manuscript emerged out of conversations with my friends and family, especially with my wife, Ina, and my brothers, Hal and Britt. At one point or another I have bounced most of my ideas about psychiatry and psychotropic drugs off Hal, who is a psychiatrist at Wake Forest University. Britt read the entire manuscript and sent me detailed thoughts related to several chapters, many of which wound up in the final version. David Gems has made several extended visits to Minneapolis after our Enhancement Technologies Group meetings, during which we spent many hours talking about nematodes, psychedelic drugs, modern primitives, and sexual fetishes. Tod Chambers has been a remarkably generous supplier of ideas about literature, culture, and identity, not only suggesting books and articles for me to read but sometimes even buying them for me and sending them in the mail. Jing-Bao Nie, my lunchtime conversation partner in Minneapolis and Dunedin, has given me many hours of insightful discussion, as has Tom Schenk. Erik Parens sparked my interest in enhancement technologies by inviting me to be a part of his project on the subject several years ago at the Hastings Center.

I wrote the bulk of this manuscript while on sabbatical leave from the University of Minnesota. I am grateful to the university for a sabbatical supplement grant, and especially grateful for the support of Jeff Kahn, the Director of the Center for Bioethics, who has done an extraordinarily effective job of making sure that those of us who spend our days at the Center are happy in our work. Four months of my sabbatical were spent at the University of Otago in Dunedin, New Zealand, where I was a Williams Evans Visiting Fellow at the Centre for Bioethics. Dunedin may be the most beautiful and hospitable spot on the planet, and the Centre for Bioethics is a remarkably fertile place for intellectual work. I am grateful to Don Evans for the invitation to visit and to the Centre faculty, staff, and students for their friendship. If Josie Johnston had not knocked on my door one afternoon, I would never have become interested in amputee wannabes, and if Annemarie Jutel had not told me that John Money's papers were in the Otago medical library, I would probably have never realized that they were there. As always, Grant Gillett and John Dawson were generous hosts as well as wonderful friends and colleagues.

I am not an anthropologist, a sociologist, or a historian, but I have carpetbagged from all these fields for this book. Genuine experts directed me to ideas and sources in these fields, including Ken DeVille, Paul Brodwin, Margaret Lock, Peter Conrad, Ray DeVries, Joe Davis, Art Frank, and Beth Haiken. David Healy and Laurence Kirmayer have given me many hours of thoughtful consultation on a variety of issues in psychiatry. Candace Myers, Anita Kozan, and Lilli Ambro helped me learn more about voice and speech-language pathology, and June Kitanaka was a helpful correspondent about Japanese identity and *taijin kyofusho*. My visit to the South Place Ethical Society in London I owe to my friend Andrew Bradstock. Rob Smith, Michael First, John Money, Paul McHugh, and Ian Hacking helped me in my research on apotemnophilia. Douglas Price spoke to me by phone about his own book on amputation, and even sent me his own translations of several articles published in languages that I do not read.

Both the title *Better than Well* and many of the thoughts the book contains I owe to Peter Kramer, who has been extremely generous with his time and his ideas. Peter has also been a helpful advisor on how to negotiate the publishing world, as have Lauren Slater, Bart Schneider, Jay Tolson, Rachel Toor, and Sian Hunter.

With a German-born wife, three German-speaking children (two of them born in Canada and the product of French and Spanish-speaking kindergartens), a Scottish education, and recent work visas stamped New Zealand, South Africa, and Canada, I sometimes feel as if my life is an ongoing clinical study in the kinds of identity questions I have written about in this book. By virtually any outcome measure that study has been remarkably successful so far, and the credit for that belongs entirely to Ina, Crawford, Martha, and Lyle.

Index

postmodernism, 46–47, 48
posttraumatic stress disorder, 176
Powell, Hickman, 181, 262–63
Premarin, 119, 281
premenstrual dysphoric disorder, 123
Prempro, 119
*Presentation of Self in Everyday Life,
The* (Goffman), 63
Presley, Elvis, 63, 303–4
Price, Douglas, 214
Price, Max, 215–16
Priest, Patricia, 87–88
Princeton University, Institute for
Advanced Study at, 289
privacy, development of, 139
Propecia, 119
propranolol (Inderal), 80
prosperity, distrust of, 101
prosthetic technologies, patients' experience of naturalness of, 2, 25–26
*Protestant Ethic and the Spirit of Capi-
talism, The* (Weber), 152–53
protest movements, 203–5
Prozac, 131, 132, 153, 156, 165
development of, 57
emotions blunted on, 74–75, 132
identity transformation through,
50–51, 52, 108
mass marketing of, 102, 119, 125
moral judgments on use of, 271, 297
OCD treated with, 123
public condemnation vs. private consideration of, 297
sexual compulsion treated with,
222–23
Prozac as a Way of Life (Chambers and
Elliott), xii
Prozac Diary (Slater), 48, 74
psychedelic drugs, 42–44, 46, 100, 180
psychiatric conditions:
cosmetic improvement for, 121–22
criteria for diagnostic categories of,
123, 232–33
culture-bound syndromes, 71, 175,
177–78
depression, 123, 125, 156
fugue states, 174–78, 180
increased diagnoses of, 123–25
mechanistic models vs. spiritual com-
ponent of, 154–60
multiple-personality disorder, 175,
227, 228, 229–30, 231

neuroses vs. psychoses, 131
obsessive-compulsive disorder, 74,
123–24, 216
primary-care physicians' prescriptions
for, 123
support groups on, 126
as transient cultural phenomena,
227–30
see also psychopharmacology; *specific
conditions*
PsychInfo, 57
psychoanalytic theory, 48, 131
Psychopathia Sexualis (Krafft-Ebing),
214, 217
psychopharmacology:
antidepressants, xi, 50–52, 56, 57–58,
73–76, 102, 123
emotional escapism through, 295
function as focus of, 156–57
industry-driven explosion of demand
in, 120, 123–26
mass marketing of, 102, 119
self-presentation enhanced with,
122–23
for social anxiety, xv–xvi, 54–55, 56,
57–58, 75, 82, 120, 123, 125,
129, 229
tranquilizers, xv–xvi, 130–31
work ability enhanced with, 153
see also specific medications
psychotherapy:
individual well-being as focus of,
141–42
inner truth in, 29, 48
innovative developments in, 235
in Japan, 71
as virtuous struggle, 271
public speaking, 17, 77, 79–80, 81–82,
99
Pullman, Philip, 268
Puritanism, 105, 106
purpose, of human life, 299–300
Putnam, Robert, 84

Rabbinical literature, 83
racism:
in beauty standards, 164, 166, 187,
190–93, 194, 195, 196, 203–4,
206–7
see also African Americans
Radetsky sisters, 256–57
Randolph, John, 274

tanning and, 117–18
skirts, 103
Slater, Lauren, 48, 52, 74–75
Smith, Maynard, 281
Smith, Robert, 208, 209, 211, 212, 213, 217, 234
Smith Kline, 124
SmithKline Beecham, 125
social events:
  children as center of, 227
  consumption ethic in, 106–7
  cultural differences in, 69–70
social hierarchies, identity derived from, 40–41
social phobia (social anxiety disorder), 54–59
  chronic blushing vs., 98
  diagnostic criteria of, 55
  Japanese form of, 70–73, 75–76
  medications used for, xv–xvi, 54–55, 56, 57–58, 75, 82, 120, 123, 125, 129, 229
  shyness vs., 55, 58–59, 229, 233
Solomon, Joshua, 163, 165, 171, 183, 184
Sontag, Susan, 63, 132
Soul Sister, (Halsell), 163
Souls of Black Folk, The (Du Bois), 41–42
Soupault, Philippe, 303
South:
  African-American life in, 162, 163, 164, 167, 168–70, 171
  business transformation of, 178–79
  front porches in, 150
southerners:
  accents of, 4–9, 11–14, 166
  air of abstraction in, 257
  as older women, 284
  social masks of, 69
South Place Ethical Society, 28–29, 32
speech, see voice
spinal taps, 252
sports:
  aging professionals in, 284–85, 286, 287
  competition in, 147, 262
SSRIs, see selective serotonin reuptake inhibitors
stage fright, 58, 80–81
stage performance, Japanese social anxiety vs., 72–73

status:
  recognition of, 88
  social class vs., 10–11
  speaking accents as markers of, 5, 7, 9, 11, 12
Stein, Murray, 58
Stepford Wives, The (Levin), 131–32
steroids, 36, 37–38, 40, 147, 271
Stevens, Jay, 42
Stevenson, Robert Louis, 178
Stewart, James, 164
Stewart, Lisa, 19, 24
Stewart, Martha, 24
Stigma (Goffman), 218
stimulants, 251–54, 258, 260
Storming Heaven (Stevens), 42
Struwwelpeter (Busch), 266–67, 268
Stryker, Susan, 180
suburbia, alienation in, 131–33, 144, 146, 148, 153–54, 273–74
Sue, Jean-Joseph, 214
Sullivan, Andrew, 10–11, 119
support groups, 126, 219
surgery:
  for excessive blushing, 94–95, 96, 98–99
  new procedures in, 235
  for sex reassignment, 19, 20–21, 30–31, 32–33, 52, 221–22, 230–31
  voice changes through, 21, 22
  in voluntary amputation, 208–9, 215, 220, 234–35
  see also plastic surgery
sushi restaurants, age of patrons in, 291–92
Susman, Warren, 60, 61, 62, 86
sweating, surgical procedure for, 94, 95
synthetic growth hormone, 120, 197–98, 240–41, 248–49, 261

taijin kyofusho, 71–73, 75
Takano, Ryoei, 71–72
talk shows, non-celebrity guests on, 78, 87–88
tanning, 117–18
tastes, receptivity to new experiences of, 290–94
tattoos, 113, 225, 226, 292
Taylor, Charles, 29–30, 33, 34, 40, 41, 147, 151, 152
teasing, 261–66

technology, alienation effects of,
148–51, 159
telephones, 83–84
television:
alienation effect of, 84, 85, 89
alternate reality of celebrity on,
84–86, 89–90
confessional talk shows on, 78, 87–88
intimacy of, 86
newscasters on, 91–92, 97
rapid diffusion of, 83–84
regional accents on, 5–6
social isolation and, 84
violence on, 264, 266
temporal lobe epilepsy, 178
Thatcher, Margaret, 116
theater:
of Balinese rituals, 263–64
life as, 63–64
Theory of the Leisure Class, The
(Veblen), 101, 102, 126
Thomas Cook and Sons, 178
Thoreau, Henry David, xii, 159
Three-Inch Golden Lotus, The (Feng),
247
Through the Looking Glass (Carroll),
268
Thurmond, Strom, 166
timbre, 23
Tissie, Philippe, 175, 176
Tocqueville, Alexis de, xviii–xix, 9–10,
141, 265, 295, 302–3
tourism, mass expansion of, 177–78,
179–80, 183–84
tranquilizers, xv–xvi, 130–31
transcranial magnetic stimulation, 156
transformation:
of ethnic impersonation, 161–72
morality of, 47
transient mental illnesses, 227–30
transplantation surgery, 220
transsexuals:
authentic self as goal of, 30–33
foreign travel as metaphor of, 180
gender-identity disorder diagnosis of,
221–22
sex-reassignment surgery and, 19,
20–21, 30–31, 32–33, 52,
221–22, 230–31
vocal transition developed by, 18–28
see also male-to-female transsexuals
travel:

in Bali, 180–82
as escape from boredom, 182–83
in fugue states, 174–78, 180
gender crossing vs., 180
intellectual detachment from experience of, 184–85
mass tourism developed in, 177–78,
179–80, 183–84
as pilgrimage, 170–71, 181
in racial disguise, 161–72, 180
self-discovery through, 170–71,
173–74, 181
Travis, Merle, 161
tricyclic antidepressants, 123
Trilling, Lionel, 46, 63, 83, 139
Triumph of the Therapeutic, The
(Rieff), 205–6
Trow, George, 77, 87
Turner, Victor, 218–19
Turner syndrome, 241
Twain, Mark (Samuel Clemens), 178,
267
tyramine, 57
tyranny of happiness, xiii

Ubud, Bali, 180–82
Unitarian Church, 28
United Kingdom, *see* British culture
University College London, 277
Unknown, The, 225
Upjohn Company, 124

vagrancy, 177, 178
Valium, 58, 80, 131–32, 155
Vanderbilt, Mrs. Reginald, 108
vanity, 35, 42
Veblen, Thorstein, 101–5, 106, 108,
111–12, 117, 126–27
Venus Envy (Haiken), 121
Vermeer, Jan, 139
Verne, Jules, 178
Viagra, 83, 102, 107, 119
victimization, 196–97, 198–99
Victorian era, childhood in, 237, 238,
239, 261
Vidal, Gore, 241
video games, 260
Virginia Slims, 114
virtual communities, 218
vitiligo, 167
voice, 1–25
age conveyed through, 2